CONCEPTUAL SKILLS FOR MENTAL HEALTH PROFESSIONALS

LINDA SELIGMAN

Walden University Online Instructor, Counseling Psychology
Johns Hopkins University, Faculty Associate
George Mason University, Professor Emeritus

Merrill
is an imprint of

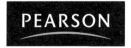

Upper Saddle River, New Jersey
Columbus, Ohio

Library of Congress Cataloging-in-Publication Data
Seligman, Linda.
 Conceptual skills for mental health professionals / Linda Seligman.
    p. ; cm.
Includes bibliographical references.
   ISBN-13: 978-0-13-223045-2
   ISBN-10: 0-13-223045-3
 1. Mental health personnel—Training of.
 2. Clinical competence.
 3. Mental health personnel and patient. I. Title.
   [DNLM: 1. Clinical Competence. 2. Psychiatry—methods. 3. Professional-Patient Relations.
   WM 21 S465c 2009]
   RC454.4.S4567 2009
   616.89—dc22

                                                                                    2007040171

Vice President and Executive Publisher: Jeffery W. Johnston
Publisher: Kevin M. Davis
Acquisitions Editor: Meredith D. Fossel
Editorial Assistant: Maren Vigilante
Production Manager: Wanda Rockwell
Production Coordination: Puneet Lamba, Aptara, Inc.
Creative Director: Jayne Conte
Cover Designer: Bruce Kenselaar
Cover image: Getty Images, Inc.
Director of Marketing: Quinn Perkson
Marketing Coordinator: Brian Mounts
Printer/Binder: R.R.Donnelley/Harrisonburg

Credits and acknowledgments borrowed from other sources and reproduced, with permission, in this textbook appear on appropriate page within text.

Pearson Education Ltd., London
Pearson Education Australia PTY, Limited
Pearson Education Singapore, Pte. Ltd
Pearson Education North Asia Ltd. Hong Kong
Pearson Education, Canada, Inc.
Pearson Educación de Mexico, S.A. de C.V.
Pearson Education–Japan
Pearson Education Malaysia, Pte. Ltd

Merrill
is an imprint of

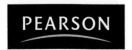

10 9 8 7 6 5 4 3 2 1
ISBN-13: 978-0-13- 223045-2
ISBN-10: 0-13- 223045-3

For my husband,
Bob Zeskind

PREFACE

This book is intended to help students, new clinicians, and more experienced clinicians in the mental health professions of counseling, psychology, and social work to develop competence in the conceptual skills of their profession. By combining the skills presented in this book with such fundamental skills as effective use of questions, reflection of feelings, eliciting and modifying dysfunctional thoughts, and behavioral-change strategies, clinicians can develop an in-depth picture of their clients and their difficulties, formulate a treatment plan that is likely to be effective, and apply treatment approaches and interventions that help people reach their goals. The fundamental skills are the building blocks of the treatment process, whereas the conceptual skills are the architectural structure that gives shape, meaning, and power to the treatment process. Ways of thinking about clients and their treatment (conceptual skills) and ways of intervening to help people (fundamental skills) are essential ingredients of mental health treatment. Mastery of both of these areas of knowledge characterizes truly skilled clinicians.

ORGANIZING FRAMEWORKS

Several organizing frameworks are used to give a clear and useful structure to this book. These include the BETA framework, many examples and case studies, and learning opportunities.

The BETA Framework

The leading theories of counseling and psychotherapy, along with their associated strategies and skills, can be organized into four broad categories that reflect their particular emphasis. This organizational framework, represented by the acronym BETA (Background, Emotions, Thoughts, and Actions) reflects the following grouping of theories:

- **Background:** Psychoanalysis, Alfred Adler's individual psychology, Jungian analytical psychology, transactional analysis, brief psychodynamic therapy, and other developmental and psychodynamic treatment systems
- **Emotions:** Person-centered counseling, existential therapy, Gestalt therapy, and other approaches that emphasize affect
- **Thoughts:** Cognitive therapy, rational emotive behavior therapy, and other theories of counseling and psychotherapy that emphasize cognitions

- **Actions:** Behavior therapy, cognitive-behavior therapy, reality therapy, brief solution-based therapy, and others that focus on modifying behaviors

The BETA framework was used to organize treatment theories in *Theories of Counseling and Psychotherapy: Systems, Strategies, and Skills,* Second Edition) (Seligman, 2006) and also was used to organize the presentation of basic clinical skills in *Fundamental Skills for Mental Health Professionals* (Seligman, 2009). This framework has been used in the present text as well, with an emphasis on skills rather than theories of counseling and psychotherapy.

The use of this organizing framework in all three books facilitates understanding of the broad range of treatment approaches and skills available to clinicians. Although each book is separate and is designed to be used by itself, any two or three of these books can easily be combined in instruction that is part of a graduate training program or other educational endeavor in the mental health professions. Following the same organizing framework allows these books to build on each other and provide learners with a comprehensive understanding of theories of counseling and psychotherapy, fundamental skills, and conceptual skills.

Most clinical skills can be logically connected to one of the elements of the BETA framework more than to the other three. For example, reflection of feeling is most strongly associated with treatment theories that emphasize emotions; modification of distorted cognitions is most strongly associated with theories emphasizing thoughts; and contracting is most strongly associated with approaches emphasizing actions. However, readers should keep in mind that most clinicians today use a broad range of interventions and do not limit themselves to those most closely aligned with their preferred theoretical orientations. As readers develop their own clinical styles, they should feel free to draw on skills presented throughout this book.

Chapters 2 through 9 of this book focus on the four elements in the BETA format, with Chapters 2 and 3 addressing skills to elicit and understand clients' background information, Chapters 4 and 5 honing in on identifying and enhancing emotions (particularly those directly related to treatment), Chapters 6 and 7 providing information on case conceptualization and other ways that clinicians understand and think about their clients, and Chapters 8 and 9 designed to help clinicians take actions, such as making referrals and giving sessions a productive structure, that contribute to effective treatment.

Descriptions, Examples, Case Studies, and Learning Opportunities

People learn in different ways, and this text offers a variety of approaches to maximize learning for everyone. When a skill is first presented in the book, a description of the skill is provided along with available and important research on the value of that skill and appropriate use of that skill. Examples and case studies are then provided to illustrate the use of the skill in practice. Finally, at the end of each chapter, exercises called Learning Opportunities allow readers to apply the learning they have gained. These learning opportunities include:

- Written exercises
- Discussion questions

- A role-play exercise
- An Assessment of Progress form, enabling readers to describe and evaluate their learning and skill development
- Personal journal questions that allow readers to apply the content of each chapter to themselves and their own lives, personalizing and making more meaningful the skills presented in the chapter

OVERVIEW OF CHAPTERS

Organized according to the frameworks described previously, the 10 chapters of this book highlight the following topics and skills:

- Chapter 1, Establishing the Foundation for Developing Conceptual Skills, discusses the importance of both fundamental and conceptual skills. It presents the BETA format, as well as some premises on which this book is based, and provides an overview of the organization of this book. In addition, this chapter introduces the Learning Opportunities, included in each chapter of this book.
- Chapter 2, Using Conceptual Skills to Understand, Assess, and Address Background: Bloom's Taxonomy, Context, Multiculturalism, and Interpretation, is the first of two chapters that focus on skills that help clinicians make positive use in treatment of clients' background information. This chapter presents a modified version of Bloom's taxonomy, a conceptual framework that is used throughout the book to help clinicians clarify their thinking about clients and their treatment. Also included in this chapter is information on effective use of interpretation, the use of context to improve understanding of clients, and the importance of multicultural competence in treatment.
- Chapter 3, Using Conceptual Skills to Understand, Assess, and Address Background: Eliciting Information, Intake Interviews, Transference, and Countertransference, describes a variety of effective approaches to gathering background information. Particularly important is the intake interview, explained and illustrated here. Information on understanding and making sound therapeutic use of both transference and countertransference completes this chapter.
- Chapter 4, Using Conceptual Skills to Make Positive Use of and Modify Emotions: Therapeutic Alliance, Role Induction, Clinician Self-Disclosure, and Clinicians' Reactions to Treatment, focuses on emotions, the second element in the BETA format. This chapter includes information on the importance of developing a sound therapeutic alliance, along with strategies to develop a positive client–clinician relationship. Ways to enhance client participation in treatment through role induction, development of client characteristics that are likely to enhance treatment, and appropriate use of clinician self-disclosure are other key topics in this chapter. Finally, this chapter addresses clinicians' feelings about their clients, helping clinicians better understand and make effective use of their own reactions.
- Chapter 5, Using Conceptual Skills to Make Positive Use of and Modify Emotions: Addressing Strong Client Emotions and Variations in Client Readiness

for Treatment, continues to emphasize the importance of emotions in treatment. This chapter uses Bloom's taxonomy and other conceptual frameworks to facilitate clinicians' efforts to help their clients modify strong and unhelpful emotions such as suicidal ideation, feeling overwhelmed in response to a crisis, and rage. This chapter also presents information on client reluctance and stages in clients' readiness for treatment, as well as ways to reduce barriers to treatment effectiveness and increase client motivation for change.

- Chapter 6, Using Conceptual Skills to Enhance Thoughts: Assessment, Mental Status Examination, Defining Memories, and Case Conceptualization, emphasizes the role of thoughts in treatment (the third element in the BETA format). This chapter provides information on both the complete and the mini-mental status examination. Discussion of assessment, using observation as well as tests and inventories, offers clinicians other approaches to understanding their clients more deeply and clearly. Defining memories provides yet another route to client assessment. Eileen Carter, a hypothetical client used throughout this book, illustrates the effective use of personality assessment, the mental status examination, and defining memories. Finally, five models of case conceptualization are presented with accompanying examples, offering clinicians a variety of approaches to better understanding clients and their strengths and concerns.

- Chapter 7, Using Conceptual Skills to Facilitate Diagnosis and Treatment Planning, discusses the importance to clinicians of the *Diagnostic and Statistical Manual of Mental Disorders* and reviews the 17 major categories in that volume. This gives readers an overview of the broad range of mental disorders that clients might present. In addition, this chapter describes and illustrates a structured approach to treatment planning, the DO A CLIENT MAP.

- Chapter 8, Applying Conceptual Skills to Actions for Positive Change: Generating Solutions, Referral and Collaboration, Structuring Treatment, and Writing Progress Notes, along with Chapter 9, describes actions that clinicians can take to improve the treatment process. These two chapters reflect the fourth element (actions) in the BETA format. This chapter provides information on giving advice to help clients find solutions to their concerns, making referrals to strengthen and enhance treatment, structuring sessions and the overall treatment process to maximize effectiveness, and using notes to track and improve progress.

- Chapter 9, Applying Conceptual Skills to Actions for Positive Change: Assessing and Terminating Sessions and Treatment and Using Research to Enhance Practice, concludes the chapters that introduce new skills. Appropriately, this chapter also talks about effective ways to conclude sessions, as well as the entire treatment process. This chapter ends with a discussion of clinicians' professional development and ways to enhance that development via research and learning.

- Chapter 10, Solidifying Conceptual Skills: Reviewing, Integrating, and Reinforcing Learning, begins with an extended intake interview of Summer Harris, a young woman who enters treatment at the urging of her parents. Readers then have the opportunity to apply many of the skills they have learned from this book to this client and her treatment. All of the Assessment of Progress forms included throughout this book are also presented in this chapter. This offers a comprehensive picture of the skills that have been described and illustrated and gives readers a final opportunity to practice, review, and rate themselves on these skills, increasing awareness of the progress and learning they have achieved. Personal journal questions conclude this chapter.

USES OF THIS BOOK

Many ways are available to make productive and effective use of the material in this book:

1. This book is ideally suited to a skills development course, extending over either one or two semesters or quarters. If its use is spread over more than one semester, then instructors might spend two classes or learning sessions on each chapter, using the first of each pair of classes for lectures and in-class demonstrations and discussion, and the second of each pair of classes for the practice group exercises.
2. This book can be combined with either my book on theories of counseling and psychotherapy (*Theories of Counseling and Psychotherapy: Systems, Strategies, and Skills*) (Seligman, 2006) or with another theories book to integrate the teaching of both skills and theories.
3. This book can be combined with my book, *Fundamental Skills for Mental Health Professionals* (Seligman, 2008) to teach an even broader and deeper array of skills. If so, the learning experience should extend over two semesters or quarters, with the first segment focusing on acquisition of fundamental skills such as open questions and reflections and the second focusing on conceptual skills such as case conceptualization and diagnosis.
4. This book can be used as a textbook for students in practicum and internship who have already had coursework in basic skill development. This book can serve as a vehicle for helping them develop and practice advanced skills.
5. Clinicians in mental health, school, or other settings can use this book on their own to review and refine their skills. Almost all clinicians can learn new skills from this book and will deepen their understanding of their clients and the treatment process as they use this text.
6. Units of this book can be selected to teach one or a group of skills in a seminar or can be incorporated into a variety of courses. Following are a few examples:
   - The information on diagnosis might be included in a course on abnormal psychology.
   - The information on the development of multicultural counseling competencies might be included in a course on multicultural counseling.
   - The information on the development of a positive therapeutic alliance might become part of an introductory course in social work, counseling, or psychology.

Feel free to innovate and experiment in your own use of this book!

ACKNOWLEDGMENTS

I am grateful for all the personal and professional support I received while writing this book. The following people made particularly important contributions to this book.

- My virtual assistant, Terri Karol, carefully checked my references, created the tables of contents, and proofread much of the manuscript. Although working with a tight deadline, she always exercised care and thoroughness.
- Diane Tuininga, Ph.D., helped me to update the research for this book and make sure that both classic and new references reflect current thinking on the topics in the book.
- Shantel Edmonds, graduate student at George Mason University, generously offered her time to conduct some additional research for this book. Her eagerness to learn and become more involved in her profession are reflected in the high quality of her work.
- Lynn Field, Ph.D., LPC, psychotherapist in private practice in Fairfax, Virginia, was deeply involved in the preliminary planning for this book. She unfailingly provided excellent research and editing skills as well as good judgment, clear feedback, and encouragement.
- Diana Gibb, Ph.D., faculty member at George Mason University and counselor in private practice, also made an important contribution to the development of this book. She carefully reviewed the manuscript and provided knowledgeable, helpful, and detailed feedback. Her understanding of graduate students and beginning clinicians helped me shape this book.
- The administrators at George Mason University provided me a study leave during which I began this book. In addition, the faculty, administrators, and staff of the Graduate School of Education at George Mason University, particularly Associate Dean Martin Ford, Dr. Gerald Wallace, and Janet Holmes, provided time and support that facilitated my work on this book.
- I am also grateful to the many students and clients I have met over the years from whom I have learned so much.
- This book would not have happened without Kevin Davis, assistant vice president and publisher at Pearson/Merrill, who invited me to write this book as well as *Theories of Counseling and Psychotherapy: Systems, Strategies, and Skills* (Seligman, 2006). He and his staff facilitated the development of this book in many ways. I am appreciative of all their assistance along the way.

- Meredith D. Fossel, editor, Content Area Methods and Counseling at Pearson/Merrill offered important information and assistance during my writing of this book.
- Special thanks are due to my family and friends, who have remained supportive through the pressures of this, my fourteenth book. My husband, Dr. Robert M. Zeskind, and my dear friend Bettie Young have been especially important to me during this time, as always, in ensuring that I have some balance in my life.

ABOUT THE AUTHOR

Dr. Linda Seligman received a Ph.D. in Counseling Psychology from Columbia University. Her primary research interests included diagnosis and treatment planning as well as counseling people with chronic and life-threatening illnesses. During her lifetime, she authored 14 books, including *Theories of Counseling and Psychotherapy: Systems, Strategies, and Skills; Selecting Effective Treatments; Diagnosis and Treatment Planning in Counseling; Developmental Career Counseling and Assessment;* and *Promoting a Fighting Spirit: Psychotherapy for Cancer Patients, Survivors, and Their Families.* She also wrote more than 80 professional articles and book chapters. In addition, she lectured throughout the United States as well as internationally on diagnosis and treatment planning and was recognized for her expertise on that subject.

Dr. Seligman was a professor in the Graduate School of Education at George Mason University in Fairfax, Virginia, for 25 years. She served as co-director of the Doctoral Program in Education, coordinator of the Counseling and Development Program, Associate Chair of the School of Education, and head of the Community Agency Counseling Program. She was later named professor emeritus at George Mason University. Dr. Seligman also served as associate at Johns Hopkins University and a faculty member in counseling psychology at Walden University, an on-line university.

Dr. Seligman was known for her extensive clinical experience in a broad range of mental health settings, including drug and alcohol treatment programs, university counseling settings, psychiatric hospitals, correctional facilities, and treatment programs for children and adolescents. She kept private practice in Bethesda, Maryland, where she provided therapy, supervision, coaching, and consultation.

Dr. Seligman served as editor of the *Journal of Mental Health Counseling* and as president of the Virginia Association of Mental Health Counselors. In 1986, her colleagues at George Mason University selected her as a Distinguished Professor, and in 1990, the American Mental Health Counselors Association designated her as Researcher of the Year. In 2007, the American Mental Health Counselors Association honored her with the title of Counselor Educator of the Year.

BRIEF CONTENTS

CONTENTS

Chapter 3
Using Conceptual Skills to Understand, Assess, and Address Background:
Information Gathering, Intake Interviews, Transference, and Countertransference   67

Chapter 8
Applying Conceptual Skills to Actions for Positive Change: Generating Solutions,
Referral and Collaboration, Structuring Treatment, and Writing Progress Notes   **235**

Chapter 1

ESTABLISHING THE FOUNDATION FOR DEVELOPING CONCEPTUAL SKILLS

Becoming a skilled and effective clinician requires learning both theory and skills. This book, *Conceptual Skills for Mental Health Professionals,* is designed to promote mastery of conceptual skills. Conceptual skills are those that influence how clinicians think about their clients, how they make sense of and understand who their clients are, and how the clients became the way they are. Conceptual skills enable clinicians to identify effective ways to help their client meet their goals and lead more rewarding and successful lives.

Important Conceptual Skills

Among the most important of the conceptual skills are

- Accurately understanding the nature of a person's difficulties, their causes and dynamics, and factors that worsen or ameliorate those difficulties.
- The ability to understand a person's strengths and self-image and how to enhance that person's awareness of those strengths.
- The ability to view people holistically, including becoming knowledgeable about relevant information on background, emotions, thoughts, and actions.
- Familiarity with models of case conceptualization that help organize and make sense of this information.
- Recognition of patterns of emotions, thoughts, and actions that suggest that people may present a danger to themselves or others, along with the clinical skills needed to avert dangerous and self-destructive behaviors.
- Knowledge of the *Diagnostic and Statistical Manual of Mental Disorders* (American Psychiatric Association, 2000), so as to be able to make accurate diagnoses.
- Development of effective and efficient treatment plans.

1

- Awareness of clinicians' own reactions to their clients and their work with them and the capacity to use those reactions to build the therapeutic alliance and enhance treatment.

These and many other conceptual skills are presented in this book. Whether you are a student or a practicing clinician; whether you are a psychologist, counselor, social worker, psychiatric nurse, or other mental health professional; and whether you work in a community mental health center, a psychiatric hospital, a private practice, a school, or another therapeutic setting, these skills should greatly enhance your ability to work effectively with a broad range of clients.

The Relationship Between Fundamental and Conceptual Skills

Conceptual skills reflect an advanced level of competence and enable clinicians to expand on and make judicious use of their fundamental or basic skills. Although fundamental skills, like conceptual skills, involve thought and judgment on the part of the clinician, they focus more on what the clinician will do and say in order to help people rather than how the clinician thinks about and understands people. Examples of important fundamental skills include:

- Making accurate and helpful reflections of feeling
- Recognizing nonverbal communications
- Making sound use of open and closed questions
- Crafting effective reflections of meaning
- Helping clients to identify, analyze, and modify their distorted cognitions
- Facilitating clients' efforts to formulate and implement behavioral-change plans
- Using imagery, systematic desensitization, relaxation, anchoring, and a broad range of other specific strategies to promote changes in people's thoughts, emotions, and actions

The Importance of Mastering Both Fundamental and Conceptual Skills

Until recently, the training of clinicians, especially at the master's level, emphasized fundamental rather than conceptual skills. However, clinicians can be fully effective only if they have competence in both conceptual and fundamental skills and can successfully integrate those skills in their work. Although fundamental and conceptual skills comprise a unit, and both are necessary learning for effective clinicians, most mental health professionals are trained in the fundamental skills first and then build on their knowledge of the fundamental skills by developing the more advanced and often more challenging conceptual skills. Just as people must learn to walk before they can dance with grace and elegance, so must we first acquire competence in the fundamental skills before we can enhance our knowledge of those skills with mastery of conceptual skills. The fundamental skills form the foundation for the acquisition of conceptual skills. Together, the two form a comprehensive treatment package that enables clinicians to provide the understanding and help that clients need.

Although the importance of conceptual skills may seem obvious, only recently has the professional literature acknowledged the considerable importance of these skills. As Duys and Hedstrom (2000, p. 8) state: "Counselors encounter conceptually complex variables when working with clients. Case conceptualization skills, understanding the flow and process of the counseling relationship, attending to multicultural dynamics, and the use of counseling theory call for increasingly complex cognitive processes." This point of view was echoed by Granello (2000), who suggested that high-level cognitive functioning allows clinicians to perform multiple professional functions, comprehend and organize a range of facts and dimensions, integrate and synthesize information, and determine similarities and differences.

Imagine that you would like to have a home built for yourself. You interview three building firms to find the one that best meets your needs. The first is well known for its excellent carpenters and electricians, but it lacks architects and designers. The second firm can prepare fine blueprints and scale models of your dream home but lacks the applied skills to execute the project. The third firm offers you the combination of skills you need. They have outstanding construction skills as well as experts who can visualize and plan the construction, providing the blueprints and guidelines the workers will need to build the home you want. Which firm would you prefer to build your dream home?

The analogy to the clinical situation is obvious. Certainly, clinicians need to have facility in such skills as asking open questions, making reflections of feeling and meaning, and using summarization and encouragers. These are the building blocks of effective change strategies. However, unless these skills are combined in coherent and clinically sound ways, they are unlikely to effect significant and lasting change. The combination of fundamental and conceptual skills characterizes outstanding clinicians and successful treatment.

Conceptual skills enable clinicians to develop a comprehensive and meaningful picture of their clients and their concerns, to organize that information in logical ways, to determine what fundamental skills to use, and to decide how to combine them into a treatment plan that is likely to be effective. The fundamental skills are essential ingredients of treatment, but the conceptual skills provide the framework that guides their appropriate use.

COMPANION BOOKS ON FUNDAMENTAL AND CONCEPTUAL SKILLS

I have written two books on skill development:

- *Fundamental Skills for Mental Health Professionals* (Seligman, 2008) includes the fundamental skills that mental health professionals in all areas of specialization need to build a therapeutic alliance and interact effectively and helpfully with their clients. This book provides a broad array of strategies and interventions to enable clinicians to initiate the treatment process, enhance a therapeutic alliance, gather information on clients and their concerns, and help people build on their strengths, improve their self-awareness, and change their self-destructive emotions, thoughts, and actions. However all of these treatment procedures are given shape, direction, and power via the conceptual skills.

- *Conceptual Skills for Mental Health Professionals,* the present book, assumes some knowledge of the fundamental skills and builds on those skills to enable clinicians to have greater competence in their work, to understand and interact with their clients in deeper and more meaningful ways, and to provide more successful treatment. In addition, clinicians with both strong fundamental and strong conceptual skills should be able to assume greater accountability for their work, to communicate more productively and wisely with managed care organizations, and to collaborate more successfully with both novice and experienced colleagues.

These two books can be used either alone or together. If they are both used, I recommend that *Fundamental Skills* be studied first, followed by *Conceptual Skills. Fundamental Skills* is designed for both beginning clinicians and those who have prior training and experience but who want to enhance their skills. *Conceptual Skills* is best used after readers have acquired at least a preliminary understanding of the fundamental skills, either from *Fundamental Skills for Mental Health Professionals* or in another way.

I have also written a third book that complements the former two. *Theories of Counseling and Psychotherapy: Systems, Strategies, and Skills* (Seligman, 2006) focuses on the major treatment approaches, such as person-centered counseling, cognitive-behavioral therapy, solution-focused brief therapy, psychodynamic therapy, and reality therapy, as well as on some innovative treatment approaches, such as eye movement desensitization and reprocessing, dialectical behavior therapy, feminist therapy, and motivational interviewing, that have demonstrated their value. Integrated and eclectic treatment systems also receive considerable attention in this book, reflecting the majority of clinicians who describe their primary clinical orientation as an integrated one. *Theories of Counseling and Psychotherapy* is designed to be used alone but can easily be combined with one or both of the previously described skills books for a unified and cohesive learning experience.

THE BETA FORMAT

The primary organizing framework, which provides the structure for all three of these books, is the grouping of clinical skills into four broad categories represented by the acronym **BETA**:

B: Background
E: Emotions
T: Thoughts
A: Actions

This grouping is based on five premises (Seligman, 2008) that follow, with accompanying discussion.

Premise 1: Similarity of Treatment Approaches

Treatment approaches are more alike than they are different. All approaches to counseling and psychotherapy include some attention to all four elements in the BETA model: background, emotions, thoughts, and actions. These are universal ingredients in all treatment processes.

The professional literature includes increasing evidence that all approaches to counseling and psychotherapy have underlying commonalities and that many of these common ingredients in treatment are associated with positive outcomes (Lambert & Bergin, 1994). Clinicians and treatment systems differ in how they conceptualize cases, the proportion of time they devote to each of the four elements in the BETA framework, and the strategies they emphasize during treatment. However, regardless of clinicians' theoretical orientations, their typical clients, the setting in which they work, and the nature of their professional specialization, mental health treatment providers use a similar array of general or fundamental skills. Among these common ingredients are the ability to form a positive and collaborative therapeutic alliance, the capacity for effective and accurate listening, communication of caring and empathy, and a talent for inspiring hope and effort among clients.

Today's clinicians, whether they are counselors, social workers, or psychologists, are more alike than they are different, sharing diagnostic systems, conceptions of mental health, treatment theories, strategies of intervention, and belief in the importance of ethical, culturally sensitive, and socially conscious treatment.

Premise 2: Categorization of Treatment Approaches

Treatment theories, strategies, and skills can be categorized and distinguished according to whether their primary emphasis is on understanding and changing the effect of past experiences (background), current feelings and sensations (emotions), thoughts and cognitions, or actions and behaviors.

Although this book is not designed to educate readers about theories of counseling and psychotherapy, the skills presented in this book are drawn from and organized according to the treatment approaches represented by the BETA model. Therefore, becoming familiar with the following, reflecting the way treatment systems are grouped in this model, should help readers better understand the corresponding grouping of skills (Seligman, 2006; Seligman, 2008).

Treatment Systems Emphasizing Background

- Sigmund Freud and psychoanalysis
- Alfred Adler and individual psychology
- Carl Jung and Jungian analytical psychology
- Freudian revisionists (ego psychologists, object relations theorists, self psychologists, and others, including Helene Deutsch, Karen Horney, Harry Stack Sullivan, Anna Freud, and Heinz Kohut)
- Brief psychodynamic psychotherapy

Treatment Systems Emphasizing Emotions

- Carl Rogers and person-centered counseling
- Existential therapy
- Gestalt therapy
- Emerging/postmodern approaches emphasizing emotions (narrative therapy, constructivist therapy, feminist therapy, transpersonal therapy)

Treatment Systems Emphasizing Thoughts

- Aaron Beck and cognitive therapy
- Albert Ellis and rational emotive behavior therapy
- Emerging approaches emphasizing thoughts (eye movement desensitization and reprocessing, neuro-linguistic programming, thought field therapy, cognitive therapy of evaluation, emotional freedom techniques)

Treatment Systems Emphasizing Actions

- Behavior therapy
- Cognitive-behavioral therapy
- Reality therapy
- Solution-focused brief therapies

Just as treatment systems can be organized according to the BETA framework, so can fundamental and conceptual skills. Of course, the organization is not as definitive as Table 1-1 may imply. The conceptual and fundamental skills presented here are used by the majority of clinicians. However, each skill is most strongly associated with the element in the BETA format under which it is listed.

TABLE 1-1   Fundamental and Conceptual Skills in the BETA Framework

	Background	**Emotions**	**Thoughts**	**Actions**
Fundamental Skills	• Open questions	• Eliciting, attending, and tracking emotions	• Eliciting cognitions	• Contracting
	• Closed questions	• Encouragers	• Classifying and assessing the validity of thoughts	• Goal setting
	• Eliciting information, especially about client's history	• Reflection of feeling/empathy, especially those that are strength-based • Summarization • Nonverbal communication	• Modifying cognitions	• Suggesting helpful tasks

	Specific Fundamental Skills	Specific Fundamental Skills	Specific Fundamental Skills	Specific Fundamental Skills
	• Earliest recollections • Lifeline • Genogram • Eliciting strengths from background • Making discussion of the past relevant	• Imagery • Focusing • New perspectives and new language • Reassurance/support • Distraction and self-talk • Use of body language to promote awareness	• Reflections of meaning • Anchoring • Reframing • Brainstorming • Making decisions and solving problems • Mind mapping • Providing information	• Empowerment • Systematic desensitization • Relaxation • Modeling/role-playing • Behavioral rehearsal • Skill development • Use of motivating language
Conceptual Skills	• Understanding context • Initiating treatment • Organizing background information • Addressing transference and countertransference • Multicultural sensitivity and awareness • Interpretation	• Establishing a therapeutic alliance • Role induction • Communicating the core conditions and providing support • Dealing with the clinician's own strong emotions • Values and judgments • Crisis intervention • Handling strong client emotions • Addressing reluctance • Clinician self-disclosure and immediacy	• Assessment • Using tests and inventories • Mental status examination • Defining the problem • Case conceptualization • Diagnosis • Treatment planning • Multicultural counseling competencies	• Stages of change • Collaboration and referral • Structuring sessions • Critical incidents • Assessment of progress • Session notes • Generating solutions • Helping people with multiple problems • Termination and periodic check-ups • Enhancing own professional development

The conceptual skills listed here are covered in this book; the fundamental skills are presented in the companion volume, Fundamental Skills for Mental Health Professionals *(Seligman, 2008).*

> ### Premise 3: The Role of Background in Development
> All people are shaped by their histories and backgrounds.

Some clinicians believe that we can best effect change in the present by focusing on early childhood issues; other clinicians pay only cursory attention to background and view a focus on present concerns as the most effective route to change. Whether you adopt one of these positions or take a stance between the two, you should always pay some attention to clients' backgrounds. This enhances the therapeutic alliance, enables us to join with clients in acknowledging the importance their histories have for them, and often helps us to identify long-standing patterns and problems that are intertwined with, reflected in, and contributing to people's current concerns. Some experiences, such as childhood physical or sexual abuse, neglectful or unreliable parenting, and a cultural background that is different from the norm, should almost invariably become an important focus of treatment. This is illustrated in the following example.

Example: The Importance of Background in Development

Jared, a 38-year-old man, sought treatment because of difficulty making commitments in both his personal and professional life. Jared and his parents are Caucasian. His parents both were born in Australia but met and married in the United States. An intelligent and attractive man, people frequently invited Jared to share activities with them. At work, too, others appreciated him; his serious demeanor and hard work had made him eligible for promotions. However, Jared nearly always turned down these opportunities, usually waiting until the last minute to do so. As a result, he had advanced little in his career and had no close relationships.

Jared's current difficulties have a direct connection to his background. His father had multiple extramarital relationships while Jared was growing up. The father made no effort to conceal these involvements but, instead, explained to anyone who would listen that this is what he had to do to remain in his unhappy marriage, which he was maintaining for the benefit of his children.

Jared recalls his mother as depressed and withdrawn during Jared's childhood, often asking the children to bring "her pills" when she was upset. The family was rarely together, although Jared's mother did attend church with the children and would read the Bible to them.

When Jared was in college, his only sibling, a younger sister, became pregnant and left home and high school to marry. Jared's father now apparently viewed himself as having completed his job as father and initiated divorce proceedings. Before the divorce was final, however, Jared's mother died of an overdose of Valium taken with alcohol. (Valium is a potent antianxiety medication that used to be widely prescribed but now is rarely suggested for ongoing treatment.)

Jared had gotten a strong message from his family experiences that people cannot be trusted, that what may be presented as responsibility and devotion may do great harm, and that neither mothers nor fathers really care about their children's needs. Jared's growing up had been so painful for him that he sought to protect himself from similar hurt by avoiding relationships.

To be effective, Jared's treatment will need to explore his background and help Jared understand and address the effect of his family messages on his current difficulties. Although his past cannot be changed, Jared's response to his past can change.

> ## Premise 4: Areas of Difficulty
> People who seek counseling or therapy generally have difficulties in one or more of three areas: emotions, thoughts, and actions. Usually, all three areas reflect impairment.

Emotions   People may experience little joy in their lives and a great deal of depression, anxiety, loneliness, anger, and other negative and painful emotions that interfere with their relationships and the choices they make in their lives. People with emotional dysfunction also often report difficulty managing their emotions; they may lose control and rage at others or avoid pleasant experiences out of fear of failure or rejection.

Example

Jared has a dysphoric mood most of the time, feeling sad and discouraged, with underlying anger. He rarely feels joyful or satisfied with himself and his life.

Thoughts   Many clinicians believe that thoughts determine emotions and actions. If people think of themselves as failures and believe that they do not have the ability to help themselves, they are likely to feel discouraged and hopeless, avoiding constructive actions that might enhance their lives. Similarly, if they believe that the world is a negative and difficult place, full of disappointments and people who care only about themselves, they will probably shy away from relationships as well as opportunities that they believe will inevitably bring only pain and loss. Distorted and unhelpful thoughts tend to further entrench themselves as people allow negative perceptions to become their reality.

Example

The previously described thoughts are typical of Jared's view of the world. His unhappy childhood, full of distorted and inaccurate messages (e.g., "My affairs help me to become a better husband and father," "Staying with my family reflects my devotion to them," "Relationships seem doomed to fail and yet we cannot survive without them") led Jared to have deep-seated negative cognitions about himself and his world, including "I have always been and always will be miserable; the best I can do is try to protect myself from some of the pain all around me."

Actions   People who seek treatment often have difficulty identifying steps they can take to help themselves. Instead, they persist in repetitive, self-destructive, and ineffectual actions that contribute to their negative emotions and distorted thoughts. Rather than trying new and more effective actions, they typically intensify their use of the same unhelpful behaviors, not recognizing the part they play in their own difficulties and unaware of any other options.

Example

Jared's actions have the goal of protecting him from pain and hurt. By avoiding significant interactions with people and remaining in a professional role where he is competent and confident, he believes that he can insulate himself from the hurt he felt throughout his youth, especially at the death of his mother. However, his actions have left him in constant conflict. Part of him longs for closeness and connections with others, and he is tempted to accept the invitations and promotions that come his way. Inevitably, however, his fear of pain wins out and he chooses the safer route, perhaps sparing himself from some hurt but also circumscribing his life in such a way as to deny himself any opportunities that might bring him the caring relationships and sense of accomplishment he craves.

Premise 5: The Importance of Identifying Strengths

All people have assets and strengths. They may stem from the person's history, emotions, thoughts, or actions. Their identification is at least as important as clarification of people's concerns and disorders.

The advent of positive psychology, developed largely by Martin Seligman (1999), sparked a rapid and welcome shift in many clinicians' perceptions of desirable treatment goals and plans. Although clinicians should continue to identify, diagnose, and understand problems and disorders that clients present, they also need to focus on clients' strengths. This can facilitate effective treatment planning, accelerate the treatment process, mobilize people's efforts to help themselves, and enhance their feelings of hope and empowerment.

Example

Jared survived great pain and loss as a young person, and his experiences increased his self-sufficiency and ability to care for himself. He supports himself well, and others seem to be impressed by both his personal and professional qualities. However, he wants to make changes in his life, to find a way out of his loneliness and life-long pain, and this motivation and his multiple strengths may well lead to a positive treatment outcome.

ORGANIZATION OF THIS BOOK

Like most people, Jared has important strengths but also significant concerns that are reflected in his emotions, his thoughts, and his actions, which clearly stem from his family background and early messages. Where to focus the treatment, both initially and after Jared has made some progress, and what approaches to use, are important decisions. Answers to those questions are determined by many factors, including

- How best to mobilize and maximize Jared's strengths.
- How to successfully develop a positive and collaborative therapeutic alliance with Jared, especially in light of his avoidance of close relationships and his mistrust of others.
- How multicultural factors such as gender, age, religion, ethnicity, and others affect Jared and his view of the world.
- The connection between Jared's background experiences and his emotional, cognitive, and behavioral difficulties.

- Which of the three areas (emotions, thoughts, actions) reflects his most prominent or troubling symptoms.
- Which of the three areas reflects symptoms that are most amenable to change.
- Jared's preferred mode of relating to the world.
- The clinician's theoretical orientation.

Chapters 2 through 9 of this book will help you better understand these factors for all clients, in order to maximize treatment effectiveness. This book presents skills for each of the four areas in the BETA model (background, emotions, thoughts, actions). Two chapters are devoted to each of the four areas in this model, as illustrated in Table 1-2. These chapters will help you formulate a clear and comprehensive understanding of your clients; build a sound therapeutic alliance with them; identify their strengths; assess whether any impairment is present in their emotions, thoughts, and actions; make an accurate diagnosis; develop a treatment plan that addresses their concerns and goals; and use your own responses to your clients, as well as your skills, in effective ways. In addition, you will have the opportunity to apply, practice, and refine your skills through role-plays, written exercises, and other learning experiences. Table 1-2 shows the overall organization of this book:

TABLE 1-2 Organization of the Book

Chapter	Element of the BETA Format	Skills Presented
2	Background	Using Bloom's taxonomy, interpretation, understanding the treatment context, multicultural awareness and competence
3	Background	Intake interviews, presenting and gathering information, transference and countertransference
4	Emotions	Developing a positive therapeutic alliance, role induction, clinician self-disclosure, therapeutic use of the clinician's feelings toward the client
5	Emotions	Dealing with strong and unhelpful client emotions, understanding and addressing variations in client readiness for treatment, dealing with client reluctance
6	Thoughts	Mental status examination, assessment, defining memories, case conceptualization
7	Thoughts	Diagnosis, treatment planning
8	Actions	Generating solutions, referral and collaboration, structuring treatment, progress notes
9	Actions	Concluding sessions and treatment, using research to enhance practice

Two additional premises that underlie the organization of this book address important ingredients in treatment. These are selection of appropriate treatment approaches and the skills and positive qualities of the clinician.

Premise 6: Treatment Planning

Although rarely is there only one right way to help people reach their goals, some approaches are clearly better than others. A treatment plan that incorporates approaches and strategies that have demonstrated their effectiveness in alleviating the symptoms and disorders in question is more likely to lead to effective, empirically supported, and efficient treatment.

This book does not seek to dictate a formula or ideal treatment approach. Rather, one of its primary goals is to equip clinicians with a broad range of treatment models and strategies that have demonstrated their effectiveness. With knowledge and competence in a range of both conceptual and fundamental skills, clinicians can build on their in-depth understanding of their clients to craft treatment plans that are likely to appeal to the clients, ameliorate their difficulties, and enable them to draw on their strengths to create more rewarding lives.

Premise 7: The Effective Clinician

Clinicians who know themselves well, who have positive and realistic self-esteem, a sound understanding of the helping professions and their own professional goals, and motivation to improve their clinical skills are more likely to achieve professional success than those who lack these attributes.

Learning the skills of counseling and psychotherapy is essential to the development of all mental health professionals. However, at least as important is the clinician's personal growth. This book is designed to facilitate both the personal and professional development of clinicians.

Learning Opportunities at the End of Each Chapter

Each chapter in this book concludes with a section titled "Learning Opportunities." This section offers readers the opportunity to process and apply the material covered in that chapter in such a way as to enhance their personal and professional development. Included in the Learning Opportunities sections are written exercises, discussion questions, role-play exercises, and personal journal questions. The benefits of these sections will be enhanced if readers take a close and truthful look at themselves as they move through this book. Particularly important are a personal awareness of their motives for entering a helping profession, their reactions to clients, the importance of the therapeutic alliance, and the power of the therapist in promoting client change.

By now, you have probably realized that becoming an effective clinician is a process that involves hard work, considerable thought, learning, and growth. It can be a rewarding process or it may be fraught with obstacles and disappointments. I hope that the learning you acquire from this book, as well as in other ways, will make your career as a mental health professional one that is both rewarding and challenging.

LEARNING OPPORTUNITIES

Although this first chapter is introductory, it follows the format of subsequent chapters and includes all four types of learning opportunities:

- Written Exercises
- Discussion Questions
- Practice Group Exercises, with an accompanying Assessment of Progress form
- Personal Journal Questions

Although fewer exercises are presented in this chapter than in later chapters, this section introduces the four types of learning opportunities that you will encounter throughout this book. In addition, this chapter provides some guidelines on how to make good use of the Practice Group Exercises, whether you are in the clinician role or the client role or have the charge of observing and providing feedback on the exercise.

Written Exercises

1. As you read the case of Jared on pages 8–10, what were your reactions? Consider your emotional responses to Jared and his parents, how you might feel as his clinician, and what you think it would be like to interact with Jared. How can you best manage and make use of your own reactions to Jared so that they promote a positive therapeutic alliance and help him make positive changes?
2. This chapter describes clinical skills as falling into two groups: fundamental skills and conceptual skills. When you think of conceptual skills, what skills first come to mind? What do you think led you to think first of these skills?

Discussion Questions

1. The BETA format, which provides the organizing framework for this book, categorizes theories and skills of counseling and psychotherapy according to whether their primary emphasis is background, emotions, thoughts, or

actions. What is your reaction to this organizing framework? How might it help you better understand the broad array of treatment approaches and strategies available? What strengths and drawbacks do you see in the BETA format?

2. This chapter presented the case of Jared. Consider the following questions raised earlier about how you might think about Jared and his difficulties as well as about ways to provide him with effective help.

- In what ways can Jared's strengths be mobilized and maximized?
- How can a positive and collaborative therapeutic alliance best be developed with Jared, especially in light of his avoidance of close relationships and his mistrust of others?
- How do multicultural factors such as gender, age, religion, ethnicity, and others affect Jared and his view of the world? You may fill in any missing information.
- What is the connection between Jared's background experiences and his emotional, cognitive, and behavioral difficulties?
- Which of the three areas reflects his most prominent or troubling symptoms?
- Which of the three areas reflects the symptoms that are most amenable to change? What information led you to that decision?
- What is Jared's preferred mode of relating to the world?
- What treatment approach seems most likely to be helpful to Jared?

Although you may not have yet learned the skills that enable you to answer all of these questions comfortably and accurately, draw on what you already do know from your training and education as well as from your personal and professional experience to discuss the answers to these questions. This should launch your efforts to draw on your conceptual skills and to think about people from a broader and deeper perspective.

3. This chapter advances seven premises that can shape how clinicians think about their profession, their roles, and their clients. Review these premises and discuss which ones seem sound and useful and why and, alternatively, which ones seem flawed and incompatible with your way of thinking about your profession.

Practice Group Exercises

Practice group exercises suggested throughout this book provide the opportunity to try out new skills, build on skills already learned, give and receive feedback, and demonstrate improvement. You have probably already experienced the benefits of clinical role-plays in other classes; they are a well-established and effective method of applying the academic material you have learned and taking your professional development to another level.

Practice group sessions can be rewarding experiences, involving shared learning and professional growth, facilitated by useful and meaningful feedback. Group members frequently develop strong and supportive relationships and benefit both personally and professionally from the group sessions.

On the other hand, practice sessions may be anxiety-provoking experiences in which people sometimes feel attacked and belittled. Our apprehensions and self-doubts may get in the way of our listening carefully to feedback and understanding it fully. We might interrupt to defend or explain ourselves and might become more concerned with being right than with learning from the feedback.

Maximizing Learning from Practice Groups

To maximize the benefits you can obtain from the Practice Group Exercises you should

- Participate fully in the group exercises.
- Record the entire practice group session (on audio or videotape) and review the tape before the next group session, listening for ways in which you might improve both your clinical skills and your participation in the group. Write down one or two changes you want to work on in the next practice session and keep them in mind.
- Adhere to the guidelines for giving and receiving feedback presented later in this chapter.
- Complete the Assessment of Progress form at the end of each chapter, beginning with the form at the end of this chapter.

Constructing the Practice Groups

I suggest that the class or training unit be divided into groups of three or four people. The composition of these groups should change no more than once, if at all, during the course or learning experience. Continuity allows participants to build rapport and trust, become familiar with each other's styles of interaction, foster positive change based on the feedback that has been shared in the group, and note and reinforce development and improvement in skills.

During each exercise, each group member usually will have the opportunity to serve as observer, clinician, and client. At a given time, one or two members of the practice group will serve as observers, depending on whether the group has three or four members. Their task is to take careful notes on the role-play, using the Assessment of Progress forms as guides. One of the observers also should assume the role of timekeeper, gently reminding the group when only two to three minutes remain in the role-play and then letting the group know when the allotted time has elapsed.

The other two members will engage in a role-play, with one assuming the role of client and the other, the role of clinician. The clinician's task, described specifically in each chapter, is to demonstrate the skills highlighted in the exercise, in the context of sound overall counseling.

The group member in the client's seat also has a challenging and potentially growth-promoting role. The client has the choice of either presenting actual concerns or role-playing a hypothetical client. More will be said on this choice and on the client role later in this section.

Practice Group Sessions

To enhance learning, practice group sessions can adopt the sequence of steps that follows. Once this pattern becomes familiar, the group will be able to move efficiently through the steps.

1. Practice group members review the exercise to be sure they have a clear and mutual understanding of the experience. Any uncertainty about the nature and purpose of the exercise is clarified within the group or with the help of the instructor.

2. Practice group members review the Assessment of Progress forms to remind themselves of their goals.

3. If this is the second or subsequent practice session, group members review, either individually or as a group, their progress thus far and identify areas of strength as well as areas needing improvement. For example, if a group member had difficulty with accurate and effective reflections of feeling in a previous session, that person should focus on both the new skills to be practiced in the session and the skill of reflecting feelings that needs improvement.

4. Determine group members' initial roles. In the first group meeting, initial roles can be chosen by preference. View the three or four possible roles as a sequence and, if possible, progress through all roles in each meeting so that each member has the opportunity to experience each role:

- Clinician
- Observer 1/timekeeper
- Client
- Observer 2 (for groups with four members)

For each subsequent group session, assume the role in the sequence that comes next after the one you first took in the previous session. In other words, if your initial role in the previous group was the clinician, begin the second session as observer 1, then become the client, then observer 2 (for four-member groups), and finally the clinician. For the third practice session, you first assume the client role. This rotation ensures that the same person does not repeatedly begin or end the session as the clinician (both of which have advantages and disadvantages) and that each person has approximately the same amount of time in each of the three or four roles over the course of the practice group's meetings. This rotation also ensures that, for four-person groups, a person will not have to assume client and clinician roles one after the other, a potentially stressful sequence. Sufficient time should be allowed for each exercise, if possible, so that group members have the opportunity to assume all four roles.

5. Engage in the first iteration of the skill development exercise.

6. Initiate feedback with the person in the clinician role describing and assessing his or her own performance. That person should address the following:

- Brief overview of the role-play experience
- Strengths of clinician and session
- Assessment of the clinician's ability to demonstrate effectively the skills highlighted in the exercise as well as overall skills

- Identification of areas needing improvement or causing the clinician discomfort or concern and suggestions for skill development
- Questions the clinician might have for the group about his or her skill development

7. The person in the client role should provide feedback next, followed by the person or people in the observer role. Each should address the following, with the "client" also providing information about his or her reactions to the clinician's interventions and interactions:

- Overall reaction to the experience
- Identification of effective verbal and nonverbal interventions
- Assessment of the clinician's strengths and ability to demonstrate effectively the skills highlighted in the exercise as well as overall skills
- Ways the role-played session could have been even more helpful

8. While receiving feedback, the clinician should make sure he or she has a clear understanding of the feedback and takes notes on the Assessment of Progress form on important feedback and information that will promote skill development.

9. The clinician then summarizes the group feedback, checking his or her understanding of the feedback received, and identifying specific areas of strength as well as areas needing improvement.

10. Practice group members then change roles, moving on to the next role in the sequence, and the preceding steps are repeated.

The Nature and Importance of Helpful Feedback

One of the most important determinants of the value of practice group sessions is how group members give and receive feedback. Giving feedback can be a challenge, but it is also an art that can be learned and that can contribute greatly to clinicians' skill development. Participants should avoid dominating the group and should allow ample time for others to contribute their perceptions and ideas. They should offer feedback in a way that is empowering and open to discussion and is not harsh, demeaning, or demoralizing. Suggestions are most helpful if they are specific, easily understood, and readily implemented. Giving and receiving feedback effectively can greatly enhance the value of the groups. These skills also can be used productively in many other personal and professional settings.

Giving Feedback

Following are some examples of feedback given to clinicians:

> **Unhelpful Feedback:** You acted like you were the client's mother and really talked down to her. I think you have some mother issues that need attention.
> **Unhelpful Feedback:** I was bored during this session. The session didn't go anywhere, just talking heads philosophizing about life.
> **Helpful Feedback:** You have so many good ideas on how to help her; I'm impressed by your creativity. But Camille doesn't respond well when you give her

advice. I noticed that, when you gave her advice, you spoke more loudly and sat with your arms and legs crossed. She didn't really listen to your suggestions and just went on talking about how hard her life was. You might be able to build a stronger therapeutic alliance with Camille if you intervened less often, softened your tone of voice and your eye contact, and tried to work more collaboratively with her. You might ask her what she sees as the next steps in her efforts to help herself and enable her to find some new and more effective strategies that she can really own. Remember how she seemed to cheer up last week when you gave her some options? Perhaps that is a strategy you can use again. What do you think about what I've said?

The differences between the helpful and unhelpful examples are probably clear to you. The clinicians in the first two examples speak in vague and critical terms without offering specific examples or suggestions. The focus is on the clinician or the session rather than on the interventions. In addition, the language is insulting and unprofessional.

On the other hand, the third speaker begins and ends with positive feedback, is specific, focuses on interventions and strategies rather than on the clinician or the client, asks for the recipient's reactions to the feedback, and suggests specific ways to improve. The feedback is respectful and professional, yet it points out areas that might benefit from change.

The following guidelines will help you to provide useful feedback:

- Feedback should be gentle, supportive, respectful, and professional.
- Feedback should focus on strengths first, then address areas that need improvement, and then conclude in a positive way.
- All feedback should be specific so that the recipient can readily grasp the information. Pinpoint times in the session when the clinician made particularly effective and noticeably weak interventions.
- Feedback should focus on the clinician's words and behavior, not the person.
- Feedback should focus on a few important areas; avoid inundating the clinician with information.
- Feedback should include specific but tentative suggestions for improvement.
- Feedback should be linked to goals and previous skill development exercises and experiences.
- Understanding of and reactions to feedback should be checked out with the recipient and discussion should be invited.

Receiving Feedback

Listening to feedback and making good use of helpful suggestions are at least as challenging as giving sound feedback, especially for people who may doubt or devalue their abilities. Hearing objective, clear, specific, and useful feedback is one of the best ways to learn new skills and improve your effectiveness as a clinician. Over the course of your training, you will receive feedback from many sources. The following information will help you make good use of the feedback you receive from others about your skills.

Let's look at common types of responses to the helpful feedback in the previous example:

> *Response 1:* I was going to ask for her input as soon as I finished telling her what I thought she should do next.
> *Response 2:* She always gets so philosophical whenever I try to get her to focus on her problems; I didn't want her to get off track again.
> *Response 3:* Thank you for pointing that out.
> *Response 4:* It didn't occur to me that she might be uncomfortable about my giving her advice. What made you think about that?
> *Response 5:* That's a good point. Maybe I was scared we would just keep going around in a circle. How might I have worked more collaboratively with her?

Despite the high quality of the feedback, the five respondents have very different reactions. The first two seem more concerned with defending their interventions than they are with acquiring new learning. The second respondent even blames and disparages the client. Response 3 is a neutral one; it is hard to determine whether that person really absorbed and thought about the feedback. The fourth respondent is having difficulty understanding the feedback, and that is a common reaction. Asking for clarification is appropriate and can help the clinician decide whether the feedback is meaningful and useful. Respondent 5 seems most likely to benefit from the feedback; that person has clearly heard the feedback, tries to understand what led him to take too much control over the session, and then seeks to learn even more by asking for additional help. Responding to feedback in that way is most likely to promote skill development.

Let's go back and look at one of the examples of unhelpful feedback, followed again by some responses.

> **Feedback:** I was bored during this session. The session didn't go anywhere, just talking heads philosophizing about life.

> *Response 1:* I guess you're right. I didn't realize the session was unproductive. I wonder if I really have what it takes to be a good clinician.
> *Response 2:* Maybe so, but not every session can be full of brilliant insights and life-changing behaviors. Remember that session you had when you and the client spent about 20 minutes talking about what she should cook for her mother-in-law's visit?
> *Response 3:* OK. Anybody have comments on anything else?
> *Response 4:* You probably have a good point, but the way you're talking to me isn't helpful. It just makes me feel angry and put down. Let's try to come at this in a different way.

Although the person providing feedback here may be on the right track, the delivery is far from growth-promoting and is likely to elicit self-blame and defensiveness from the recipient. Response 1 reflects those feelings of self-blame, whereas response 2 is a defensive and attacking one. Response 3 is probably the most common reaction to the type of feedback illustrated in this example. The person may well have some strong reactions to the feedback but pushes those feelings away, at least temporarily, and changes the subject. Making a response like the fourth one is not easy; it calls for courage, honesty, and the ability to take a risk. However, the fourth response, offering a straightforward reaction to the unhelpful nature of the feedback, is most likely to promote skill development and personal growth for both the giver and the receiver of feedback.

The following guidelines for responding to feedback can help you maximize the learning you receive from this process:

- *Be aware of and address any discomfort you experience when hearing negative feedback.* Of course, try to listen to the feedback objectively and focus on what you can learn from it. However, you also might be doing what Albert Ellis called "awfulizing" and magnifying a minor or occasional error or omission. Try to put critical feedback into perspective, balancing it with all the positive feedback you have received. Also, be sure you are clear on the substance of the feedback. If the discomfort continues, discuss the feedback and your reactions with a supervisor, professor, trusted colleague, or therapist.
- *Avoid being defensive and attacking in response to negative feedback.*
- *Write down the feedback you receive.* This can help you obtain a balanced and accurate picture of the feedback. Reviewing what you have written affords you the opportunity to think over the feedback, assess its value, and, if necessary, obtain more information later so you can understand and use the feedback in helpful ways.
- *If you believe the delivery of feedback is confusing, harsh, or attacking, be courageous and state how the delivery or content of the feedback could have been made more helpful.*
- *Be aware of and address any discomfort you experience when hearing positive feedback.* Both positive feedback and negative feedback can make us uncomfortable. Our self-doubts might lead us to believe that people are just praising our work to avoid hurting our feelings or we might feel like an impostor, concealing our shortcomings from others. We might even think that we cannot live up to the positive images people have of us and might feel anxious and uneasy when others are impressed by our skills. These are all common responses to positive feedback. Again, writing down the feedback you receive and discussing it with trusted colleagues can help you appreciate your strengths.
- *Be sure you have a clear understanding of both the positive feedback you receive and the suggestions for improvement.* Restate the feedback you receive to be sure you have heard it correctly. Ask for examples and, if people have not offered specific ways for you to improve your skills, ask what you might have done differently and how you might improve your work.
- *Keep track of your goals and the progress you make toward those goals.* The Assessment of Progress forms provided in each chapter will help you accomplish

this. Seeing yourself moving forward can be empowering and rewarding and can encourage further improvement.

- *Focus on your strengths and improvements, but continue to set realistic goals for yourself.* You will probably feel successful and satisfied in this field if challenge and growth are exciting prospects to you and if you continue to promote your own learning and development in realistic ways.

Role-Playing a Client

Just as skills and strategies can help you succeed when you role-play a clinician, so are there skills that can help you enjoy and learn when role-playing the client. These skills can also enable you to help the other learners in your practice group when you are in the client role.

As a client, you will be talking about concerns or issues that are likely to benefit from some help. You usually have the opportunity to choose whether to present concerns that you are experiencing in your own life or to assume a persona and talk about problems that are not really your own. You might role-play one of your clients, someone you know, or an imagined client. You might even take on the role of someone in a novel, film, or television program that is familiar to you, or you may role-play a famous figure in history. Of course, if you portray an actual person, you must change any identifying information to protect the confidentiality and privacy of that person. In addition, taking on the role of a well-known historical figure or media personality presents the risk that the role-play will become silly, if, for example, you take on the body language and attitude of Elvis Presley or Bill Clinton. Both choices, role-playing yourself or role-playing an actual or hypothetical client, have benefits and drawbacks.

Role-Playing a Hypothetical Client

Benefits

- There is little risk that the person in the client role will become hurt or upset.
- You can feel free to present more severe issues and concerns.
- Group members can observe and discuss freely how a clinician might treat such a challenging problem or client.

Drawbacks

- The clinician might not be able to provide a realistic presentation of the client.
- The clinician or the other group members might not take the problem or person seriously.
- The group members might become more involved with the intricacies of a melodramatic story than with their skill development.
- The clinician will not have the opportunity to see the interventions actually make a difference in the client's life.

Presenting One's Own Concerns

Benefits

- Presenting actual concerns makes the exercise more realistic.
- The person in the client role may experience some personal growth as a result of this process.
- Clinicians can assess the effect of their interventions by looking at changes in clients and their targeted concerns over time.

Drawbacks

- Clinicians may be reluctant to ask personal questions of their colleagues.
- The person in the client role may become upset or hurt during the process.
- If group members present their own serious concerns, that may affect how the other participants view them and can interfere with the development of trust and rapport in the practice group.
- Presentation of serious personal concerns by a group member also can create dilemmas for other members. Should they share this information with the instructor? Do they have an obligation to help the person outside of class? Should they avoid giving critical feedback to a group member who is in crisis?
- Group members who present their own concerns may find themselves feeling uncomfortable with their level of self-disclosure. They may inadvertently disclose more than they originally intended, or they may feel reluctant to answer appropriate yet personal questions posed by the clinician.

Instructors may want to recommend whether people in the client role present their own concerns or those of a hypothetical client. If instructors leave this decision up to the individual group members, that decision should be made with care and deliberation. People who present their own concerns in practice group sessions can minimize the risks of that decision through careful selection of the issues they present.

Select concerns that focus on you rather than on another person, that seem amenable to change, and that are not painful or difficult for you to discuss. Present concerns that are specific, meaningful, and important but that are unlikely to feel overwhelming, either to you or to the clinician. Focus on current issues, rather than past wounds, and avoid important issues that you are currently addressing in therapy. Instead, bring up concerns or decisions that are common, that are likely to be shared by some of the other learners, and that you would not mind becoming public information.

The following are categories of concerns that are probably suitable for discussion in practice group sessions.

- Making decisions about professional goals and direction
- Finding more balance in your life
- Improving and building current relationships
- Changing habits or behaviors, such as exercise, food choices, use of leisure time, reducing clutter, or devoting more time to academics

- Improving interpersonal skills, such as parenting, initiating conversations, and making requests of others
- Coping with current issues, such as a relocation, an unrewarding relationship, or a minor conflict with a family member
- Dealing with relatively minor disappointments and fears, such as failure to receive a promotion, loss of contact with an old friend, or fear of flying

The following are concerns that probably should *not* be the focus of role-plays in the practice group:

- Serious drug or alcohol problems
- Suicidal ideation
- Severe depression or anxiety
- Traumatic experiences
- Issues that date back to childhood
- Life-threatening illness
- Loss of contact with reality
- Uncontrollable anger
- Sexual or physical abuse
- Conflicts with instructors or students who may be known to others in the group

When you are working in your practice group, remember that you are in control of yourself. You can reveal as much or as little as you choose. Although I encourage you to be helpful to the other group members, you, like all clients, should collaborate with the clinician in setting the agenda for your sessions. You have the right to let the clinician know that you choose not to discuss certain areas of your life. Be sure to take care of yourself so that your experience as a client is a rewarding one.

Confidentiality

Maintaining the confidentiality of the practice group is essential. This needs to be clearly stated as a ground rule for the group. Only if group members are confident that information about their lives or their performance in the practice group will not be shared with others inappropriately can they feel comfortable engaging in the exercises in such a way as to promote personal and professional growth.

Exceptions to the guideline of confidentiality may exist, and these should be stated and explained before the first practice session. Instructors or supervisors responsible for this learning experience may want group members to provide written or oral feedback on their own performance in the group and on that of their colleagues. Even if this is a part of the group experience, I encourage supervisors and instructors to promote a group atmosphere that is conducive to collaboration, openness, and empowerment. Emphasis should be on people's self-evaluations rather than on how others evaluate them.

Although I strongly encourage group members to present concerns that are not highly charged, the direction of a session is often unpredictable. Unanticipated worrisome issues may emerge. As in the real world of counseling, social work, and psychology, clinicians are permitted to break confidentiality if clients present a danger to themselves or to others. However, this is not a decision to be made lightly; breaking confidentiality usually should be done only after consultation with a colleague or supervisor. If you believe that someone in your practice group presents a danger, or if you believe that the concerns presented by a group member require professional help, you should discuss this matter with the group member and then with your instructor or supervisor. This guideline, too, should be clearly stated before the group begins its role-plays so that all participants understand the circumstances under which confidentiality may need to be broken.

Practice Group Exercise

The practice exercise in this chapter, the first in the book, has several purposes:

- Introducing the participants to the format of the practice group exercises.
- Beginning to develop some rapport and comfort among the group members.
- Providing the opportunity for participants to give each other feedback following the guidelines in this chapter.
- Establishing a baseline for skill development.
- Initiating the process of identifying skills both strong and those that need development or improvement and formulating plans for change.

Form into your practice groups following the instructions presented earlier in this chapter.

Participants as Clients

When each participant is in the client role, he or she should begin with a brief description of the client to be role played, including age, gender, physical appearance, and presenting concerns. The participant should remain in the role of that client throughout the day's role play.

Participants as Clinicians

The participant in the clinician role should conduct an initial interview with the role-played client, focused on establishing a positive therapeutic alliance and determining answers to the questions presented later in this section. Although the clinician will make considerable use of questions, these should be integrated with other interventions that communicate empathy and active listening, and most of the following questions should be broken down and explored rather than being asked as stated here.

Questions   As the basis for the role-plays, the person in the clinician role can use a modified version of the questions raised in this chapter about Jared, exploring the following questions with the role-played client over the course of this initial interview.

- In one or two sentences, how would you describe the nature of your difficulties? What is your understanding of what led to the development of your concerns?
- What are your most important strengths and assets, and how can they be mobilized and maximized?
- What are the highlights of your background?
- How do multicultural factors such as gender, age, religion, ethnicity, and others affect you and your view of the world?
- What emotional, cognitive, and behavioral patterns, strengths, and difficulties are characteristic of you?
- What are the connections between your background experiences and your emotional, cognitive, and behavioral patterns, strengths, and difficulties?
- Which of the three areas (emotions, thoughts, actions) reflects your most prominent or troubling symptoms?

Participants as Observers

While in the observer role, participants should take notes on the clinician's demonstration of skills, following the topics on the Assessment of Progress form later presented in this chapter. Observers should feel free to embellish and go beyond the categories in the form, as long as they emphasize strengths and prepare to provide useful, specific, and constructive feedback.

Timing of Exercise

Ideally, at least 15 minutes should be allowed for each role-play. Another 5 or 10 minutes should be allowed for feedback following each role-play.

Assessment of Progress Form 1

1. Identify at least two strengths demonstrated by the clinician, indicating the interaction with the client or the intervention that exemplified each strength.

   a. _____

   b. _____

2. What efforts did the clinician make to initiate a positive therapeutic alliance with the client? How effective were they?

   _____

   _____

   _____

3. Describe how the clinician approached the process of obtaining information from the client. Consider the types of interventions the clinician used (e.g., open question, closed question, encourager), the pacing of the session, the mix of interventions used by the clinician, and nonverbal communications. How successful was the clinician in obtaining the information in the questions provided for this role-play?

   _____

_____

_____

_____

4. List two ways in which the clinician might have improved upon his or her use of clinical skills and the process of the session:

a. _____

b. _____

Personal Journal Questions

The fourth and last type of exercise included in the Learning Opportunities at the end of each chapter is the Personal Journal Questions. I encourage you to keep your responses to these questions together, in an actual written journal or a computer file. In this way, you can review all of your journal responses and have a record of some of the introspection and insights that grew out of your involvement in this learning experience. Be sure that, before you begin to respond to the Personal Journal Questions, you have a clear understanding from your instructor as to who will have access to your responses to these questions. Will these responses be only for your eyes, or will they be turned into your instructor? The level of confidentiality of these responses may affect what you choose to write in your journal, because some of these questions ask for self-disclosure and information on your own background. Be sure to take care of yourself and, if others will have access to your journal responses, write only what you are comfortable sharing. However, I hope that the journal will provide you an opportunity to gain self-awareness and think through some challenging personal and professional issues.

Here is your first set of Personal Journal Questions.

1. What thoughts and feelings do you have as you begin to read this book and participate in the associated class or training experiences? What do you hope you will gain from these experiences? What concerns do you have about these experiences? How can you address those concerns so that they do not interfere with your learning?

2. Assume that you are your own client. Respond briefly to each of the following questions, as they pertain to you:
   a. In one or two sentences, how would you describe the nature of the client's difficulties? What is your understanding of what led to the development of the person's concerns?
   b. What are the client's most important strengths and assets, and how can they be mobilized and maximized?
   c. What are the highlights of the client's background?
   d. How do multicultural factors such as gender, age, religion, ethnicity, and others affect the client and that person's view of the world?
   e. What are the client's emotional, cognitive, and behavioral patterns and difficulties?

f. What are the connections between the client's background experiences and his or her emotional, cognitive, and behavioral patterns and difficulties?

g. Which of the three areas reflects the client's most prominent or troubling symptoms?

h. Which of the three areas reflects the symptoms that are most amenable to change?

SUMMARY

This chapter introduced many of the concepts that are essential to your understanding and effective use of this book. These concepts include:

- The division of clinical skills into fundamental and conceptual skills and the differences and similarities between the two
- The BETA format, in which theories of counseling and psychotherapy as well as treatment strategies are organized according to whether their primary emphasis is on background, emotions, thoughts, or actions
- A set of premises about the clinician, the client, and the mental health treatment process

In addition, this chapter included information on the four types of learning opportunities provided at the end of each chapter in this book. Particular attention was paid to the effective use of the practice group sessions as a learning tool and a discussion of how participants can make best use of role-plays and the process of giving and receiving feedback that accompanies them.

Chapter 2 begins the presentation of conceptual skills that focus on background. Among others, these skills include a framework for improving understanding of clients, ways to gather information in meaningful ways, and the importance of emphasizing clients' strengths in clinical work.

Chapter 2

USING CONCEPTUAL SKILLS TO UNDERSTAND, ASSESS, AND ADDRESS BACKGROUND

BLOOM'S TAXONOMY, CONTEXT, MULTICULTURALISM, AND INTERPRETATION

OVERVIEW

This chapter focuses primarily on conceptual skills related to assessing and addressing background. When people come into counseling or psychotherapy, they are not blank slates; their lives do not begin when they start treatment. Rather, they bring with them a lifetime of experiences, emotions, and ideas. Even if you are a school counselor working with four-, five-, and six-year-olds, the children you counsel have already formed attachments to their caregivers that will affect the relationships they will have throughout their lives. They have already learned ways to get attention, to meet their needs, and to control their bodies and their emotions. They already have self-images and can talk about what they want to be when they grow up. Adult clients, of course, bring with them a far more extensive range of experiences.

Current thinking in counseling and psychotherapy has increasingly recognized the importance of the work of John Bowlby (1978, 1988). Bowlby, an object relations theorist, believed that there is a strong correlation between people's early attachments to their caregivers and their later emotional development and relationships.

These findings and many others suggest that, to understand clients well and to determine the best ways to help them, clinicians should take a holistic view of people that encompasses their background, development, family of origin, and experiences. The many important aspects of people's lives and the precipitants of their seeking help provide a context that informs and improves the treatment process. Particularly important is understanding people's cultural contexts and worldviews. In addition, an appreciation of people's important relationships is useful in enabling clinicians to identify and address their characteristic ways of interacting with others as well as any transference reactions they may have to the clinician. This also is useful in helping clinicians to understand any countertransference reactions that they have toward their clients. All of these topics and more will be explored in this chapter and the next, both of which focus on background.

This chapter presents the following conceptual skills relevant to understanding and helping people deal with both background and current issues:

- *Using a taxonomy to organize and analyze client information:* A modified version of Bloom's taxonomy is presented and its use is illustrated in several ways.
- *Understanding the context of treatment:* Motivation, source of referral, place, time, purpose, presenting concerns are important aspects of context.
- *Using interpretation to promote insight.*
- *Developing multicultural awareness and competence.*

CLARIFYING CONCEPTUAL SKILLS USING BLOOM'S TAXONOMY

Conceptualizing clients and their treatment can be broken down into a series of steps. One useful framework that delineates the series of steps is derived from a taxonomy of educational objectives, developed by Bloom, Engelhart, Furst, Hill, and Krathwohl (1956) and applied to counselors by Granello (2000). I have made some further modifications and adaptations to this taxonomy so that it better meets the needs of developing clinicians.

The modified version of Bloom's taxonomy includes two key elements, *content* and *process*, with process subdivided into six conceptual skills or steps. The taxonomy is shown in Table 2-1, with each step reflected by a question that represents the conceptual processes undertaken at that point. Further explanation of each step, accompanied by an illustrative example, follows.

TABLE 2-1   Modified Version of Bloom's Taxonomy

Content
What are the facts?

Process
How do the facts promote understanding of the person and how to help him or her?

• Comprehension	What do I know and understand about the facts?
• Organization	What principles, categories, and generalizations help me to understand this information?
• Analysis/Synthesis	How are these facts related, and what inferences can I draw about their connections?
• Interpretation	What does all this mean (underlying significance), and what sense does all this make?
• Application	What approaches seem most likely to be effective in building a sound therapeutic relationship with this client and helping this person achieve his or her treatment goals?
• Evaluation	How effective has my treatment been, how could I make it even more effective, and what can I learn from this experience?

Content

The content is the answer to the question, "What are the facts?" By making effective use of fundamental skills such as open and closed questions, reflections of feeling and meaning, and encouragers, clinicians can elicit important information about their clients. Clinicians in search of content are almost like reporters, gathering and clarifying information so that they can become familiar with the important people and experiences in a client's life, the chronology of that person's history, and the salient thoughts, emotions, and actions that characterize the client. In seeking content, clinicians also seek knowledge of relevant terms, categories, and patterns (Miller, Sadler, Mohl, & Melchiode, 1991).

Example

A young woman named Shana presents with symptoms of very low weight and purging. A clinician focused on content will gather such information as the duration and severity of Shana's symptoms, her family and cultural background, any family history of eating and other problems, her current life situation, her strengths, effective and ineffective strategies she has used to help herself, and the diagnostic criteria and types of eating disorders.

Process

Once clinicians have obtained the content or information they need, they can process the information so that it will be useful to them, guiding and informing the direction of treatment. Processing is divided into the following six steps.

Comprehension   In this step, clinicians answer the question, "What do I know and understand about the facts?" This is the most basic level of understanding, making use of information without necessarily relating it to other information or recognizing its implications. Clinicians check out their understanding of the information they have received to be sure they correctly heard and grasped the content that clients provided. Summarizing and paraphrasing are particularly useful in ensuring accurate comprehension.

Example

In early sessions with Shana, the clinician might identify the important aspects of Shana's background, such as her history of self-destructive relationships and her strong bond with her father, and determine what additional information may be needed. Clinicians make sure to attend to assets and positive experiences as well as the client's difficulties. An intake interview is a powerful way to obtain this information. Clinicians may also refer the client for a physical examination or administer a mood inventory to deepen their knowledge and understanding of this person.

Organization   Next, clinicians answer the question, "What principles, categories, and generalizations help me to understand this information?" To make sense of the information they have obtained, clinicians need to organize that information into meaningful categories. Categories might include developmental milestones, family background, characteristic emotions, cognitive patterns and intellectual abilities, habits and behaviors, strengths, physical health, social relationships, and career history. Eliciting information in a systematic way during an initial session or intake interview facilitates the process of organizing client information.

Example

The clinician might draw the following generalizations about Shana. She has a history of sabotaging and avoiding relationships, especially with men. She has been in a series of disappointing jobs that have made little use of her strong abilities and education. She evades questions about her physical health and has not had a physical examination in three years. Her family background reflects a dysfunctional structure; the client reports that her father doted on her and paid little attention to her mother. The client was triangulated into her parents' conflicted relationship and did her best to mediate between them. Shana has significant strengths: She completed college, seems to be of above-average intelligence, has strong verbal skills, and recognizes that she needs to make changes.

Analysis and Synthesis   Clinicians now need to answer the question, "How are these facts related, and what inferences can I draw about their connections?" Analysis entails identifying patterns: repetitive experiences, behaviors, or ways of feeling and acting in response to life events. Comparing and contrasting client responses and life experiences facilitate analysis and lead to clarification of organizing principles (Granello, 2000). Synthesis entails integrating information from disparate sources such as interviews, client records, clinician observation, inventories, and discussions with others who are familiar with the client. This step further contributes to the clinician's efforts to develop a holistic picture of the client, draw generalizations, and develop hypotheses to promote understanding of the client and ways to help that person.

The processes of analysis and synthesis enable clinicians to make a multiaxial diagnosis, reflecting the clinician's understanding of both the client and the *Diagnostic and Statistical Manual of Mental Disorders* (*DSM-IV-TR*) (American Psychiatric Association, 2000). These processes also enable clinicians to develop a preliminary case formulation, an understanding of the dynamics of the case, and possible reasons why clients are having the difficulties they are experiencing.

Example

The clinician perceives connections between Shana's family structure and dynamics and her difficulties in interpersonal relationships and self-esteem. Her unhappy role in her family, combined with her enmeshed relationship with her father, has led her to avoid intimate peer relationships. Family messages influenced her to view herself as immature and incapable of functioning at a high level, leading to her unhealthy eating, underemployment, and self-doubts. Despite all this, Shana did graduate from college and has lived on her own for nearly a year. Her diagnoses include both an eating disorder (anorexia nervosa) and long-standing depression (dysthymic disorder).

Interpretation   In this next step, clinicians answer the question, "What does all this mean, and what sense does all this make?" Interpretation involves giving a deeper meaning to the information that has been provided, looking at the underlying significance and effects of the client's experiences and reactions. Interpretations should not be viewed as facts but rather as hypotheses or "hunches" that might explain the client's difficulties. These hypotheses or hunches can then be explored with the client and confirmed, revised, or discarded.

Example

Shana's eating disorder seems to reflect an effort to maintain the safety of her "little girl" role in her family and her enmeshed relationship with her father. She fears intimate relationships, both because of their sexual aspects and because they remind her of her parents' unhappy marriage. Her emaciated appearance helps her avoid seeming mature and sexual and becoming involved with her peers. In addition, her purging gives her a sense of control that she lacks in other areas of her life.

Application   In the previous step, clinicians developed in-depth understanding of their clients and the dynamics of their difficulties. Now, clinicians are ready to answer the question, "What approaches seem most likely to be effective in building a sound therapeutic relationship with this client and helping this person achieve his or her treatment goals?" Drawing on all they have learned about a client, as well as their academic and experiential learning, clinicians apply this knowledge to the development of sound treatment plans and interventions. Essential to the success of this step is a solid grounding in clinical skills, such as diagnosis and treatment planning, and familiarity with a broad range of treatment approaches.

Example

The clinician recognizes that development of a sound therapeutic relationship with Shana needs to be a gentle and gradual process, helping her to reduce her fears of closeness and self-disclosure. Treatment should combine psychodynamic, cognitive, and behavioral strategies. This should enable the client to gain insight into the background factors that contributed to her disorder, change her distorted cognitions about herself and her relationships, and modify her unhealthy eating and interpersonal behaviors.

Evaluation   In this final step, clinicians answer the questions, "How effective has my treatment been, how could I make it even more effective, and what can I learn from this experience?" Once a treatment plan has been implemented, clinicians should constantly monitor its effectiveness. If the client seems to be responding to treatment, collaborating in the treatment process, completing all or most agreed-upon tasks, and making gains, the treatment plan is probably an effective one. On the other hand, if client reluctance is growing, the client does not seem committed to or engaged in the treatment process, or the client is deteriorating rather than progressing, changing the treatment plan is probably indicated. This typically necessitates a return to earlier stages of this taxonomy, perhaps gathering more background information, seeking alternate interpretations for the client's actions, or revising the hypotheses and case formulation.

Example

The clinician observed that, although Shana gained insight into the connections between her family background and her current difficulties, she was still reluctant to make behavioral changes. Additional attention needed to be paid to the client's fear of becoming an adult and having people expect more from her. Further work on skill development, and more time spent on modifying her cognitive distortions, seemed likely to accelerate the process of behavioral change. Drawing on her intellectual strengths might provide a safe and productive avenue for Shana to gain some objectivity and reduce her fear of change.

This chapter, like many of the following chapters in this book, draws heavily on this taxonomy to facilitate the development of clinical conceptualizing skills. It offers a systematic way to make sense of information about clients and move from information gathering to diagnosis to treatment planning to assessment of treatment effectiveness. The Learning Opportunities at the end of this chapter offer the opportunity to apply the modified version of Bloom's taxonomy to a client.

INTERPRETATION AND INSIGHT

Perhaps the most challenging step in following the taxonomy is interpretation, understanding the meaning and importance of information obtained from a client. Interpretation happens on two fronts: in the mind of the clinician and in the therapeutic interactions between the client and the clinician.

Regardless of their therapeutic orientation, nearly all clinicians try to make sense of their clients, to understand their motives and wants. We might think of this as a sort of internal interpretation in which clinicians ask themselves questions such as, "I wonder what led my client to deceive his wife again after they had worked so hard to get their marriage back on track?" and "What sense can I make of my client's self-doubts when she has had so many successes in her life?" Questions such as these, as well as the clinician's answers to such questions, will inevitably influence the treatment process, whether or not these interpretations are shared with the client.

Depending on the clinician's theoretical orientation, the nature of the client's concerns and strengths, their therapeutic alliance, and the treatment plan that guides their work, interpretation may be an important part of the client-clinician interaction. Clinicians may share their interpretations with clients so that the client can consider whether the interpretations are accurate and consequently the client can develop greater insight, self-awareness, and better choices. Usually, treatment is even more productive if clinicians can facilitate clients' efforts to formulate their own interpretations. This typically leads to more accurate and helpful insights, as well as clients' growth and empowerment.

The Process of Interpretation

Interpretation is a process that is intended to give people a new frame of reference, a different and usually deeper understanding of themselves and their lives. Interpretation often links past and present, drawing on past experiences to shed light on present emotions, thoughts, and actions. Interpretation goes beyond what people have stated or perceived and gives them new perspectives and explanations. In other words, they gain greater insight into themselves and their lives. This can enable them to reconceptualize their lives and to present a revised and more helpful, narrative of their experiences. At least as important are the changes in clients emotions, thoughts, and behaviors that insight can facilitate.

On the other hand, interpretation can undermine the treatment process and detract from the therapeutic alliance. Poorly timed or intrusive interpretations can make people feel misunderstood and ashamed, can lead them to mistrust and doubt their clinicians, and can leave clients feeling unsafe and vulnerable. Consider the following examples that reflect the use of effective and ineffective interpretations and also facilitate comparison of interpretations with other types of interventions.

Example

> **Client statement:** It didn't bother me at all when my fiancée broke our engagement. I always expected it to happen anyway so it was no surprise.

Examples of Clinician Responses

- Restatement: It didn't bother you at all when your fiancée broke your engagement?
- Paraphrase: You weren't upset when your fiancée broke your engagement because you had anticipated she would do that?
- Encourager: No surprise?
- Open question: What led you to expect her to break the engagement?
- Closed question: When did this happen?
- Reflection of feeling: Perhaps you even felt relieved when what you anticipated finally happened.
- Requesting a client interpretation: I wonder if you see any connection between your reaction to the end of your engagement and your past relationships with women.
- Helpful clinician interpretation: I wonder if your mother's abandonment of you has led you to expect that all women will leave you.
- Helpful clinician interpretation: And yet I know you hoped this relationship would work out for you. Could you be protecting yourself from pain by convincing yourself that the end of the relationship was inevitable?
- Helpful clinician interpretation: Sometimes when we expect something to happen, we inadvertently take steps to make it happen. I wonder if in some way you created a sort of self-fulfilling prophecy. What do you think about that idea?
- Unhelpful interpretation: You are clearly in denial of your true feelings, perhaps because you have never fully dealt with the pain of losing your mother.

As you can see, unlike other types of interventions, interpretations offer new perspectives on people's experience. Interpretations are designed to encourage people to take a closer and deeper look at their feelings and perhaps gain greater insight and self-awareness. The first three interpretations presented, though they are strong statements, are gently phrased and allow the client the opportunity to think about and perhaps reject or elaborate on the ideas. The last interpretation, however, sounds accusatory and is likely to make the client feel uncomfortable and perhaps even angry. Interpretations are powerful tools, but they must be used with great care and sensitivity.

Questions About the Process of Interpretation

Think about your reactions to the previous examples and respond briefly to the following questions:

1. Of all the client responses presented, which would you use and why?
2. How would you compare the helpful interpretations to the other types of interventions?
3. Which interventions seemed most likely to be helpful and why?

Perhaps the depth and strength of the interpretations appealed to you and seemed to offer you a vehicle for using your own insight and intellectual abilities to help people. On the other hand, you may have found the interpretations to be intrusive and viewed them as pressuring the client. How much or how little use you make of interpretations is up to you, but interpretation is a tool that should be familiar and available to all clinicians.

Differing Viewpoints About Interpretation

Clinicians differ in terms of the importance they ascribe to interpretation and insight and about the place they believe these interventions have in treatment. Freud and his followers were the first and most vocal proponents of interpretation and insight. They viewed insight as the ultimate goal of psychotherapy and used interpretation liberally to help clients achieve greater insight. Modern clinicians who practice from a psychoanalytic or psychodynamic framework generally continue to place great importance on interpretation and insight.

Many clinicians, however, do not share that perspective. Cognitive, behavioral, person-centered, and solution-focused therapists, for example, typically minimize the role of interpretation in their work and, instead, emphasize exploration of present thoughts, emotions, and actions.

Despite this variation, nearly all clinicians recognize that, at least occasionally, interpretation can be a helpful addition to the treatment process. Current clinical thinking seems to be that, although interpretation may be a necessary part of treatment, it is a starting point and usually is not sufficient to accomplish the changes in emotions, thoughts, and actions that are generally the goals of modern counseling and psychotherapy.

Effective Use of Interpretation

Many types of interpretations are available. Clinicians' personal style and theoretical orientation, the specific client, the presenting concerns, the nature of the therapeutic alliance, the goals of treatment, and the topic of the interpretation all influence the type of interpretation that is most appropriate. Interpretations may be especially helpful under several specific circumstances:

- When treatment has reached an impasse.
- When a client keeps repeating the same harmful patterns and behaviors.

- When present emotions, thoughts, or actions do not seem to make sense on the surface.
- When the client seems to be overreacting to an event or interaction.
- When the client has strong emotional reactions to the clinician that do not seem to be based in present reality.
- When the present is a clear repetition of the past.

Interpretations can stem from a variety of perspectives; some of these follow, with examples.

- **Feminist/gender-based interpretation:** "It sounds like your role as a woman is very different from that of your mother. I wonder if that is creating some conflict for you."
- **Developmental interpretation:** "You seem to be saying that, when most of your friends were asserting their independence and establishing strong connections with their peers, you and your father continued to be each other's primary sources of support. I wonder if that has a lot to do with your being a sort of late bloomer, just beginning to establish your independence as you approach 30."
- **Multicultural interpretation:** "I wonder if at least part of the reason for the conflict you are having with your daughter has to do with cultural issues. You came to the United States in your late 20s and still view yourself as Vietnamese, while she was born in the United States and ascribes little importance to the traditional Asian values that still are so meaningful to you."
- **Psychodynamic interpretation**: "Some clinicians view depression as anger turned inwards. Could it be that your depression reflects anger you have toward yourself or someone else?"

Formats for Effective Interpretation   Language is an important factor in determining the effectiveness of interpretations. Consider the following examples, which provide some helpful formats for the delivery of interpretations.

- **Hunches:** "I have a hunch that you enjoy all the attention you receive when you are sick and can't go to school. Maybe that makes it hard for you to get well. What do you think about that?"
- **Noting themes:** "I've noticed a theme of men mistreating you that keeps coming up in our conversations. You've talked about your father's verbal abuse, your math teacher's criticism of your work, your physician's lack of caring when you are in pain, your supervisor's failure to praise your work, and several of your boyfriends who seemed neglectful. What do you make of that pattern?"
- **Noting connections:** "Your strong reaction to your teacher's inability to attend your recital reminds me of the feelings you had as a child when your parents separated and your father stopped coming to your soccer games. I wonder if you see any connection there."

- **Noting discrepancies and differences:** "You have had many disappointing relationships with family and friends. It strikes me that this relationship seems to be different for you, perhaps because you have more control now. What is your reaction to that?"
- **Reframing:** "You have described yourself as a 'hopeless workaholic' but you derive great satisfaction from your work. Perhaps you are really actualizing your potential."

Illustration of an Effective Interpretation   Let's look at a simple illustration of how interpretation, leading to greater insight, can enrich clients' lives and facilitate positive change.

Flo had been raised in a spiritual family; a bedtime prayer was an important ritual in her family. As she moved into her teenage years, one of the ways she asserted her independence was by refusing to participate in the family prayers. She felt comfortable with her decision and rarely gave it a second thought.

Fifteen years later, however, Flo sought treatment for depression following the birth of her first child. Despite considerable evidence to the contrary, Flo persisted in believing that she was not doing a good job as a mother. Exploration of Flo's feelings for her child and her role as a mother shed no light on her self-doubts as a parent. The clinician then shifted to the past, looking for patterns and connections, and asked Flo about her family of origin, especially the mothering she had received.

Based on information from this conversation, the clinician made the following interpretation:

> Flo, it sounds like in nearly all respects you are emulating the positive qualities you saw in your own mother and in your vision of how a mother should be. In light of that, it is puzzling that you are so dissatisfied with yourself as a mother. One piece I do hear that is missing from your parenting style is an emphasis on spirituality. You talked about your own family's nightly prayer and how that lost its importance for you as you moved into adolescence. But I'm wondering if that weren't more important than you realized and perhaps is what is missing for you now in your role as a mother.

Now that she had an adult perspective, Flo was able to recognize the importance of the nightly prayer in unifying her family and providing a sense of security and belonging. Because Flo had not been providing her daughter the same spiritual foundation she had gained from her family, she had a sense that something was missing and that she was an inadequate parent. Through discussion with her husband, Flo was able to create a personal prayer that was compatible with the beliefs she and her husband shared. Establishing a nightly ritual of saying this prayer with her current family enhanced Flo's perception of herself as a mother and helped her create in her new family the sense of closeness and security she had in her family of origin.

This example reflects many of the characteristics of the positive use of interpretation in counseling and psychotherapy. Important characteristics of helpful interpretations follow.

Characteristics of Effective Interpretations

Clear and Relevant Purpose-   Interpretations should:

- Be presented with a clear and relevant purpose in mind
- Be designed to help people resolve their presenting concerns
- Help people make sense of their emotions, thoughts, and actions
- Promote awareness of patterns and connections
- Encourage a greater sense of self-control and direction
- Facilitate change, not just promote insight

Effective Delivery-   Interpretations should:

- Focus on the present and possible current explanations before moving to the past.
- Be combined with empathic interventions to provide support and encouragement and reduce any threat presented by the interpretations.
- Be used sparingly.
- Be carefully timed so that the client is receptive rather than resistant.
- Be elicited from the client as much as possible.
- Be gently suggested, not forced; insights should not be rushed.
- Always be checked out with clients; clinicians should give them the opportunity to react to, modify, accept, or reject the interpretation.
- Be revisited and explored as appropriate to ensure that they are meaningful and useful to clients.

The Learning Opportunities at the end of the chapter offer you the experience of developing some interpretations. In addition, you will have the opportunity to critique and improve on interpretations made by others.

APPLYING CONCEPTUAL SKILLS TO CONTEXT

Now that you have some understanding of the modified version of Bloom's taxonomy, as well as of interpretation, an important step in the process section of the taxonomy, we turn our attention to using these tools to improve understanding of people's contexts.

The term *context* has many meanings. It can refer to the circumstances of people's lives when they seek treatment; their views of the world; or their ethnic, cultural, and spiritual origins, to mention just a few meanings of the term. This chapter demonstrates ways to apply conceptual skills to context, with particular attention to people's multicultural contexts. The knowledge you have gained of interpretation in the previous section should help you gain a deeper appreciation of the importance of context, both in our daily lives and in our clinical work.

Have you ever wondered what leads a person to pick a particular day and time to make a call for help? Have you discussed with clients how they decided to call your particular agency, how they heard about your services, and what expectations they have for the treatment process? Finding answers to questions such as these can enable you to better understand a client's context and frame of reference when beginning treatment. This information is important in helping clinicians initiate treatment in positive ways, quickly identify interventions that are likely to be helpful, and begin development of a sound therapeutic alliance.

Examples of Context for Seeking Treatment

Consider the following responses when the clinician asks four 12-year-old girls, "What led you to want some help from me now?" Based only on these brief replies, you will probably begin to form some impressions of these clients. Ask yourself the following questions as you read the four client replies.

- Which one would you be most interested in seeing for treatment? Why?
- Are any of these girls someone you would not want to have as a client? Why?
- What differences are there likely to be in the ways you would begin to work which each of these clients?

Client 1: My parents said that if I didn't stop talking back to them, I would need to see a shrink. Our pastor recommended you, but you can't stop me from telling my parents what's on my mind.

Client 2: We moved here last month and I haven't really made any friends yet. I've been feeling pretty lonely and keeping to myself a lot. My parents thought it might help me to talk to someone. My school counselor suggested I see you. Can you help me?

Client 3: Something happened last week, but it's too hard to talk about.

Client 4: I don't know. Is that clock on your desk really a tape recorder, and are you taping everything I say?

The presenting problems, the apparent motivation toward treatment, the source of referral, the goals, and the openness and emotional health of each client is different. Those differences reflect part of the initial context for treatment. That context is likely to have a great impact on the development of the therapeutic relationship and the nature and effectiveness of treatment.

Ingredients in Treatment Context

The context of treatment generally includes the following ingredients.

- **Demographic characteristics of the client:** When client and clinician first meet, they typically know little about each other. The clinician's information about the client may be limited to demographic information and a first impression that provides some knowledge of gender, age, ethnic/cultural background, and appearance. Paperwork completed by the client may provide additional information on such matters as presenting concerns, family composition, place of residence, and medical history. Of course, the clinician will acquire a better understanding of the client and more information on the client's background and context as treatment progresses.

- **Source of referral:** How did the client learn of the clinician and/or the agency? Was it from a telephone directory? A friend or colleague? A lawyer, physician, or other mental health professional ? A member of the clergy? A managed care organization? The Internet? How and what a client is told about a clinician or agency when given a referral is likely to affect the client's expectations, motivation, and attitude toward treatment.

- **Choice of clinician:** Did the client take time to learn about the clinician's credentials or to talk to several clinicians before making an appointment? Or did the client make a choice based on limited information, perhaps because of participation in a managed care program, the need for a reduced fee, confidence in the referral source, lack of interest in investing time in finding a suitable clinician, or another reason?

- **Treatment facility:** Sometimes the client's choice of a treatment program or clinician provides information about that client's treatment preferences. For example, the woman who seeks help from an agency focused on women's issues may be struggling with concerns related to her role as a woman and may feel more comfortable in a setting where most people are female. The African American man who drives many miles from his suburban home to an urban treatment program focused on the needs of African Americans may feel a strong bond with others of his ethnic and cultural background, or he may be seeking to reconnect with his cultural origins. The client's choice of both clinician and treatment facility typically provide useful information about that client.

- **Precipitant for seeking services:** What led the client to seek treatment at this particular time? Had considerable thought and planning preceded the contact, or was it made impulsively or under pressure, perhaps in response to a heated argument, a disappointing experience, or a threatened failure?

- **Motivation**: Are the nature and source of the client's motivation strong and intrinsic, reflecting the client's genuine wish for help and change? Or is the motivation extrinsic, coming from a concerned parent, a dissatisfied partner, a critical supervisor, or even a court order?

- **Presenting problem(s):** The reasons that people initially give for seeking treatment are referred to as their *presenting problems*. These may reflect their own interest in self-improvement (e.g., "I feel sad and tired much of the time") or a concern someone else has about them (e.g., "My wife says I should drink less and spend more time with the family"). The presenting problem may turn out to be the client's most important concern, or it may be only the first step toward identifying more urgent or fundamental difficulties. Some people are initially reluctant to discuss personal concerns with a stranger, so they present with a more acceptable but less compelling problem. Others are unaware of the real nature of their difficulties. For example, the man who is profoundly depressed and having suicidal thoughts may be more comfortable focusing on his problem in falling asleep, whereas the young woman who was sexually abused as a child may initially focus on her disappointing peer relationships.

- **Strengths and assets:** From their initial contact with a client, clinicians should be alert to the presence of strengths and assets that they can help develop further and access in treatment. Even an initial telephone conversation and introductory meeting can enable clinicians to spot such strengths as intelligence, curiosity, verbal abilities, self-care, sense of style, organizational skills, and support systems.

Eight Elements in the Context of Seeking Treatment

To summarize, eight elements are important in providing understanding of the context of someone's initial request for clinical services:

1. Demographic characteristics of the client
2. Source of referral
3. Choice of clinician
4. Treatment facility
5. Precipitant for seeking services
6. Motivation
7. Presenting problem(s)
8. Strengths and assets

Case Examples

Contextual information for a case is presented here to promote understanding of these factors. This information is organized and discussed according to the steps in Bloom's modified taxonomy, continuing our use of this framework to facilitate sound application of conceptual skills. Following this illustration, you will have the opportunity to process a second case. Both cases are drawn from the examples of the 12-year-old girls presented on page 40.

> *Client 1/Jolie:* My parents said that if I didn't stop talking back to them, I would need to see a shrink. Our pastor recommended you, but you can't stop me from telling my parents what's on my mind.

Content (What are the facts?)

Demographic Characteristics: Jolie is a 12-year-old Caucasian female. She is an only child, living with both parents in a suburb of a large metropolitan area. She is tall and slender. Her hair is very dark, and at her initial session she was dressed entirely in black. Jolie has multiple piercings in each ear and studs in her nose and her tongue.

Source of Referral: Jolie's parents brought her for treatment at the suggestion of her school counselor.

Choice of Clinician/Treatment Facility: Jolie's parents sought help from a social worker at a community mental health center in their town. The family's pastor recommended the therapist as being "skilled in treating difficult adolescents."

Precipitant for Seeking Treatment: Treatment was sought after Jolie had several unexcused absences from school, which led to an argument between Jolie and her parents. Jolie reportedly threatened to run away with her boyfriend if her parents "kept trying to control my life."

Motivation: Jolie's overt motivation seems to be reflected in her statement, "My parents said that if I didn't stop talking back to them, I would need to see a shrink. Our pastor recommended you, but you can't stop me from saying what's on my mind." This statement suggests that Jolie is angry at being brought in for treatment and unmotivated to engage in the treatment process. Although Jolie's parents sought treatment for her, they stated that they hoped she would not need too many appointments because their busy work schedules made it difficult to bring her to the appointments.

Presenting Problems: Jolie's parents expressed concern about her falling grades, her unexcused absences from school, and her threats and verbal arguments with them. They reported a sudden decline in Jolie's behavior about seven months ago. Jolie, herself, reported no difficulties except for being "nagged by my parents."

Strengths and Assets: Jolie had been an above-average student until recently, so she probably has good academic skills. She is outspoken, determined, and apparently seeking more independence and self-direction, qualities that can be strengths. Her parents are concerned about Jolie and recognize that she needs some help.

Process

Comprehension (What do I know and understand about these facts?):   Both the school counselor and Jolie's parents are concerned about the negative changes they have observed in Jolie, which began rather suddenly about seven months ago. These changes are worrisome and suggest that she needs help. At least at this point, however, Jolie denies needing help.

Organization (What principles, categories, and generalizations help me understand this information?):   Changes in Jolie show up in all aspects of her life. This becomes clear when the initial facts are viewed in terms of the BETA (background, emotions, thoughts, actions) framework, discussed in Chapter 1. A review of her background suggests that her current symptoms are uncharacteristic of Jolie and reflect a negative change. Her parents seem confused by this and are not using effective strategies to address these changes in Jolie. They seem reluctant to invest much time and effort in helping her. Family dynamics and relationships may well be a contributing factor in this situation. Emotionally, Jolie expresses anger and resentment. Her thoughts reflect a rejection of family and school and a focus on herself and her peer relationships. Behavioral changes are reflected in a change in appearance (piercings, dressing in black), unexcused absences from school, a decline in school performance, and argumentativeness.

Analysis/Synthesis (How are these facts related, and what inferences can I draw about their connections?): The contrast between Jolie's usual attitudes and behaviors and her current patterns is telling. Parents, teachers, and school counselor all agree that Jolie changed about seven months ago. Other young people with a similar history, adopting dress and behaviors like Jolie's, are often involved in harmful use of drugs and alcohol. Sexual activity may be another factor and is not unusual in young people who manifest sudden negative changes. Jolie's symptoms reflect a diagnosis of oppositional defiant disorder as well as a possible substance use disorder. Underlying depression also is often present in young people who manifest symptoms such as those that Jolie evidences.

Interpretation (What does all this mean, and what sense does this make?): Jolie is rejecting the guidance and direction of parents and school personnel. Instead, she is strongly affiliating herself with a peer culture and appears to be making unwise choices in relationships and behaviors. Jolie may be motivated by a poor sense of self and a strong desire for peer approval. Intense involvement with a boyfriend at her young age suggests both a need for affirmation and an other-directedness. These negative attitudes and behaviors may, at least in part, have resulted from Jolie's failure to find adequate role models, closeness, and affirmation in her family. The following hypotheses need further investigation:

- Jolie has a poor sense of self and low self-esteem, leading her to seek external validation.
- Difficulties in Jolie's family relationships are contributing to her withdrawal from her family and to her negative behavior.
- Jolie is involved in use of drugs and/or alcohol.
- Jolie is engaging in a harmful sexual relationship.
- Other factors, such as depression and academic problems, may be further compounding Jolie's difficulties.

Interviews with Jolie, her parents, and her teachers will be the primary source of information. A drug/alcohol screening and mood disorders inventory can provide further information.

Application (What approaches seem most likely to be effective in building a sound therapeutic relationship with Jolie and helping her make positive changes in her emotions, thoughts, and actions?): The clinician must take account of Jolie's reluctance to engage in treatment and her apparent resentment of authority figures. Time must be taken to develop a rapport with Jolie and earn her trust so that she comes to believe the clinician can help her evaluate her life and make positive changes.

At this early point in treatment, reality therapy seems likely to be an effective treatment system; this approach emphasizes the development of rapport and typically works well with young people who are acting in self-destructive ways. It emphasizes assessment and modification of thoughts and actions, both of which are problem areas for Jolie. If Jolie does become more motivated over the course of treatment, some exploration of background might help her understand the factors that contributed to her current difficulties. In addition, family counseling is likely to be helpful.

Evaluation (How effective has my treatment been, how could I make it even more effective, and what can I learn from this experience?):   In this initial stage of treatment with Jolie, evaluation should focus primarily on the development of a collaborative client-clinician relationship. An essential ingredient in successful treatment with Jolie is promoting her engagement in treatment as well as her understanding of the client and clinician roles. As treatment progresses, evaluation will focus on the effectiveness of reality therapy and other interventions in effecting positive change in Jolie's emotions, thoughts, and actions.

Now let's look at an application of the modified Bloom's taxonomy to another of the 12-year-old girls presented on page 40. This client, Henye, is very different from Jolie, and so is her taxonomy.

Client 2/Henye: We moved here last month and I haven't really made any friends yet. I've been feeling pretty lonely and keeping to myself a lot. My parents thought it might help me to talk to someone. My school counselor suggested I see you. Can you help me?

Information on content is provided for this client. Your task is to complete the subsequent six steps in the modified Bloom's taxonomy. In developing your analysis, don't worry if you do not yet have training in diagnosis and in theories of counseling and psychotherapy. Base your processing on the coursework you have already completed in your field and on your own understanding of human development and the treatment process.

Content

Demographic Description: Henye, like Jolie, is a 12-year-old girl. She and her parents and 17-year-old brother lived in France for the past seven years. Her mother, a faculty member at a university in France, is currently spending a year at a university in the southeastern United States. The family arrived in the United States about a month ago, three months after the school year began. Henye is somewhat shorter than average for her age but appears well nourished and athletic. She is casually and dressed in jeans and a white blouse.

Source of Referral: Henye and her parents agreed that some counseling might help her to feel more comfortable with the family's relocation. Her parents requested referrals from Henye's school counselor as well as from two staff members at the university where her mother is currently employed.

Choosing a Clinician: Henye's parents conducted brief telephone interviews with three clinicians who had been recommended and selected the one who had the most experience with young adolescents.

Treatment Facility: Henye's parents chose a psychologist in private practice, believing that Henye would be more comfortable in a setting that was relatively small and quiet, compared to a community mental health center. Henye's parents let the clinician know that they would like to be kept informed about Henye's treatment and made some specific suggestions of how they thought the clinician might help Henye.

Precipitants for Seeking Treatment: Both before and after their move, Henye and her parents talked about the challenges the family might face when they came to the United States. Her parents had not been concerned about Henye's adjustment until the family watched a television program together about France. Henye became tearful and told her parents that she wished they had not come to the United States.

Motivation: Although therapy was a new experience for Henye, her parents explained the process to her and helped her see how it might be beneficial to her. Her parents had marital counseling that helped them in the past and were hopeful that treatment would ease Henye's adjustment to the United States.

Presenting Problem(s):   Henye and her parents were concerned about Henye's adjustment to the United States, particularly her ability to form peer relationships. Her parents described her as a "quiet girl" whose primary interest was in sports, especially running and swimming. Henye also was very attached to her pets, now being cared for by relatives in France.

Strengths and Assets: Henye is aware of and able to talk about the challenges she has encountered in relocating to the United States, especially her longing for friends, her separation from her pets, and her rewarding life in France. She seems to be introspective and articulate. She is willing to meet with a therapist and is eager for some help. In addition, her parents themselves had a positive experience with therapy and are supportive of Henye's receiving some professional help.

Process   You now have information on the context of Henye's treatment and are ready to process that information. Using Bloom's taxonomy, as illustrated with the earlier case of Jolie, complete the following steps, either in writing or via discussion.

1. Comprehension (What do I know and understand about these facts?)
2. Organization (What principles, categories, and generalizations help me understand this information?)
3. Analysis/Synthesis (How are these facts related, and what inferences can I draw about their connections?)
4. Interpretation (What does all this mean, and what sense does this make?)
5. Application (What approaches seem most likely to be effective in building a sound therapeutic relationship with Henye and helping her make positive changes in her emotions, thoughts, and actions?)
6. Evaluation (How effective has my treatment been, how could I make it even more effective, and what can I learn from this experience?)

The preceding section took a circumscribed view of context, focusing primarily on people's presenting concerns, strengths, family situation, and motivation for treatment at the time they begin counseling or psychotherapy. In this section we expand our perspective, taking a broad view of people's contexts. We now consider the multicultural variables that characterize our clients, as well as ourselves as clinicians. These variables include gender, age, abilities, and relationship status as well culture, ethnicity, religion and spiritual beliefs, and socioeconomic status.

Over the past 20 years, appreciation of and attention to the importance of diversity and multicultural competencies and sensitivity have had powerful effects on the professions of counseling, social work, and psychology. Several factors have contributed to this result. First is the growing numbers of people in minority or underrepresented groups. According to Sue, Arredondo, and McDavis (1992), well-known researchers in multicultural counseling, by 2010, "racial and ethnic minorities will become a numerical majority" (p. 278). More than 10% of the population of the United States are immigrants, many of whom have experienced considerable stress, oppression, and economic and political difficulties (Yakushko & Chronister, 2005). Accompanying this numerical growth of people from diverse backgrounds has been a growth in power; Derald Wing Sue, Patricia Arredondo, Courtland Lee, and others from underrepresented groups have become increasingly vocal and persuasive about the importance of multicultural competencies for mental health professionals. Their position has been strengthened by the writings of Allen Ivey, Paul Pedersen, and others who take the position that effective counseling and psychotherapy require all clinicians to understand and make positive use of diversity in their work.

The Evolution of Multiculturalism

How clinicians view multiculturalism has changed and evolved over the past 50 years. The mental health literature from the 1950s and 1960s presents clinicians as being color-blind. Diversity and cultural differences were largely ignored, as were clients' contexts; the focus of treatment was primarily on people's inner experiences rather than their contexts. This color-blindness was viewed as desirable and as reflecting open-mindedness and lack of prejudice.

This perspective changed in the 1970s, when clinicians realized that they were doing people a disservice by ignoring their multicultural backgrounds. Although some writers, such as Derald Wing Sue, took a broad perspective and discussed the importance of understanding people's worldviews, most focused on the special needs of a particular ethnic group. Articles and book chapters addressed such topics as counseling African Americans and counseling women.

Although certainly some attention to the particular characteristics and special needs of multicultural groups is necessary, many clinicians viewed literature that was narrowly focused on a specific multicultural group as contributing to feelings of differentness and separateness, perpetuating an "us and them" perspective. Consequently, during the 1980s and early 1990s, attention shifted away from specific groups to the importance of taking a broader perspective of diversity, emphasizing understanding and appreciation of cultural context and of individual differences. Multicultural competencies emphasized the importance of attending to not only cultural, ethnic, and religious characteristics but also gender, age, sexual orientation, abilities, and socioeconomic status.

Multicultural Competence in the 21st Century

Understanding of diversity continued to advance in the late 1990s and the early part of the 21st century. Now, multiculturalism and multicultural competence are broadly defined. According to Constantine and Ladany (2000), multicultural counseling competency "has been defined as the aggregate of counselors' attitudes/beliefs, knowledge, and skills in working with individuals from a variety of cultural (e.g., racial, ethnic, gender, social class, and sexual orientation) groups" (p. 155). Constantine and Ladany go on to state that those with high levels of multicultural counseling abilities and sensitivity "recognize the importance of considering cultural issues in the context of therapeutic tasks such as case conceptualization" (p. 162). For this reason, this text emphasizes the importance of multicultural competence.

Multicultural counseling in this century has not only taken a broad perspective, it has also sought to strengthen and empower people who may have been disenfranchised because of their religious beliefs, cultural background, sexual orientation, different abilities, or other characteristics. As Robinson (1997) stated:

> Multiculturalism means willingly sharing power with those who have less power. . . . Multiculturalism uses unearned privilege to empower others. . . . Within a multicultural framework, differences are honored and celebrated through the conscious process of unlearning learned prejudices . . . With multiculturalism, differences are valued and are viewed as indispensable to a healthy society. (p. 6)

In addition to these changes, the focus of multicultural treatment has shifted away from a narrow focus on the client. It now takes a perspective that encompasses not only the context and characteristics of the client but also the characteristics, attitudes, and skills of the clinician and the relationship between the client and the clinician. It also views multicultural competence as an evolving and ongoing process.

Another Perspective on Multicultural Competence

Readers should keep in mind that some controversy currently surrounds this topic, although the importance of understanding and appreciation of diversity, as well as multicultural competency, are emphasized in this chapter. Some clinicians believe that all competent clinicians can deal effectively with diversity and multiculturalism and that mental health professionals do not need a separate set of multicultural competencies to improve their work (Goh, 2005). This is an issue that merits thought and discussion. Consider both positions as you read the section of this chapter on multicultural competencies.

The Multiculturally Skilled Clinician

Sue, Arredondo, and McDavis (1992) identify three important dimensions of a culturally skilled clinician: (1) beliefs, (2) attitudes, and (3) knowledge and skills. They describe a culturally skilled clinician as

- One who is "actively in the process of becoming aware of his or her own assumptions about human behavior, values, biases, preconceived notions, personal limitations, and so forth" (Sue et al., 1992, p. 481). Such clinicians have knowledge of their own assumptions as well as of their own racial and cultural heritage and multicultural characteristics; they understand how diversity and multicultural variables affect them, both personally and professionally (Arredondo, 1999, p. 107). In addition, they understand how "oppression, racism, discrimination, and stereotyping" affect people in all aspects of their lives.
- One who "actively attempts to understand the worldview of his or her culturally different client without negative judgments" (Sue et al., p. 481). Culturally skilled clinicians are aware of their own culturally based perceptions and can be nonjudgmental in comparing their worldviews with those of their clients. In addition, they understand the effects that social, economic, and political constructs can have on people and their self-images and know that these constructs can promote negative societal and individual circumstances such as poverty, powerlessness, and stereotyping (Arredondo, 1999).
- "In the process of actively developing and practicing appropriate, relevant, and sensitive intervention strategies and skills in working with his or her culturally different clients" (Sue et al., 1992, p. 481), culturally skilled clinicians take steps to eliminate stereotyping and discrimination in the way clients and others are evaluated, tested, described, and treated by mental health professionals, organizations, and society as a whole.

In addition, Arredondo, Rosen, Rice, Perez, and Tovar-Gamero (2005, p. 156) suggest that clinicians pay attention to three clusters of variables as they strive to identify and understand the effects that multicultural variables have had on a person. These three clusters are

1. Age; gender; race, culture, language, and ethnicity; physical and mental abilities; sexual orientation; and social class.
2. Education; career development and military experiences; relationship status and experiences; health habits and beliefs; and interests and leisure activities.
3. Social, political, historical context (e.g., people who were young adults during the Vietnam War era had a different social, political, and historical context than those who were young adults during the quieter 1980s and those who are now young adults during the conflicts in Iraq and Afghanistan).

The Process of Becoming a Culturally Skilled Clinician

Becoming a culturally skilled clinician involves attending not only to the individual client but also to yourself and to the social, political, and cultural contexts and multicultural variables that affect both you and your clients. It entails careful treatment planning that matches treatment approaches and interventions to the clinician's understanding of the client's cultural context and worldview. In addition, it involves going beyond a multicultural focus and obtaining a full and in-depth understanding of clients.

Application of Bloom's Taxonomy to Eileen Carter

The companion volume to this book, *Fundamental Skills for Mental Health Professionals* (Seligman, 2008), introduces a client named Eileen Carter. Whether or not you have read that book, this section provides enough information about Eileen Carter for you to see how a combination of the modified Bloom's taxonomy and a focus on multiculturalism can deepen your understanding of people.

Two versions of the taxonomy are presented here, both focused on Eileen. The first provides general information, with some attention to multicultural factors. The second emphasizes multicultural factors and their effects on Eileen.

Content (What do I know and understand about the facts of this client's life?)

Demographics: Eileen Carter is a 24-year-old married African American woman. She has a four-year-old son, Charles Jr. She and her family live in a two-bedroom townhouse that they rent. Eileen has been a full-time homemaker for the past four years but has recently begun taking college courses.

Presenting Concerns: Eileen's presenting concerns focus on marital difficulties and her wish to continue her college education. According to Eileen, her husband Charles is opposed to her attending college and has refused to provide child care and financial support as well as emotional support for this venture.

Prior Psychological Difficulties: As a teenager, Eileen developed a problem with drugs and alcohol. Her misuse of alcohol continued until she became pregnant with her son. She reports several prior relationships with men in which she was emotionally and physically abused. She had two abortions before meeting her husband.

Current Life Situation: Eileen's primary relationships are with her husband and son. She has some contact with her mother and two brothers. She reports no leisure activities other than playing with her son. Eileen works part-time in telephone sales from her home.

Cultural, Religious, and Socioeconomic Background: Eileen is African American and was brought up to have Christian beliefs. She has a strong faith in God and values her cultural heritage.

Family of Origin: Eileen is the second of three children in her family of origin. She has two brothers, one four years older than she and one four years younger. She reports little closeness in her family. She perceives her father, an electrician, as having been "alcoholic" and her mother, a beautician, as "detached." Her father died suddenly when Eileen was 10 years old. After that, Eileen spent about six months in foster care before being reunited with her family. The family is described as "ships passing in the night," with little closeness or intimacy. Especially after the father's death from a heart attack, financial difficulties and the mother's efforts to earn money and meet her own emotional needs led to feelings of estrangement in the family. Family messages encouraged the children "not to cause problems" and to minimize their dependence on the family.

Current Family: Eileen takes great pleasure in her son. She reports wanting her marriage to improve and is troubled by the conflicts between her husband and herself.

Developmental History: Eileen reports an unremarkable development. Her parents rarely discussed Eileen's early years, and she has little recollection of her childhood.

Social and Leisure Activities: Eileen has no close friends and, other than her husband and son, is fairly isolated. She expresses an interest in making friends but has taken few steps to make that happen. Similarly, although she expresses an interest in such leisure activities as dancing, listening to music, and visiting museums, she engages in few leisure activities.

Career and Educational History: As a child and adolescent, Eileen had little interest in school. She was a satisfactory student in elementary school, but her performance declined after the death of her father. She left school at 16 and received a GED two years later. Her feelings about college are quite different, and she is enthusiastic about continuing her education. Eileen's work history has been sporadic. Prior to her marriage, she worked in bars and nightclubs, either as a waitress or a dancer. She has been primarily a homemaker since her marriage, doing some telephone sales work from her home.

Medical History: Eileen reports high cholesterol that is being treated with medication (Lipitor). She has had two abortions and gave birth to one child.

Health-Related Behaviors: Eileen has greatly reduced her consumption of alcohol and no longer uses harmful drugs. She smokes one to two packs of cigarettes a day but plans to reduce her consumption of cigarettes. She gets little exercise. Her high cholesterol has prompted her to pay some attention to her diet, but she states that her diet still needs some improvement.

Process

Comprehension (What do I know and understand about these facts?):   Eileen has had serious difficulties in the past (dropping out of school, drug and alcohol misuse, abusive relationships, two abortions), but she has dealt effectively with many of her concerns. She has many strengths that enabled her to come this far, including her motivation and determination, her cultural heritage, her love for her son, her enthusiasm for college, and her wish to improve her marriage.

Organization (What principles, categories, and generalizations help me to understand this information?):   Eileen's concerns can be organized in the following way.

- **Problems with impulse control:** Early and continuing use of drugs and alcohol, unwise choices in relationships, three unplanned pregnancies.
- **Relationship difficulties:** All of Eileen's important relationships, except her relationship with her son, have been either abusive, distant, or conflicted. She lacks role models for healthy relationships.
- **Issues related to goals and direction:** Until recently, Eileen had little sense of direction. She sought comfort in relationships that did not meet her needs. However, the birth of her son and her college coursework provided her with a positive sense of direction for the first time in her life. Her faith in God and her valuing of her cultural heritage also are positive elements that might further enhance her sense of direction.
- **Low self-esteem:** Eileen has little sense of self; she has only limited awareness of her development, her strengths, and her values.

Analysis and Synthesis (How are these facts related, and what inferences can I draw about their connections?):   Eileen's family background seems to have been devoid of closeness, warmth, affirmation, and support. Particularly after the death of her father, she received little positive parenting. Emulating the behavior of her mother and seeking to reduce her own loneliness, Eileen placed great importance on having a man in her life. Her need for love led her to involve herself in unhealthy and abusive relationships. She numbed her feelings with drugs and alcohol, at least in part because of the family history of alcohol misuse. She had no image of healthy relationships and had no positive female role models to help her make use of her potential and develop in healthy ways.

By the time Eileen met her husband Charles she was beginning to realize the self-destructive nature of her choices. Because he was not physically abusive and offered her marriage, she viewed him as a better choice than her earlier relationships. However, Charles's apparent need to be in charge and to have Eileen in a subservient role ultimately led to conflicts between them.

Interpretation (What does all this mean, and what sense does all this make?):   Eileen's lack of nurturing and positive role models throughout her childhood seem to be strongly related to her subsequent difficulties. She lacked a sense of self-worth, leading her to seek value vicariously through her relationships with men who initially appeared powerful but who, in fact, were abusive. Nevertheless, Eileen's strong dependency needs led her to move from one unhealthy relationship to another, seeking a fantasized relationship that might compensate for the loneliness and lack of attachment she had experienced throughout her childhood. Her father's early death probably contributed to her efforts to replace him in her life with a romantic relationship.

Although Eileen does not recognize symptoms of depression in herself, she has probably been experiencing a long-standing underlying depression, characterized by hopelessness, helplessness, and guilt. Sexual relationships, as well as drugs and alcohol, probably masked that depression, but it must be kept in mind and addressed in her treatment.

Eileen's marriage to Charles does seem to represent a move toward health as she matured. Although her marriage has difficulties, they are not of the magnitude of those in her earlier relationships. Her pregnancy and the subsequent birth of Charles Jr. were turning points for Eileen. Giving birth to a child may have helped to assuage some of Eileen's guilt for her two abortions. Her decision to greatly reduce her consumption of alcohol while she was pregnant seems to reflect a sincere effort to "do things differently this time." For the first time, when Charles was born, Eileen perceived herself as having an important role and being fully loved and accepted by another human being. This enabled Eileen to value herself more, leading to her enrollment in college. Her initial success in college contributed further to her sense of empowerment, and Eileen began to envision a different and more rewarding life for herself, one in which she was valued both by herself and by others.

Unfortunately, as Eileen became less dependent on her husband and developed a greater sense of self-efficacy, conflicts emerged in her marriage. According to Eileen, Charles sought to curtail her involvement in college. Despite Charles's objections, Eileen has persisted in her efforts to continue her college education and is trying to pass on her new-found love of learning to her son.

From a diagnostic point of view, Eileen probably has a dysthymic disorder (long-standing underlying depression) along with a prior history of substance abuse and both physical and emotional abuse. She probably also has dependent personality traits.

Application (What approaches seem most likely to be effective in building a sound therapeutic relationship with Eileen and helping her achieve her treatment goals?): Eileen's treatment might focus productively on the following areas:

- **Emotions:** The clinician should further assess for the presence of depression and employ interventions designed to reduce depression and promote self-confidence and self-efficacy. Eileen is likely to have a strong need for acceptance and support in treatment and needs help in learning to form healthy, close, and caring relationships with other adults. Her strong religious faith and the value she places on her cultural heritage might be used to further enhance her self-esteem. Finding positive female role models in the African American community might be particularly useful to her.
- **Thoughts:** Despite her recent progress, Eileen is still struggling with many of the dysfunctional thoughts that contributed to her difficulties throughout her life. These thoughts might include, "I must have a man to take care of me and make me feel important," "I am unlovable," "I have little to offer in a relationship," and "I should put others' needs ahead of my own."

- **Actions:** Particularly important is helping Eileen find a way to continue her education and succeed in her coursework. In addition, she would probably benefit from help with communication skills, enabling her to dialogue more successfully with her husband and develop some friendships. Eileen's health habits also need attention; she wants to reduce or eliminate her use of cigarettes, she needs to incorporate exercise into her life, and she needs to improve her diet. If conflict increases between her and Charles or if she has difficulty finding a way to continue her education, Eileen might once again turn to alcohol to numb her feelings; preventive interventions are needed to help Eileen maintain her sobriety. Parenting skills might be helpful to her as well, in light of her own lack of good parental role models.
- **Treatment:** Eileen is likely to benefit from treatment that has a practical and present-oriented focus, but also pays attention to her painful history, especially her attachment and developmental difficulties. Cognitive and behavioral approaches should be emphasized. Cognitive therapy would focus on modifying the dysfunctional thoughts that have led Eileen to make so many self-destructive choices. Behavioral interventions would emphasize finding ways for Eileen to continue in college, develop better communication and parenting skills, and build a fuller life for herself, including friends and leisure activities as well as better health habits. A detailed multiaxial diagnosis and treatment plan for Eileen are provided later in this book.

Evaluation (How effective has my counseling been, how could I make it even more effective, and what can I learn from this experience?): Once treatment with Eileen has been implemented, monitoring her progress is essential. Eileen has a long history of emotional difficulties and, although she currently seems to be moving in a positive direction, regression clearly is a possibility. Mutually agreed-on goals that are clear and measurable will facilitate frequent assessment of progress and help ensure that Eileen continues to move forward.

Application of a Multiculturally Oriented Version of Bloom's Taxonomy to Eileen Carter

Now that you are acquainted with Eileen Carter and have reviewed the application of Bloom's modified taxonomy to this client, we shift our attention to the relevant multicultural aspects of this woman. The following topics and questions, organized according to the format of Bloom's taxonomy but oriented toward understanding background and multicultural factors, demonstrate the richness and usefulness of gaining multicultural understanding of people.

Content (What multicultural variables characterize the client?)

Eileen is a 24-year-old African American woman who grew up in a lower-middle-class neighborhood in a mid-Atlantic state in the United States. Her father died when she was a child. Despite her mother's efforts to earn enough money to support the family, it was a struggle to provide for the family's basic needs, and they had to apply for public assistance. Because she was so overburdened, Eileen's mother was able to maintain little involvement with her community and her church.

Eileen is currently married to an African American man and has one child. They live in a middle-class suburb of a large city.

Eileen was raised in the Protestant religion. Although religious observances were not a big part of her family life, her parents communicated a strong belief in God. Eileen has been more strongly drawn to her religion as an adult but has not been attending church.

Process

Comprehension (What implications have these variables had for the client?): Most of the families in Eileen's childhood neighborhood and most of the children who lived nearby and attended school with Eileen were African American. Consequently, Eileen felt comfortable in her elementary school. However, her middle and high schools were dominated by children from Jewish and Italian backgrounds, many of whom seemed to have a stronger educational foundation than did Eileen.

Shortly before Eileen entered middle school, her father's death caused a precipitous decline in family finances and led her mother to return to work after placing her children in foster care for six months. The family was now poorer than others in the neighborhood and, as far as they knew, they were the only family receiving public assistance. Many of the mothers in Eileen's neighborhood were employed outside of the home, and some were single parents; however, this was unusual among the young people in Eileen's middle and high schools, and teachers seemed to assume that all students came from financially comfortable two-parent families with mothers who stayed at home. This pattern was reflected in the literature that was read in school.

Eileen's gender further contributed to her difficulties. Her mother had different expectations for Eileen than she did for Eileen's brothers; Eileen was expected to do the housework that her mother no longer had time to do, while her brothers were encouraged to play with their friends and complete their schoolwork. Throughout her childhood years, her parents had paid more attention to her brothers' academic and athletic successes than they did to Eileen's, a common gender-based attitude for parents at that time. In addition, Eileen had few role models of achieving women; other than her teachers, who reportedly paid little attention to Eileen, she only saw women who stayed at home with children or who worked in low paying, unrewarding jobs.

Eileen felt increasingly out of place and different from her peers. She became less involved and interested in school; her use of drugs and alcohol and her early sexual involvement began. As an attractive young woman, she found that she could obtain the attention and sense of importance she craved via her relationships with men.

On the surface, Eileen seems to fit in well in her current environment. She and her husband live in a townhouse in a neighborhood that includes people from a wide range of ethnic and cultural backgrounds. Most are families with young children. Some of the mothers are employed outside of the home, while others are at home with their children. However, Eileen feels that she doesn't belong in this setting because she perceives her background as being very different from those of the others in the neighborhood.

Organization (What are the central themes or topics that characterize the effects the client's social, political, economic, and cultural background has had on him or her?): The following central themes and topics characterize the effects that Eileen's background has had on her:

- Feelings of differentness and not belonging
- Lack of close ties with her neighborhood, her culture, and her church
- Low self-esteem and the perception that she had few options, linked, at least in part, to early messages about her gender, her race, and her socioeconomic status
- A perception that men are more powerful and superior to women and that women must have a man in their lives to complete themselves
- A wish to become more identified with and connected to her religion and her cultural roots

Analysis and Synthesis (What meaning do these central themes have for the client now? What is her or his worldview?): As a girl and young woman, Eileen's cultural, ethnic, and socioeconomic background combined to lead her to feel different from and inferior to her peers. Her self-esteem suffered, and she came to believe that her sexuality and her relationships with men were the only ways she could find a place for herself and gain some affection and prestige.

Being a child of the 1980s also contributed to Eileen's difficulties. The women's movement had gained momentum, and Eileen received some messages that women could aspire to educational and professional success. However, few of the women around her reflected this picture of women. In addition, her male peers, who meant so much to her, tended to disparage the women's movement and advocated a secondary and subservient role for women.

In terms of her worldview, Eileen believes that the appropriate role for an African American woman is to become a wife and mother and put her own needs after those of her family. She believes that success for women is measured by how they are viewed by others, especially by the men in their lives. Eileen perceives life as difficult and joyless, especially for people with less money than those around them, and she thinks nothing can be done to change that.

Interpretation (How have the dynamics and development of the client's difficulties been shaped by multicultural factors in his or her background and present life?): Although Eileen is currently leading a comfortable middle-class life, the effects of her social, cultural, ethnic, and socioeconomic background have stayed with her. In fact, the contrast between the context of her life during her adolescent years and her current context has contributed to her confusion regarding her appropriate role.

Eileen's family and multicultural backgrounds led her to have experiences and attitudes that had a profound negative effect on her. Her feelings of not belonging, her low self-esteem, her devaluing of her ethnic and gender identity, and her lack of role models all influenced her decisions to neglect her studies in middle and high school, to drop out of school as soon as possible, and to become other-directed, deriving her tenuous sense of self from her sexual relationships.

Now that Eileen has matured, she has achieved a somewhat greater sense of belonging and importance. Much of that stems from her role as mother of a son. Eileen's current context, including her marriage to an African American man, her middle-class lifestyle, and her contacts with other women, has somewhat enhanced her self-esteem and given her the courage to begin college. This step is important for Eileen because it represents a departure from the worldview she held for many years and from the worldview of her family and childhood neighbors. For the first time, she is making independent choices that enhance her self-esteem and increase her awareness of her strengths.

However, Eileen's feelings about these choices are conflicted. Part of her perceives herself as a fraud and doubts her ability to succeed in college. That perspective is strengthened by her husband's objections to Eileen continuing her education and Eileen's own belief that she owes her primary loyalty to her husband and son rather than to herself. Her guilt about her past is another limiting factor, leading her to feel ashamed and out of place when she ventures into school or church or even socializes with others whom she perceives as better than she.

The healthy, growing part of Eileen longs to continue her education, to find in college a place where she can achieve in a way that is right for her and where she has a sense of accomplishment and belonging. She wants to make friends, affirm her cultural and religious heritage by joining a church, and have personal goals that include, but go beyond, creating a loving home environment for her family.

Application (What are the treatment implications of this analysis and interpretation?): Consideration of multicultural factors in Eileen's background is important not only in understanding her but also in the choice of clinician and the development of a treatment plan. Eileen seems most likely to benefit from a clinician who provides her with a role model and contributes to her feelings of competence and power. Consequently, a woman, perhaps an African American woman, is a good choice for Eileen's clinician. Also important is the establishment of a collaborative therapeutic relationship that encourages Eileen to take charge of her life, make wise and thoughtful decisions, and appreciate her many strengths. The clinician's communication of caring, support, and acceptance will contribute further to empowering Eileen.

Eileen is likely to benefit from a treatment approach that helps her understand the effects that multicultural factors have had on her. At present, she blames herself for the unrewarding choices she made in her relationships, her limited education, and even her treatment of her body. Although taking responsibility for one's choices is an important part of healthy development, Eileen's profound self-blame is not promoting healthy development. Rather, it is holding her back and making her feel that she cannot do anything right and will never find feelings of accomplishment and joy in her life. Perhaps by understanding how ethnic, social, gender, political, cultural, and economic factors in her background all contributed to the poor choices she made, Eileen could reduce her feelings of self-blame and low self-esteem. That might enable her to believe that, now that she has matured and sought help, she can make far more rewarding choices.

At the same time, extensive analysis of her past does not seem likely to be helpful to Eileen. She has some decisions she must make fairly rapidly. She sought counseling primarily because she wanted to improve her present life. Some exploration of her background can help Eileen understand herself better, but that should not be the primary focus of her treatment. Instead, she needs help in using her increased knowledge of the effects that multicultural factors have had on her development, as well as her understanding of her worldview, to make positive changes in the present.

Evaluation (To what extent and in what ways has treatment helped the client to understand the effects of multicultural factors on her or his worldview and development? How has that understanding been reflected in changes in the person's emotions, thoughts, and actions?): Although a final evaluation cannot be done because Eileen's treatment has not yet been completed, a clinician working with Eileen might look for the following signs of positive change (Arredondo, 1999):

- Eileen can describe important multicultural factors, both in her background and in her present life.
- She has knowledge of ways in which those factors shaped her development.
- She can identify societal factors such as stereotyping and discrimination that contributed to her difficulties. She is alert to the presence of those factors in her current life and has ways of successfully addressing their negative effects, both for herself and for others.
- She reports feeling greater self-esteem and enhanced empowerment.
- She can articulate both her past and present worldviews and can identify positive and helpful changes in her worldview.
- She reports greater feelings of well-being and a greater sense of joy in her life; feelings of shame and differentness have been reduced and replaced with an awareness of herself as a capable person.
- Eileen is now making thoughtful and positive choices that will enable her to move forward with both her family goals and her personal goals.
- She has improved relationships with family, friends, and associates.

Improving the Clinician's Multicultural Competence

The questions that were used to enable us to understand and address the effects of multicultural factors on Eileen Carter can be rephrased so that they promote awareness of your own multicultural dimensions and competence. Consider the following questions with reference to yourself.

- **Content:** What multicultural variables characterize your background as well as your present life?

- **Process**
  - **Comprehension:** What implications have these had for your life?
  - **Organization:** What are the central themes or topics that characterize the effects these multicultural variables have had on your life?
  - **Analysis and Synthesis:** What meaning do these central themes have for you now? What is your worldview?
  - **Interpretation:** How have the dynamics and development of your joys and difficulties been shaped by multicultural factors in your background and in your present life?
  - **Application:** What are the treatment implications of this analysis and interpretation? In other words, what could you do, either on your own or through therapy, to make positive changes in your emotions, thoughts, and actions via increased understanding of your own multicultural characteristics and worldview? Also, what does this information suggest about the types of treatment approaches and interventions that are most likely to appeal to you, both as a client and as a clinician?
  - **Evaluation:** To what extent and in what ways would treatment be likely to help you to understand the impact of multicultural factors on your own worldview and development?

Implications for Practice

The process of looking at both yourself and Eileen through a multicultural lens has probably increased your awareness of the importance of multicultural factors and competencies. Like many of us, you may have realized that this is a neglected area of learning for you. It is also possible that you realized that you have characteristics of what Srebalus and Brown (2001, p. 48) called "unintentional racists," people who practice or tolerate racism, usually without understanding that they are engaging in stereotyping or discrimination themselves.

Ferreting out and moving toward the elimination of those attitudes in ourselves and in others is a challenging process. However, we are likely to have success in improving our multicultural awareness and competencies if we can

- Be aware of our own heritage and background and the effects they have on us, our interactions with others, and our work as mental health professionals.
- Be open to learning about and participating in cultures that differ from our own.
- Focus on the strengths and contributions of diversity.
- Be honest and realistic about our own reactions and experiences and be willing to explore and address our own stereotypes and bias.
- Be aware of issues of power and privilege.
- Recognize our limitations.
- Notice ways in which we are both similar to and different from others.
- Remain curious, interested, and surprised.

This chapter has introduced an array of conceptual skills related to understanding and making therapeutic use of a client's background information. These include the following:

- Using the modified Bloom's taxonomy to facilitate case conceptualization and analysis
- Making helpful interpretations
- Understanding the importance of context
- Developing multicultural awareness and competencies
- Using Bloom's taxonomy to facilitate understanding of the effects and importance of multicultural factors in both our clients' lives and our own lives

The following exercises provide an opportunity to apply the skills you have learned in this chapter. Included are written exercises, discussion questions, practice group exercises, an assessment tool to use in your practice groups, and questions and activities to address in your personal journal.

Written Exercises/Discussion Questions

1. What do you see as the advantages and disadvantages of using a framework such as the modified Bloom's taxonomy to organize and increase your understanding of your clients? Are there ways in which you might improve on this format? If so, how might you do that?
2. Interpretation is a powerful tool for clinicians. Some clinicians view it as essential to effective treatment, whereas others believe that interpretations are unnecessary and detract from people's efforts to improve the present condition of their lives. Discuss or write about your perspective on interpretations, particularly how you believe they should be used to enhance treatment.
3. Your client is an 18-year-old woman known as Nati, a high school junior, who sought treatment at a community mental health center at the suggestion of her school counselor. When counseling was suggested to Nati, her initial reaction was negative and she seemed hurt by the suggestion that she might need help. However, after the purpose of counseling was clarified for her, Nati cautiously agreed to some counseling.

   About a year ago, Nati's family immigrated to the United States from their home in Africa to seek medical treatment for Nati's younger sister, who had developed cancer. The family had been relatively affluent in Africa, but Nati's parents had difficulty finding professional jobs in the United States. Consequently, they worked long hours at low-paying jobs. Nati became the primary caregiver for her sister, age 8, and her twin brothers, age 10. Nati has been performing poorly at school, appears fatigued and depressed, and has not made friends with other students.

Analyze the contextual information provided, using the modified Bloom's taxonomy. Be sure to include information on all of the following elements in Bloom's model:

- Content
- Process

  - Comprehension
  - Organization
  - Analysis/Synthesis
  - Interpretation
  - Application

4. Multicultural counseling competencies are very important in finding effective ways to help Nati. In her native land, women's primary role is that of wife and mother; domestic skills, especially the ability to bear and care for children, are highly valued. When Nati's parents gave her responsibility for her younger siblings, they told her that this experience would improve her prospects for making a good marriage. Address the following questions in relation to Nati, using the information provided in both this question and Question 3:

- What multicultural variables are relevant to this client?
- What implications do these variables have for understanding Nati?
- What are the central themes or topics that characterize the effects that Nati's social, political, economic, and cultural background are likely to have had on her?
- What meaning are these central themes likely to have for her now? What conflicts or issues are likely to arise for Nati in the United States in light of these themes?
- What do you think that Nati's worldview is like? How do you think that might have changed since her immigration to the United States?
- How have the dynamics and development of Nati's difficulties probably been shaped by multicultural factors in her background as well as in her present life?
- What are the treatment implications of this analysis and interpretation?

5. Develop an effective interpretation you might make to Nati, focused on the conflict she is experiencing between the values inherent in her family and background and those reflected in her current social environment.

Practice Group Exercise: *Conceptual Skills Focused on Background*

Divide into your practice groups, as described in Chapter 1. Be sure that you are familiar with the structure and process of the practice group exercises, particularly if this is the first meeting of your group.

The practice group exercises in this and the following chapters will build on your knowledge of fundamental clinical skills through the addition of conceptual skills. While learning and practicing your conceptual skills, you will have an opportunity to further refine your fundamental skills. Be sure to record your practice sessions (on audio or video tape), both for the group's review and for your own review of your session. I recommend that you record not only the practice session but also the subsequent discussion. This will enhance your efforts to improve your skills.

The practice exercise in this chapter covers the following *conceptual skills:*

- Ability to understand and apply the modified Bloom's taxonomy
- Demonstration of multicultural awareness and competencies
- Ability to make effective and helpful interpretations

In addition, the following fundamental skills will enhance your ability to participate effectively in this exercise:

- Appropriate use of open and closed questions
- Ability to use a range of interventions
- Ability to elicit essential information

Practice Group Exercise

For this exercise, one person will initially assume the role of clinician and the other will assume the role of a client. (The other one or two group members will serve as observers.) For purposes of this exercise, the person in the client role should assume the persona of an individual with multicultural characteristics that are important in both understanding that person and making sense of that person's presenting concerns. Examples of such people include

- A man who had been hospitalized for schizophrenia, now stabilized on medication, who must seek employment.
- A child from a biracial family background who is confused about her identity.
- A Jewish woman whose parents strongly disapprove of her relationship with a man from Saudi Arabia.
- A gay man who is uncertain whether to tell his conservative father about his sexual orientation.

If multicultural dimensions in your own life have affected your current concerns, you may choose to be yourself when you are in the client role. However, be sure that you are comfortable talking about the issues you present and that those issues are not too complex for you to discuss briefly with other learners. If you choose to assume a role for this exercise, you can act as if you are one of the people described previously, present the concerns and issues of someone you know (of course, being sure to conceal that person's identity), or be creative and make up a client who interests you.

The person in the clinician role will conduct an interview focused on exploration of both presenting concerns and multicultural variables. In addition, the clinician should make at least one interpretation, ideally related to the connection between the client's presenting concerns and that person's multicultural background and characteristics.

The interviewer also should try to make good use of the fundamental or basic skills, especially open and closed questions. In addition, the clinician should seek to demonstrate the multicultural competencies discussed in this chapter. These include maintaining awareness of your own assumptions, actively seeking to understand the multicultural background and worldview of the client and the effects these factors have had on that person, and making sure that the interview is free of stereotyping and discrimination.

Timing of Exercise

If possible, allow a total of approximately two hours for this exercise, with each of the four role-plays and their discussion taking 30 minutes. If you do not have this much time, do only two role-plays, one for each dyad. The drawback of this version is that each person will have the opportunity to be either client or clinician but will not be able to try out both roles.

- Allow 20 minutes for each role-played intake interview.
- Take about 10 minutes to provide feedback to the person in the clinician role. Be sure to begin the feedback process with the person in the clinician role focusing on his or her own performance. Focus on strengths first, and offer concrete suggestions for improvement. Like all the practice exercises in this book, this should be a positive learning experience, not one that makes people feel criticized or judged. Feedback should focus on the areas listed in the following accompanying Assessment of Progress form.

In addition, during the feedback process, spend a few minutes responding to the following questions, related to the effects of the client's multicultural characteristics on the treatment process.

- What multicultural variables are relevant to this client?
- What implications do these variables have for understanding the client?
- What effect is this client's social, political, economic, and cultural background likely to have had on him or her?
- In light of this, what central themes, conflicts, or issues are likely to arise in the course of this person's treatment?
- What do you think this client's worldview is like?

Assessment of Progress Form 2

1. Describe the types of interventions the clinician used during this interview.

   _____

   _____

   _____

   _____

   a. Should a particular type of intervention have been used more or used less?

   _____

   b. How effective was the balance of open and closed questions?

     _____

   c. How well were other interventions integrated with the questions?

     _____

2. What was the flow of the interview like? What made it flow well? What would have made it flow more smoothly?

     _____

     _____

     _____

     _____

3. How effective were the clinician's efforts to gather information on:
   a. The client's presenting concerns?

     _____

   b. Important multicultural variables in the client's life?

     _____

4. What might have made the clinician's efforts to gather that information more successful?

     _____

     _____

     _____

     _____

5. What interventions or clinician attitudes demonstrated multicultural competencies? What improvements, if any, might the clinician have made in how he or she elicited and addressed multicultural characteristics?

     _____

     _____

     _____

6. Did the clinician make at least one interpretation? If so, comment on the timing and effectiveness of that interpretation.

     _____

     _____

     _____

7. Summary of feedback, including identification of at least two strengths and one area needing improvement:
   a. Strengths:

     _____

     _____

   b. Areas needing improvement:

     _____

Personal Journal Questions

1. Identify at least two multicultural variables that have been important in your own development. Write about ways in which these dimensions made you who you are.
2. Have you ever felt that people were discriminating against you or seeing you in stereotyped ways? Write about how that felt and how you handled that situation.
3. Do you believe that the fields of counseling, social work, and psychology pay too much, too little, or appropriate attention to multicultural issues? Write briefly in response to this question.
4. Listen to the recording of the role-played interview in which you participated. Respond to the following questions about that role-play.
   a. List one or two interventions you made or heard another person make that seemed particularly effective.
   b. List one or two interventions you made or heard that you think should have been changed. How might you have improved on these interventions?
   c. What do you view as your greatest clinical strengths at the present time?
   d. List two or three goals you currently have to improve your clinical skills.
5. What is the most important thing you learned from this chapter and its exercises?

SUMMARY

This chapter focused on using conceptual skills to promote understanding of people's backgrounds. A modified version of Bloom's taxonomy was introduced to provide a framework for understanding and making therapeutic use of background information. This chapter paid particular attention to deepening understanding of people's contexts, developing multicultural awareness and competencies, and effective clinical use of interpretation.

Chapter 3 continues our focus on conceptual skills associated with background. Included in that chapter are a discussion of intake interviews, gathering and presenting information in meaningful ways, and understanding and making effective therapeutic use of transference and countertransference.

Chapter 3

USING CONCEPTUAL SKILLS TO UNDERSTAND, ASSESS, AND ADDRESS BACKGROUND

INFORMATION GATHERING, INTAKE INTERVIEWS, TRANSFERENCE, AND COUNTERTRANSFERENCE

OVERVIEW

Chapter 2 introduced the use and application of conceptual skills to explore and understand people's backgrounds. That chapter presented a modified version of Bloom's taxonomy, along with several ways in which it could be applied, particularly in enhancing understanding of context and multicultural background. Chapter 2 also presented information about the use of interpretation.

Chapter 3 continues our focus on conceptual skills to enhance knowledge and productive use of background information. The emphasis in this chapter is on describing and illustrating ways to gather information to enhance the treatment process and the therapeutic alliance as well as to deepen and broaden both the client's self-awareness and the clinician's understanding of the client. An intake interview is included in this chapter to exemplify what is probably the most important approach to gathering background information. An analysis of this interview, according to the modified Bloom's taxonomy, provides additional knowledge about both productive ways to process intake interviews and helpful ways to use the taxonomy. In addition, this chapter presents information on transference and countertransference, client and clinician reactions to each other that typically stem from background and that can be processed in worthwhile ways using conceptual skills. Like all of the chapters in this book, this chapter concludes with Learning Opportunities that provide review, application, and practice of some of the knowledge and skills presented in the chapter.

EFFECTIVE INFORMATION GATHERING

Information gathering during treatment is probably most intensive during the first few sessions, when clinicians are just beginning to get acquainted with their clients, but clinicians obtain information throughout the treatment process. This information gathering deepens their understanding of topics and issues that have been discussed and expands their picture of their clients by providing information about new experiences and concerns.

Guidelines for Effective Information Gathering

The following guidelines can enhance the process of information gathering:

- Clinicians should have a purpose in mind when asking for information and should be able to articulate that purpose. They should not simply ask a series of routine questions or go on "fishing expeditions" without direction, goals, or at least hunches.
- Information gathering should benefit both the client and the clinician. It should not be guided by clinicians' curiosity or their personal need to explore further a particular problem or incident. Appropriate motivations for information gathering include improving the therapeutic alliance, clarifying the diagnosis, formulating an effective treatment plan, and enriching understanding of clients so that clinicians can be more sensitive to clients' needs, more aware of their strengths and difficulties, and more able to help them.
- Information gathering should be individualized and should grow naturally from the client–clinician dialogue. Although clinicians do need to obtain some demographic and other basic information at the start of treatment, that often can most easily be done by having the client complete some forms, thereby streamlining the intake process and maximizing the time that can be used to discuss issues that are important to the client.
- Open rather than closed questions should be emphasized. Open questions allow the opportunity for the client to provide a broad range of information, whereas closed questions typically request a brief reporting of facts. Instead of asking a client a series of closed questions, one open question usually yields more relevant information. Particularly useful are questions beginning with "What" and "How," which usually initiate open questions, rather than with "Where" or "When," which generally signal closed questions. Questions beginning with "Why" usually are undesirable because they can make the client feel uncomfortable, under scrutiny, and even attacked.
- Questions should be integrated with other interventions such as reflections of meaning and feeling as well as encouragers. This smoothes and softens the information gathering process, promotes the therapeutic alliance, and helps clients feel understood and involved.
- Clinicians should emphasize client strengths and encourage hope through the information gathering process as they do throughout the entire treatment process.
- Clients should be engaged in the information gathering process and should understand clinicians' reasons for requesting information.

Following are some strategies that can accomplish these goals.

- Ask the client's permission to discuss highly charged areas. For example, the clinician might ask, "I know it is difficult for you to talk about the abuse you experienced. How would you feel about discussing it with me now?"

- Explain why you are seeking information whenever the reason may not be evident. The clinician might say, "Up to now, we have focused on the concerns that brought you into treatment. It would help me to put them in context by getting some information about your background. Can we take some time now and talk about your background and family history before getting back to the current issues in your family?" Or the clinician might explain, "Often people have patterns in their relationships. Perhaps looking at some of your other important relationships would help us understand the conflict you are having now with your partner." Strategies for effective interpretation, presented in Chapter 2, can help you to draw connections among pieces of information so that the client can understand your interest in obtaining more information about some topics.

- Explain why you are not seeking information whenever the reason may not be evident. You might say, "You mentioned that your conflict with your supervisor reminds you of conflicts you used to have with your father. It might be helpful for us to talk further about your father, but I'd like to put that on the shelf for the moment so we can continue our exploration of your interactions with your supervisor. How do you feel about that?"

- Allow the client the opportunity to introduce new topics and take charge of the dialogue. The clinician might say, "We've covered a great deal of ground today, but I wonder if there is anything we've missed that you want to be sure we talk about or discuss in more detail before we finish our session for today," or "You have brought in quite a few concerns today—your thoughts about continuing your education, your conflict with your supervisor, and your recent disagreement with your partner. Where would you like to begin?"

From the initial session onward, clients should derive clear benefit from the information gathering process. They may increase their self-awareness, gain pride in all they have accomplished, acquire new perspectives and a clearer and more accurate picture of their lives, and obtain information and insights that will help them make wiser choices and set more meaningful goals.

Examples of Information Gathering

Review the following examples of unhelpful and helpful information gathering, which illustrate the principles we have discussed.

Unhelpful Information Gathering

Clinician: Do you have a college degree?
Client: No.
Clinician: How far did you get in school?
Client: I started college but dropped out in my sophomore year.
Clinician: Why did you do that?
Client: I wasn't doing very well… it seemed like a waste of time. Now I regret that choice.
Clinician: Did you ever continue your education?
Client: Not in any formal way, but I read a great deal about areas that interest me.
Clinician: But you never tried to go back to college?
Client: No.

Helpful Information Gathering

Clinician: What is your educational background like?
Client: I started college but dropped out in my sophomore year.
Clinician: You sound sad as you say that.
Client: Yeah, I do regret that. I wasn't doing well and so it all just seemed like a waste of time and money. Now that I'm older, I've discovered I really enjoy learning about topics that interest me. And, of course, it would have helped my career to have that college degree.
Clinician: So you have a different picture of education now that you are more mature. What have you done about that shift in your perception?
Client: I've done lots of reading on my own, but never continued my formal education. It just feels too late for that.
Clinician: We can talk further about that, but you did pursue your education independently. What are some of those areas of interest to you?

What differences do you see between the two dialogues? Notice the overall tone and intensity of the interviews as well as the client and clinician statements, the types of interventions, and the probable effects of the two dialogues.

Did you notice that the second clinician used a much greater variety of interventions, communicating interest in and empathy for the client? That clinician also emphasized strengths, used primarily open rather than closed questions, and probably contributed to the development of the therapeutic alliance. Notice how the second clinician paid attention to the client's efforts at self-education and left open the possibility of continued formal education.

COLLECTING BACKGROUND INFORMATION/INTAKE INTERVIEWS

Intake interviews are the primary vehicle for obtaining background information on clients. Understanding the context in which a client sought treatment (discussed in Chapter 2) can help to focus and guide the intake interview. Obtaining some background information early in the treatment process is an essential ingredient of effective treatment. It can facilitate understanding of clients' self-images, the reasons for the development of their symptoms, the effects those symptoms have had on their lives, and the clients' strengths and coping skills, along with many other important pieces of information. The intake interview is an ideal vehicle for beginning to gather background information. Regardless of the clinician's theoretical orientation, knowing how to plan, conduct, and process an intake interview is an important clinical skill.

Goals of the Intake Interview

During the intake interview, both client and clinician form impressions of each other. Those initial impressions typically affect the therapeutic process strongly. Sometimes treatment lasts for only a single session, either because the client leaves treatment prematurely or because only one session seems indicated. In a meta-analysis, Bloom (1981) found that 30–35% of people treated at family counseling agencies, 25–30% of those seen at community mental health centers, and 15% of people seen at university counseling centers received only one treatment session. These findings emphasize the importance of clinicians progressing quickly toward helping clients accomplish their goals.

Treatment goals can be divided into two categories, those that enhance the therapeutic relationship and those that help the client gain self-awareness, effect positive changes, and attain goals. Of course, both categories are important to the success of treatment, and the two often overlap. Although the intake interview is designed primarily to facilitate understanding of the client and initiate client growth and positive change, it also promotes development of a sound client-clinician alliance. The following list includes the typical goals of an intake interview and initial session.

Promote the Therapeutic Alliance

- Introduce the client to the treatment facility and establish the ground rules for the treatment process.
- Begin developing rapport, trust, and openness between the client and the clinician.
- Help the client understand the roles and responsibilities of the client and the clinician and the need for the client to participate actively in the treatment process.
- Initiate collaboration between the client and clinician.
- Assess and begin to increase client motivation and reduce barriers to positive change.
- Enable the client to appreciate the help that treatment can provide.

Increase the Clinician's Understanding of the Client as Well as the Client's Self-Awareness

- Determine the suitability of the client and his or her concerns for the agency's and clinician's services.

- Gather any additional demographic and multicultural information that may be needed initially.
- Conduct a preliminary inventory of the client's presenting concerns and symptoms.
- Determine any urgent issues, particularly whether the client is in any danger or presents any danger to the self or others.
- Begin to identify the client's strengths and goals.
- Obtain sufficient information for a mental status examination (discussed in Chapter 6).
- Obtain sufficient relevant background information to enable the clinician to understand multicultural issues, conceptualize the case, make a preliminary diagnosis, and develop an initial treatment plan.

Chapters 2 and 3 focus primarily on those objectives that increase understanding of the client, including conducting a preliminary inventory of the client's presenting concerns and symptoms; obtaining, processing, and interpreting relevant background information; identifying and addressing transference and countertransference; and demonstrating multicultural awareness and competence. This chapter also illustrates the application of Bloom's taxonomy to the intake interview. Later chapters will teach the skills that are needed to accomplish other goals of the intake process.

Procedures for Conducting Intake Interviews

Procedures for conducting intake interviews vary, depending on the nature and purpose of the mental health facility, the theoretical orientation of the clinician, and the nature of the client. However, three approaches are often used to gather background information.

1. The intake process is separate from the treatment process and is overseen by a clinician who may or may not subsequently provide the client's treatment. Such an intake interview may be conducted by one clinician or by a group of treatment providers who interview the client during this process, perhaps including a mental health counselor or psychologist, a psychiatrist, a social worker, and a vocational rehabilitation specialist. The intake process is designed primarily to assess the client's suitability for the agency's services and to develop an initial diagnosis and treatment plan. This model is especially common at community mental health centers and specialized mental health agencies such as rehabilitation programs and substance-use treatment programs.

2. The first few sessions of the treatment process are devoted to a formal intake procedure. Once enough information has been obtained from that process to develop a diagnosis and treatment plan, treatment generally continues with the same clinician who conducted the initial interview. This model is often used in private practice settings as well as in other clinical settings.

3. Treatment begins immediately, with little attention paid to a systematic gathering of background information. Such information will be elicited as needed to further the treatment process. This model is particularly common in settings that emphasize brief, present-oriented treatment such as counseling programs in schools and colleges, crisis intervention centers, and career counseling centers.

Steps in the Intake Process

When preparing to conduct an intake interview, and during that process, the clinician typically goes through the following steps, regardless of which of the three approaches to intake interviews is being used.

- **Decide what information is needed:** Just as interview procedures vary, so does the information elicited during that process. Discussion of presenting concerns and symptoms is almost always part of the process. However, other topics included in the interview depend on such factors as the nature of the treatment facility, the clinician's theoretical orientation, and the client's symptoms and concerns. A list of potential intake topics (e.g., work history, family background, medical history) is presented later in this chapter to facilitate selection of those topics that are important to cover in a given interview. To streamline the process, clinicians should have in mind the categories of information they want to obtain from an intake interview.
- **Decide how to gather information:** A dialogue between the client and clinician is usually the primary approach to gathering intake information. However, clinicians may also rely on questionnaires, inventories, client records, and other informants such as a parent or partner to provide information. The client's permission should almost always be obtained before seeking information from others, especially if the client is an adolescent or adult and does not present a danger.
- **Decide how to record the information:** Few clinicians can retain all the detailed information that clients provide in an initial interview. Consequently, note taking or tape recording is generally used to facilitate the clinician's later review and processing of the information. Most clinicians prefer note taking, because subsequent review is less time-consuming than listening to a recording. In addition, a small percentage of clients are uncomfortable with the process of tape recording, but it is rare for a client to object to note taking during the session. Of course, clients' informed consent should be obtained before any record of client information is made. Clients are more likely to agree to note taking or recording procedures if the clinician explains that these approaches aid the clinician's efforts to identify and understand experiences and issues that are important to the client and can make the treatment process more effective and efficient.
- **Obtain the information:** A varied array of interventions typically is useful in conducting a successful intake interview. Open questions are usually the

most important and common of these, with some use being made of closed
questions to gather specific factual information. Paraphrase and summarization also are important to ensure accurate listening and understanding
of what the client is communicating. Accents and restatements are useful in
maintaining the flow of the interview. Reflections of feeling and meaning
also have important roles in the intake process; these interventions can
contribute greatly to the establishment of a positive therapeutic alliance
and smooth the flow of the interview.

- **Review the information for gaps:**   Sometimes omissions are as telling as
  the information that people do provide. When clinicians review information obtained from an intake interview, they should compare that information to the categories of information provided later in this chapter and take
  note of any omissions or imbalances. For example, the client may talk at
  length about his mother but say little about his father, or he may say a great
  deal about his leisure activities but neglect to talk about his work. Subsequent discussion of these gaps may prove especially fruitful.
- **Process the information:**   The modified Bloom's taxonomy (Bloom et al.,
  1956) will once again be used to illustrate the processing of information
  gleaned from an intake interview. However, the clinician's school or agency
  may prefer another approach to processing intake data. Any systematic approach to making sense of the information can be used as long as it enables
  the clinician to obtain a clear understanding of clients and their concerns
  and to formulate accurate diagnoses and sound treatment plans.

Example of an Intake Interview

The following intake interview was conducted with Rosa Ishak, a 22-year-old
woman who sought help at a community mental health center. The referral was
made by Rosa's college advisor. Assume that, prior to the intake interview, Rosa
completed forms that provided demographic information and she was oriented to
the treatment process. Rosa is nearly six feet tall and appears to be about 100
pounds overweight. She has a dark complexion and dark brown hair. She is casually dressed in an oversized T-shirt that reads "Keep On Truckin'" over a picture of
two large trucks crashing into each other. She wears jeans and combat boots. An
emblem on her jacket reads "My IQ is bigger than my age. Is yours?" In contrast to
her appearance, she speaks in a soft, gentle voice with a slight Southern accent.
She waits for the therapist to tell her where to sit and glances frequently at the
therapist but without making direct eye contact. A transcript of the highlights of
the interview follows.

> *Clinician:* Rosa, we've already spoken about the counseling process, about
> confidentiality, and about some other guidelines. I wonder if you would like
> any more information on the sort of help I can offer you.
> *Client:* No, I been in counseling before.
> *Clinician:* What was that for?

Client: Oh, lots of stuff. Once when my Mom kicked my Dad out, she wanted me to see a counselor, I guess to be sure I was ok. And then when I was diagnosed with ADD.

Clinician: Sounds like you have been through a great deal, including family conflicts and having an attention-deficit disorder.

Client: Yeah, but I didn't find out I has ADD 'til I was about 11 or 12. Before then they thought I was just a bad, dumb kid, but they finally figured out that it wasn't my fault that I couldn't sit still. I tried but I couldn't help myself. They gave me some medicine and that helped some. I graduated from high school on time, first one in my family to finish high school. Pretty good, huh? I'm not hyper anymore but I still have trouble paying attention. That's a big issue at school.

Clinician: The ADD is still a concern for you, but you sound proud of graduating from high school on schedule. We'll certainly talk more about all that. But first, what brings you in for some help now?

Client: Well, I'm going to college now. I only take two or three courses a semester because of the ADD and because I have to work to help out at home and pay my expenses. I've passed some of my courses but I ain't a real good student. I have this counselor in disability services who has been real nice and tried to help me, but she said maybe I should have more help than she could give me so she sent me to you. I really want to finish my associate's degree but I've been at it for four years and I'm just now off academic probation for the first time and done with my remedial courses.

Clinician: So college is very important to you but it's been a real struggle.

Client: Yeah, you got it. But it's like everything is a struggle. It's real important to me and my Mom that I finish my degree. That's her dream, to have me finish college.

Clinician: So both you and your Mom are hoping you can complete your degree. It sounded like there are other challenges in your life too. What else is going on?

Client: Well, it's not just the courses. I just don't fit in at school. I drive an hour to get to school; it's in this suburb, real different from where I live. Most of the other students live near school, but there ain't any other schools near where I live. The other students don't have to work, their parents pay for their books and courses, and they just hang out all the time. I work in the rec center so I get to watch it all. It's like nobody can see me there. All they ever say to me is, "How much is a Coke?" or "When can I use the pool table?" Nobody even knows my name. And they're all thin and nearly all of them are Caucasian... it's like they can't see anybody who looks different.

Clinician: It sounds like you feel pretty invisible there.

Client: I never thought about it like that, but I guess you're right.

Clinician: We'll talk more about this too, but I'd like to get the whole picture of your life. What is your home and family situation like?

Client: That ain't so great either. I told you my mom kicked my dad out. I was about seven then. She says he was drinking and running with other women and she couldn't stand it anymore. I don't remember him too well, haven't seen him since. My mom says I look like him, tall and big and dark-skinned. He's African American and my mom is Caucasian. Her family came here from Mexico. But I guess I got mainly my father's genes. Things weren't too bad when it was just my Mom and me. Not much money but we managed. Then about two years later my mom gets it in her head that I needed a dad and so she gets married again. Big mistake! Can you believe she marries a guy from Indonesia; I'm still not even sure where that is. And he's Moslem, get that! I don't know what I am now, Caucasian or African American or Asian? Christian or Moslem? What a mess. Anyhow, so my Mom's new husband adopts me and we're supposed to be one happy family, except he doesn't give a—about me. He wants his own kids, especially a son. He and my mom have two daughters, my half-sisters, and then Mom quits making babies. No son, no happy husband. Ain't that a joke. So Mr. Ishak, as I like to call him to my Mom, isn't around much anymore. He drops by every once in a while to give my Mom a check and see his daughters. They look like him, real thin like those models who never eat, not like me. My Mom has really had it tough. She wants me to finish college and so I'm tryin' my best to do that and to help her out with money too.

Clinician: It sounds like you're very devoted to your mother and that you two have been through a great deal together.

Client: Yeah, she's been great to me, really the only person who ever has. But I can't even talk to her about what's going on.

Clinician: Can't talk to her?

Client: No. Last year, a guy asked me out for the first time. He was African American, from Africa, and he really seemed to like me. He would call me every night to say good night and once he paid to take me to the movies like a real date. I thought my Mom would be happy when I told her, but as soon as she found out he was African American, she went ballistic and said that I shouldn't trust him. I didn't know what to do so I just stopped answering his calls. I still miss him.

Clinician: That was a real loss for you, but it sounds like you felt you needed to respect your mother's wishes. What other people are important to you?

Client: I told you about my advisor in the disabilities office. And in high school I had a teacher who was really hot and he tried to help me. He was a man but he taught cooking. I was in a vocational program and he told me he thought I could do better; he even helped me fill out my application for college. But I haven't seen him in four years.

Clinician: But a couple of people have believed in you and that meant a great deal to you.

Client: Duh, wouldn't anybody feel that way?

Clinician: Yes, I think so. What else is important to you?

Client: I really do like to cook and I'm pretty good at it, just like my Mom. I know I should watch my weight but it makes me feel good to cook at home and I cook for the snack bar at the rec center. I make these great cheese steaks! I'll bring you one sometime.

Clinician: So cooking is a real strength you have. How about some others?

Client: I think I'm really good with kids. I'm in this program to train me to be a aide in a preschool. I've done baby-sitting in my neighborhood and then for my sisters and I really get along with little kids. I understand them and can always make them laugh when they're upset or missing their Moms.

Clinician: So getting along well with children is another strength you have. It also sounds like you have a great deal of determination to reach your goals.

Client: Yeah, I guess you could say that. I could just get a job near home at a pizza place or a laundry and live an easier life but I don't want to do that.

Clinician: I hope you feel proud of the hard work you have done. I'd like to ask a little more about your childhood, what important memories you have about that time of your life.

Client: I already told you about my parents breaking up. The other kids were ok about that; lots of them had only one parent. But I got teased a lot because of my weight and the ADD. I must have been pretty tough to have in class. For awhile, my Mom took me to church, but then someone told her not to bring me anymore because I made too much noise and spoiled the service. We just stopped going.

Clinician: Those reactions from other people must have been pretty painful for you. You mentioned church; what place do religion and spirituality have in your life now?

Client: I think there's a plan for us. I can see myself someday living in a big house, having a husband and a bunch of kids, maybe even running a restaurant and cooking my special dishes. I just don't know how to get from here to there. I know a want a college degree, but I guess I ain't real sure how that will help me. Sometimes I get really down and feel pretty hopeless about everything.

Clinician: Do you ever feel so bad you think about hurting yourself?

Client: Do you mean, am I gonna kill myself? No, I never feel like that. I have a friend who's pretty depressed and she uses drugs and alcohol to help her; I don't even do that. I just make believe I feel fine and keep moving.

Clinician: It sounds like we're starting to identify some goals that are important to you. We have lots more to talk about, but our time is drawing to a close so we'll have to put some topics on a list for next time. Is there anything else you want to be sure to talk about today or to mention before we schedule our next appointment?

Client: No, I guess not. You didn't tell me what I should do yet, but I guess we can talk more about that next time. I sure did talk a lot though; it seems like you got my whole life story all at once.

Clinician: You did share a great deal about yourself. How do you feel about that?

Client: It's different. I don't talk about myself much but it felt ok. Well, I'll tell you more of my story next week and then maybe you can tell me what I should do.

Processing the Intake Interview

The following analysis of the interview with Rosa Ishak processes the information from the interview according to the modified Bloom's taxonomy. Notice that strengths are highlighted when they are relevant.

Content (What are the facts?)

Rosa Ishak is a 22-year-old single biracial woman who is tall and approximately 100 pounds overweight. Her biological father is African American and her mother is Caucasian and comes from Mexico. Rosa has not seen her biological father since she was seven years old. She lives with her mother and two half-sisters, with occasional visits from her adoptive father, who is Moslem and from Indonesia. Rosa is a sophomore at a community college about an hour from her home. She works at the college recreation center. She sought help at the suggestion of her college advisor and is struggling with academic, family, interpersonal, and intrapersonal concerns.

Process

Comprehension (What do I know and understand about the facts?)

- **Presenting Concerns:**   Rosa presents a range of academic, family, interpersonal, and individual concerns. Her progress in college has been slow; she has failed some courses, although she passed others, but she needed four years to complete her freshman-year requirements. Rosa was diagnosed with attention-deficit/hyperactivity disorder (ADHD) when she was 11 or 12 years old, and the ADHD seems to have interfered with her academic progress. Rosa also reports discomfort with her racial and religious identity, her self-image and weight, and her relationships with her peers. In addition, she experiences some depression.

- **Prior Psychological Difficulties:**   Rosa has numerous long-standing difficulties that go back to her childhood. These include her ADHD, her academic difficulties, the many changes and racial differences in her family, including having two fathers, being biracial, her weight, and her family's economic situation. She reported being teased by her peers because of some of these difficulties, and she received criticism from authority figures such as her minister. However, she values the encouragement and support she received from her high school cooking teacher and from a counselor at the college.

- **Current Life Situation:**   Rosa seems to have a close relationship with her mother and generally feels loved and appreciated by her, although her mother may have some difficulty with Rosa being biracial and may be pressuring Rosa to complete college. Rosa seems to accept her half-sisters and sometimes cares for them, but also seems envious of their appearance. Rosa attends college and works part-time there to pay her expenses and help her mother financially. Rosa did not report involvement in leisure or social activities.

- **Cultural, Spiritual, and Socioeconomic Background:**   Rosa is biracial and seems confused about her identity. She resembles her biological father, who is African American, but she has been raised by her mother, who is Caucasian. The Moslem and Indonesian background of her adoptive father adds another element that is disturbing to Rosa. Her religious education has been limited and she had negative experiences at church. However, Rosa seems to have faith that God will help her to achieve her dreams. The family has had considerable economic difficulties but that is now slightly improved, with the addition of Rosa's income and some help from her adoptive father.

- **Family of Origin:** Rosa is the only child of her biological parents. Her mother reportedly "kicked her father out" because of his involvement with alcohol and his extramarital relationships. Her mother remarried and has two daughters, ages 9 and 11, from her second marriage. Her mother has been the one constant in Rosa's life, and her mother's love and values seem very important to Rosa.

- **Developmental History:** Rosa reportedly has ADHD and has been overweight since childhood. She had academic difficulties throughout school, as well as impaired peer relationships. However, she did begin baby-sitting when she was fairly young and describes herself as being very good with young children.

- **Social and Leisure Activities:** Rosa reports that she enjoys cooking and caring for young children, and she views herself as skilled in both areas. She interacts with her peers well enough to work at the recreation center but reports no close friendships or leisure activities.

- **Career and Educational History:** Rosa is a sophomore at a community college. She has struggled to get this far in her education but seems determined to complete her associate's degree. She has had a successful work experience at the college recreation center, where she has been employed since beginning college, although she perceives other students as ignoring her at her job.

- **Medical History:** Rosa appears to be approximately 100 pounds overweight. She also has been diagnosed with ADHD and has taken medication for that disorder for many years.

- **Health-Related Behaviors:** Although Rosa reports that her biological father misused alcohol, she denies any use of alcohol or harmful drugs. She enjoys cooking and does not seem motivated to change her diet to promote weight loss, although she is apparently uncomfortable with her weight.

Organization (What principles, categories, and generalizations help me to understand this information?): Rosa's concerns can be organized in the following way.

- **Problems with self-esteem and self-image:** Rosa seems to have a negative view of herself that encompasses her physical appearance, her academic abilities, her social skills, and her racial identity. She does view herself as working hard to succeed at college and as being skilled in cooking and in interacting with young children.

- **Relationship difficulties:** Other than her relationship with her mother, all of Rosa's relationships seem to have been disappointing. She perceives herself as an observer and outsider and, although she seems to long for closeness and acceptance, she does not know how to achieve that goal.

- **Issues related to goals and direction:** Rosa seems eager to complete college and make a better life for herself, in terms of both relationships and a career. However, her goals are unclear; the symbol of the college degree is more important than what it will enable her to accomplish. She envisions herself having a home and family of her own and perhaps running a restaurant, but she has no clear path to get from her present situation to the one she desires.

Analysis and Synthesis (How are these facts related, and what inferences can I draw about their connections?): Many factors in Rosa's background have come together to leave her feeling confused and inadequate. In a variety of ways, she is different from her own family, the other college students, and her neighborhood peers. This is reflected in Rosa's conflicted presentation of herself: She assumes a tough style of dress but has a gentle manner and dreams of having a loving family of her own. Although she can recognize some of her strengths, she focuses on her shortcomings and differences. She has chosen a path (attending college in a suburban community) that seems likely to highlight her shortcomings rather than build on her strengths and help her overcome her difficulties.

Multicultural factors play a strong role in Rosa's development. These include her biracial heritage, her lower socioeconomic background, her culturally complex family, her weight, her diagnosis with ADHD, and her lack of a solid spiritual grounding. She is not able to integrate these disparate aspects of herself into a positive self-image and is left feeling fragmented and confused.

Interpretation (What does all this mean, and what sense does all this make?): Despite the efforts of her apparently loving mother, Rosa has never gotten the help she needs to help her develop a positive and cohesive sense of self, to establish clear goals and direction, and to build on her strengths and individuality. She wants acceptance and belonging and, with her mother's encouragement, has chosen a college degree as the symbol that she hopes will bring her success and enable her to become more like other young women her age. Whether or not college is a wise choice for Rosa, that choice seems to grow out of a confused picture of herself and may have further exacerbated her negative self-image and sense of differentness.

Rosa's persistence in college and work are a testimony to her strengths and determination to build a more rewarding life. However, she is struggling with failure experiences as well as underlying sadness.

Rosa may be enmeshed with her mother, the only person who stayed with her and gave her the love and care she needed, and may be overly influenced by a need to please her mother. This seems to be reflected in Rosa's persistence in college, her continuing residence with her family, and the influence of Rosa's mother on Rosa's choices of friends. Although, of course, this close mother–daughter bond needs to be protected, Rosa needs to individuate and appreciate her own strengths and differences.

From a diagnostic perspective, Rosa seems to have not only ADHD but also dysthymic disorder, an enduring mild-to-moderate depression. Rosa probably also has weak social skills and may have some social anxiety that limits her efforts to build relationships.

Application (What approaches seem most likely to be effective in building a sound therapeutic relationship with Rosa and helping her achieve her treatment goals?):   Rosa's treatment might focus on the following areas.

- **Emotional:**   The clinician should further assess for the presence of depression and employ cognitive-behavioral and other interventions designed to reduce depression and promote self-confidence and self-efficacy. Rosa probably will have a strong need for acceptance and support in treatment and needs help in learning to form healthy, close, and caring relationships with others. She does have some sources of pride and strength, and these should be nurtured.
- **Thoughts:**   Rosa struggles with many dysfunctional thoughts that have contributed to her difficulties throughout her life. These thoughts might include, "I am unlovable," "I have little to offer in a relationship," and "I am different from others and those differences are all undesirable." Again, cognitive-behavioral interventions are indicated.
- **Actions:**   Particularly important is helping Rosa identify goals that will be meaningful to her and likely to lead to success. She needs to review her decision to attend college, determine whether this is the right choice for her, and, if so, to strengthen her intrinsic motivation and develop a clearer idea of how she will benefit from continuing college. Part of this process is determining realistic career goals that are likely to be rewarding to Rosa. She also will probably benefit from help with socialization and communication skills, enabling her to initiate conversations with other young adults and hopefully develop some friendships. Rosa's health habits need some attention, although this issue must be handled with great care in light of Rosa's already negative self-image. If she is motivated, she might benefit from incorporating exercise into her life and improving her diet. Perhaps her interest in cooking could be used as a way to initiate discussion of healthy eating.
- **Treatment:**   Rosa is likely to benefit from treatment that has a practical and present-oriented focus, but that also pays attention to her history and especially the multicultural variables that are so important in her life. Cognitive and behavioral approaches should be emphasized. Cognitive therapy should focus on modifying the dysfunctional thoughts that hold Rosa back and make it difficult for her to appreciate herself and her distinctive characteristics. Replacing self-defeating thoughts with positive ones could facilitate her efforts to build relationships and establish rewarding and realistic goals. Behavioral interventions should emphasize helping Rosa bring more balance in her life so that she has friends and leisure activities as well as responsibilities. Treatment might also help Rosa to develop better health habits.

    Medication for ADHD, and perhaps also for depression, should likely be part of Rosa's treatment. Medication is likely to strengthen the effects of Rosa's counseling.

Evaluation (How effective has my treatment been, how could I make it even more effective, and what can I learn from this experience?): Once treatment with Rosa has been implemented, monitoring her progress is essential. Her ADHD, her history of rejection and complex family relationships, and her depression are all risk factors that may lead Rosa to become discouraged, to view treatment as one more drain on her time and energy, and to stop treatment prematurely. Mutually agreed-on goals that are clear and measurable will facilitate frequent assessment of progress and help ensure that Rosa continues to move forward. A strong and trusting therapeutic alliance can also make a difference in encouraging Rosa's continued involvement in treatment. The teacher and advisor who provided Rosa some help and affirmation are both very important to her, suggesting that such a relationship with her clinician could have similar positive results.

TRANSFERENCE AND COUNTERTRANSFERENCE

As you can see from the discussion of Rosa's treatment, the therapeutic alliance plays an important role in determining the progress and outcome of treatment. Chapter 4 provides further information about the development and importance of a sound therapeutic alliance, but in this chapter we pay particular attention to transference and countertransference. These processes are discussed here because they are connected to the backgrounds of both the client and the clinician. Understanding those backgrounds, as well as the signs of transference and countertransference, can enable clinicians to determine when transference reactions are affecting treatment. With that knowledge, they can either address the barriers and emotional responses that may result or understand and employ transference and countertransference reactions to enhance treatment.

The concepts of transference and countertransference stem from the work of Freud and other early psychodynamic and psychoanalytic therapists. Among today's clinicians, psychodynamic and psychoanalytic therapists, with their emphasis on the importance of background, probably pay the most attention to transference and countertransference. Most clinicians, however, regardless of their theoretical orientation, are aware of these patterns and the possible need to address their effect on treatment.

Definitions of Transference and Countertransference

Transference and countertransference can be defined as perceptions of or reactions to another person that are determined primarily by a projection onto that person of past relationships and experiences rather than by the actual characteristics or actions of that person. The term *transference* describes the process of clients projecting onto their clinicians reactions and characteristics that stem largely from the clients' early relationships. *Countertransference* reactions involve clinicians projecting onto their clients reactions and characteristics that stem largely from the clinicians' early relationships.

For example, a man who had a seductive and abusive mother manifested transference in many of his relationships; he mistrusted nearly all women, including his therapist, and viewed them as seeking to exploit or take advantage of him. This prevented him from collaborating successfully with his therapist.

Countertransference was evidenced by a psychologist whose father viewed any disregard of the rules, particularly lateness, as a personal insult to him. The clinician became annoyed when one of his clients was sometimes late for appointments, not recognizing that an attention-deficit/hyperactivity disorder made it difficult for the client to meet her commitments.

Although some clinicians believe that transference and countertransference reactions are uncommon, many clinicians and theoreticians believe that they are widespread. According to Strean (1994),

> All patients—regardless of the setting in which they are being treated, of the therapeutic modality, or the therapist's skill and years of experience—will respond to interventions in terms of transference. It is important for clinicians of all persuasions to recognize that the most brilliant statement in the world will be refuted by a patient who is in a negative transference. It is equally important for clinicians to recognize that the most inaccurate statement in the world will be positively accepted if the patient is in a positive transference. (p. 110)

Understanding and Addressing Countertransference

Freud and other early psychodynamic clinicians described countertransference as the interference of the unconscious in the therapist's ability to understand a client. This definition has now been broadened to include any emotional reactions that clinicians have to their clients, especially those that are not related directly to the reality of the client's presentation. You may be surprised to learn that clinicians have reactions that are counterproductive and often distorted, but countertransference reactions are common. The challenge for clinicians is to recognize and deal effectively with countertransference reactions, making sure that these reactions are not harmful to clients or to the treatment process.

Teyber (1997) provided a useful list of common signs of countertransference reactions that are likely to impede the therapeutic process. Countertransference may be present when clinicians

- Become anxious and change the subject.
- Withdraw and become silent.
- Become directive and authoritative.
- Provide clients with unrealistic reassurance.
- Create excessive distance between themselves and their clients.
- Rescue clients when they are capable of helping themselves.
- Engage in frequent and excessive self-disclosure.
- Have strong emotional reactions to a client.
- Overidentify with the client.
- Demand that a client make a particular decision or behavioral change.

Taken to an extreme, countertransference reactions can lead clinicians to ignore appropriate professional boundaries and establish friendships or even sexual relationships with their clients. I have seen the damage done to clients whose previous therapists established intimate relationships with them, focused the sessions on the therapist's difficulties rather than those of the client, became angry with clients who did not progress rapidly or follow their advice, or frequently lost control of their emotions in the sessions. Clearly, clinicians must be alert to and deal effectively with their countertransference reactions.

Does this mean that clinicians should not have any emotional reactions to their clients or that they should not form a bond or work collaboratively with their clients? Of course not! That would certainly be countertherapeutic. As discussed in the next chapter, communicating caring, support, hopefulness, and interest to clients can greatly enhance the treatment process. In addition, clinicians' reactions to clients' demeanor and behaviors can be used to provide clients feedback on how others might perceive them. For example, clients who are chronically late for appointments, who behave in angry and aggressive ways both in and out of sessions, and whose poor physical self-care is evident would probably benefit from a clear but gentle statement of the clinician's reactions to those behaviors. The clinician might also provide some information on the reactions those behaviors are likely to elicit from others.

Distinguishing between countertransference reactions and appropriate and helpful responses to clients can be challenging. The following additional guidelines, focused primarily on self-awareness, can help clinicians become cognizant of their own countertransference reactions.

- Keep Teyber's signs of countertransference in mind.
- Know yourself. Be aware of common patterns of reaction that you have toward people. For example, do you typically feel competitive with people about your age who seem more successful than you are? Do you feel judged by people who remind you of one of your parents? Awareness of patterns such as these can help you anticipate and curtail countertransference reactions.
- Recognize your own strong beliefs about how people should lead their lives. For example, would you disapprove of someone who decided to have an abortion, would you feel angry toward an adolescent who began smoking marijuana, would you rejoice when someone in a long but troubled relationship finally decided to marry, or do you believe that marriages cannot recover from infidelity? Reactions and beliefs such as these may interfere with your objectivity and your goal of helping people make decisions that are best for them.
- Monitor yourself whenever you are tempted to engage in a possible boundary violation, such as buying a gift for a client, calling a client for no particular reason, giving a client extra time in sessions, reducing a client's fee, or meeting a client away from the office. These behaviors may be professional and appropriate, but they may also be clues to the presence of countertransference.
- Seek supervision or consultation with a colleague whenever you find yourself having a strong or puzzling response to a client. Another person with

more objectivity may be able to help you sort out your reactions, determine whether countertransference is indeed present, and take steps to ensure that treatment continues in a productive direction.

Additional information on identifying and addressing countertransference reactions can be obtained from the discussion of transference that follows.

Understanding Transference

Transference is probably easier to identify than countertransference, if only because people typically have more objectivity in assessing someone else's behavior than their own. In addition, most clinicians try to understand patterns in their clients' lives and may focus particularly on the connection between early relationships and current relationships. That link can facilitate the identification of transference reactions.

Signs of Transference

Clues to the presence of transference are similar to those that signal countertransference. Especially telling are a client's strong emotional responses to the clinician, particularly those that seem unwarranted or that repeat ways in which the client characteristically responds to people.

Transference, like countertransference, can be either positive or negative. One of my clients, a lonely young woman, thanked me repeatedly when I asked for her help in closing a heavy window in my office. She viewed this as a sign that I appreciated her strength and trusted her enough to ask for her help with this simple task. Another client became enraged with me because I kept her waiting while I took an emergency telephone call. My explanation and assurances that I would add on the time to the end of her session only angered her further; she interpreted this as a sign that I did not respect her busy schedule. Both women overreacted and manifested behavior that reflected how they related to people in other settings. The first woman worked hard to ingratiate herself with others and, in so doing, often overwhelmed and frightened them by her need for closeness. The second woman, on the other hand, believed that nearly everyone in her life took advantage of her and exploited her. Although she had experienced considerable mistreatment in her life, her automatic reactions of anger and resentment sabotaged her efforts to establish healthy and mutually rewarding relationships.

Addressing Transference

Clinicians differ greatly in their thinking about the appropriate response to transference. Clinicians who have a traditional psychoanalytic orientation, for example, typically believe that transference should be encouraged and that its analysis and working through is an essential ingredient in successful treatment. Clinicians practicing transactional analysis and brief psychodynamic psychotherapy acknowledge the importance of transference but pay only limited attention to that process during treatment. On the other hand, clinicians whose theoretical orientation is cognitive-behavioral or person-centered may agree that transference exists but pay little or no attention to that process during treatment unless transference interferes with progress. Regardless of theoretical orientation, clinicians' ability to identify and process effectively both transference and countertransference reactions are important therapeutic skills.

How do you think I should have handled the transference reactions of the two women described previously? I gently shared with the first woman that her efforts to connect with people could backfire and push them away. We looked for similar examples that reflected this pattern, and she was able to recognize that, in fact, a less effusive reaction on her part could actually help her build better relationships. I did not share my perceptions with the second woman out of concern that I would do further damage to our therapeutic alliance. However, I made a mental note of what I observed and looked for less threatening examples to discuss with her in subsequent sessions.

Application of Bloom's Taxonomy to Transference

The modified version of Bloom's taxonomy can be used to help clinicians understand and address transference and countertransference reactions. The reactions of Rosa Ishak, presented earlier in this chapter, illustrate this.

Content (What are the facts?)

Rosa's counselor began to feel uncomfortable with some of Rosa's positive and negative reactions to her and wondered whether transference might be present. Her processing of Rosa's reactions follows.

Process (How do the facts promote understanding of the person and how to help him or her?)

Comprehension (What do I know and understand about the facts?): Rosa manifested both positive and negative reactions to her counselor, a woman about 30 years older than she. Rosa was extremely respectful toward the counselor, followed up on any suggestions the counselor made, and expressed strong appreciation for the counselor's time and attention. At the same time, Rosa was sometimes withdrawn and seemed mistrustful of the counselor.

Organization (What principles, categories, and generalizations help me to understand this information?): The counselor sought meaningful patterns in the timing of Rosa's positive and negative responses. The positive reactions occurred during and after sessions in which the counselor's interventions could be viewed as praising Rosa and giving her suggestions as to how to succeed in college and develop better relationships. Rosa also seemed especially gratified when the counselor listened to Rosa's descriptions of her interpersonal interactions. These often seemed more suited for discussion over lunch with a girlfriend, but Rosa had no close peers with whom to process her interactions and to learn what are normal and expectable reactions for a young woman. The negative reactions arose especially when the counselor tried to engage Rosa in making her own decisions rather than suggesting what might be the best alternative. Rosa became particularly guarded and retreated into generalizations (e.g., "People with a college degree make more money") rather than talking about herself and her feelings when the counselor tried to explore Rosa's motivation for attending college.

Analysis/Synthesis (How are these facts related, and what inferences can I draw about their connections?): Rosa's only close relationship has been with her mother, who tends to tell Rosa what to do and believes strongly that Rosa should complete at least a two-year college degree. Rosa also has had positive interactions with a teacher and an advisor, both in authority and advice-giving positions. Rosa has been wounded by many of her other relationships, including her peers who teased her, the two fathers who failed to give her the love and attention she craved, and the teachers and minister who disapproved of her behavior and contributed to her low self-esteem. As a result, Rosa responded well to the counselor when she reminded Rosa of her mother and of the helpful teacher and advisor. On the other hand, when the counselor did not fit this image, Rosa became mistrustful and self-protective, probably trying to ward off any messages or information that might communicate that she was not doing the right thing. The positive transference reflected Rosa's view of the counselor as a friend and perhaps even a surrogate mother. However, any hint that the counselor was not fully supportive and approving led Rosa to react with mistrust and to put up barriers between herself and her counselor.

Interpretation (What does all of this mean, and what sense does all of this make?): Rosa's close relationship with her mother, her perception that most people are hurtful and untrustworthy, and her longing for approval and support led her to have transference reactions to the counselor. When the counselor acted in ways that were reminiscent of Rosa's mother or of the girlfriends she wanted to have, Rosa had positive reactions, whereas any counseling interventions that seemed to question Rosa's decision to attend college or failed to give her support and direction elicited a negative reaction. Rosa seemed to want her counselor to affirm and praise everything that Rosa was doing and thinking, especially when it reflected advice she had gotten from her mother. This probably reflected Rosa's potentially enmeshed relationship with her mother as well as her self-doubts, other-directedness, and need for external validation.

Application (What approaches seem most likely to be effective in addressing this issue?): Gentle exploration of Rosa's transference reactions could help the therapeutic alliance, the treatment process, and Rosa's efforts to form healthy relationships. Working collaboratively, Rosa and her counselor could identify times when Rosa had strong emotional reactions to the treatment process and then link these to Rosa's relationship with her mother, her self-doubts, her need for unconditional approval, and her expectation that people often are hurtful and untrustworthy. Exploration of other relationships Rosa has had would probably indicate that her transference reactions affected those relationships as well, perhaps interfering with her efforts to develop friendships at school. Treatment could then focus on helping Rosa anticipate, identify, and curtail such reactions; build her self-esteem and self-confidence; develop the communication skills she needs to nurture relationships more effectively; and develop a relationship with her mother that allows Rosa more independence and self-direction.

Evaluation (How effective has treatment been, how could it be even more effective, and what can be learned from this experience?): Monitoring Rosa's reactions to the discussion of transference is essential. If it is not done with great care and considerable support, discussion of this topic may prove threatening and painful to Rosa, who might perceive her counselor as criticizing her. This, in turn, may lead Rosa to terminate treatment prematurely. Engaging Rosa in exploring her reactions to the counselor may help her to feel empowered and less vulnerable, thereby facilitating discussion of the highly charged topic of transference.

The modified version of Bloom's taxonomy can also be used to help clinicians better understand and address their countertransference reactions. The Learning Opportunities provide an opportunity to apply the taxonomy to a clinician's countertransference reactions.

LEARNING OPPORTUNITIES

This chapter, like Chapter 2, presented conceptual skills that focus on collecting and making sound therapeutic use of background information. The new skills presented in this chapter include:

- Gathering information in ways that are meaningful and helpful to clients
- Conducting an intake interview
- Better understanding clients by making effective use of background information obtained through an intake interview
- Understanding and making therapeutic use of transference and countertransference

These skills and their presentation built on the learning introduced in Chapters 1 and 2 and continued to use the modified Bloom's taxonomy as a tool for organizing, analyzing, and making sound use of background information. In addition, this chapter, like the previous chapter, emphasized the importance of developing a sound therapeutic alliance, identifying and reinforcing clients' strengths, and integrating a range of fundamental and conceptual skills in clinical work.

The following exercises provide the opportunity to apply the skills that have been presented in this chapter.

Written Exercises/Discussion Questions

1. Chapter 2 presented information on Eileen Carter, a 24-year-old married African American woman, who has a traditional marriage. She does not

work outside the home and is focused on caring for her child. Her clinician is a Caucasian woman, age 36, who has a doctorate. She has always been a strong supporter of women's rights. She and her husband value an egalitarian marriage and, at present, he is the primary caretaker of their two young children.

    a. What transference issues seem most likely to arise here?

    b. What countertransference issues seem most likely to arise here?

    c. How would you suggest that Eileen and her therapist address both transference and countertransference issues?

    d. In what ways, if any, do you think that transference and countertransference reactions can be used positively in Eileen's treatment?

2. Clinicians vary greatly in terms of the importance they place on identifying and analyzing transference reactions in treatment. Discuss your ideas on the most helpful ways to address transference in treatment. In what ways will your attention to and processing of transference be affected by the client's presenting concerns, that person's motivation toward treatment, the severity and urgency of the client's difficulties, and the setting in which treatment takes place?

3. Either write out an intake interview with a hypothetical client or have two of the students (or the instructor and one student) role-play an intake interview. What did you learn from the role-played intake interview about the following aspects of the client?

    a. Demographics

    b. Presenting concerns

    c. Prior psychological difficulties

    d. Strengths

    e. Current life situation

    f. Cultural, spiritual, socioeconomic, and other multicultural factors that affect the client

    g. Family of origin

    h. Developmental history

    i. Career and educational history

    j. Medical history

    k. Health-related behaviors

    l. Relationships

    m. Leisure activities

    n. Other relevant information

4. Process the content of the role-played intake interview conducted in response to question 3 according to the following steps in Bloom's modified taxonomy:

- Comprehension
- Organization
- Analysis/synthesis
- Interpretation
- Application

5. On pages 72–82, this chapter presented guidelines for conducting an intake interview. What additions, if any, would you make to these guidelines? What seem to you the most important guidelines to keep in mind when conducting an intake interview?

Practice Group Exercise: Conducting an Intake Interview

Divide into your practice groups, as described in Chapter 1. Be sure to record your practice sessions (on audio or video tape), both for the group's review and for your own review of your session. This will enhance your efforts to improve your skills.

The purpose of this exercise is to practice the following conceptual skills:

- Continued ability to understand and apply Bloom's modified taxonomy.
- Ability to conduct an effective intake interview.

In addition, use of the following fundamental skills will enhance your ability to participate effectively in this exercise:

- Appropriate use of open and closed questions.
- Ability to use and combine a range of interventions.
- Ability to integrate reflections of feelings and meaning into the interview.

Practice Group Exercise

In each dyad, one person will assume the role of clinician and the other will assume the role of client. Assume that this is an initial interview.

The primary task of the clinician is to conduct an effective interview, gathering enough background information to facilitate an in-depth understanding of the client while simultaneously using interventions that create a smooth flow to the interview, help the client feel comfortable, and enhance the therapeutic alliance. The person in the client role may either play him- or herself or may role-play a hypothetical client.

Timing of Exercise

If possible, allow approximately two hours for this exercise, with each of the four role-plays and their discussion taking 30 minutes. If you do not have that much time, do only two role-plays, one for each dyad. The drawback of doing this is that each person will have the opportunity to be either client or clinician but will not be able to try out both roles.

- Allow 20 minutes for each role-played intake interview.
- Allow about 10 minutes to provide feedback to the person in the clinician role. Be sure to begin the feedback process with the person in the clinician role commenting on his or her performance of the exercise, focus on

strengths first, and offer concrete suggestions for improvement. Like all the practice exercises suggested in this book, this should be a positive learning experience, not one that makes anyone feel criticized or judged. Feedback should focus on the areas listed in the following Assessment of Progress form.

Assessment of Progress Form 3

1. How well did the clinician succeed in conducting a comprehensive intake interview that would facilitate an in-depth understanding of the client? What topics, if any, were omitted or discussed too briefly? What issues, if any, received too much emphasis?

_____

_____

_____

2. What interventions contributed to making the interview effective? How might the interview have been even more effective?

_____

_____

_____

3. Describe the types of interventions the clinician used during this interview. How effective was the clinician's use of questions? How well were other interventions integrated with the use of questions?

_____

_____

_____

4. What was the flow of the interview like? What made it flow well? What would have made it flow more smoothly?

_____

_____

_____

5. Summary of feedback, including identification of at least two strengths and one area needing improvement:
   a. Strengths:

_____

_____

   b. Areas needing improvement:

_____

Personal Journal Questions

1. Many students, and even many practicing clinicians, are uncomfortable when dealing with transference and countertransference in treatment. However, these are common processes that appear in treatment as well as in our daily lives. Write briefly about a time in your life when your reactions to a person stemmed more from your early experiences than from your actual interactions with that person. What can you learn from that experience to help you to become a more effective clinician?

2. What improvement, if any, did you notice in your clinical skills if you had the opportunity to assume the role of clinician in the practice group exercise? If you did not have that opportunity, what improvement, if any, did you notice in other members of your group?

3. Put yourself into the role of a client just beginning therapy or counseling. How do you think you would feel about being the subject of an intake interview? Are there parts of your background that you would rather not share in your first meeting with a clinician? How do you think you would handle that situation?

SUMMARY

Chapter 3 continued our focus on conceptual skills associated with background. Emphasized in this chapter were meaningful and helpful ways to gather client information, conducting an intake interview, and identifying and making therapeutic use of transference and countertransference.

In Chapter 4, we shift our focus to conceptual skills associated with emotions. Included in that chapter is information on establishing a sound therapeutic alliance, role induction, clinician self-disclosure, and clinician reactions to clients.

Chapter 4

USING CONCEPTUAL SKILLS TO MAKE POSITIVE USE OF AND MODIFY EMOTIONS

THERAPEUTIC ALLIANCE, ROLE INDUCTION, CLINICIAN SELF-DISCLOSURE, AND CLINICIANS' REACTIONS TO CLIENTS

OVERVIEW

When she was three years old, my granddaughter began asking me what I do when I go to work. Seeking to synthesize what I do as a counselor and psychologist into one sentence that she could readily understand, I told her that "I help sad people to feel better." I believe that is the essence of our work. Whether treatment addresses the consequences of early attachment problems (background), dysfunctional and self-destructive cognitions (thoughts), or harmful habits and behaviors (actions), psychologists, social workers, and counselors help people feel better about themselves and their lives.

Fundamental skills that are important in helping people express and identify their emotions and in helping clinicians attend to those emotions include use of encouragers, restatements, paraphrases, summarizations, and especially reflections of verbal and nonverbal feelings. This chapter builds on these fundamental skills and helps you develop the conceptual skills you need to identify complex and challenging emotions and enable people to modify their troubling emotions.

Emotions that are present in the treatment setting can be divided into the following three groups.

1. **Emotions that clients bring into treatment:** These may include positive feelings such as love, joy, and fulfillment but, at least in the early stages of treatment, are more likely to include negative emotions such as despair, anxiety, and rage. Clinicians who are skilled at helping clients identify, express appropriately, and modify their troubling emotions are likely to make a great difference in people's lives.

2. **Emotions that clinicians bring into treatment:** Although our emotions are rarely the focus of our sessions, clinicians, too, bring emotions into the treatment room. Those emotions can have a powerful effect on the direction and success of

treatment. Emotions such as caring, optimism, and commitment to clients can greatly enhance treatment if they are expressed in helpful ways. On the other hand, we may have negative feelings toward our clients, such as disapproval, disappointment, dislike, fear, and annoyance; those emotions can undermine the best treatment plans. We also bring into our sessions emotions from our own lives; we may be tired and overworked, excited about an upcoming celebration, or angry about a recent argument. These emotions, too, have the potential to affect the treatment process. Consequently, our ability to be aware of our own feelings and deal with them constructively is an important clinical skill.

3. **Emotions that arise in response to the treatment process:** Finally, we must consider the emotional interaction of the client and the clinician. Having a shared vision of better possibilities, collaborating to make these possibilities a reality, trusting each other, and sharing the struggles and rewards of treatment can engender positive emotions in both client and clinician and serve as powerful contributors to effective treatment. On the other hand, if the client and clinician fail to develop a sound therapeutic alliance and are not collaborating effectively to achieve shared goals, both may feel discouraged. Their effort and motivation may diminish, and treatment may be ineffective.

In this chapter, we focus on ways to build a sound therapeutic alliance, including the process of role induction, strategies for clinician self-disclosure, and ways for clinicians to deal effectively with their own feelings about their clients. Chapter 5 continues to address the use of conceptual skills focused on emotion by presenting information on variations in clients' readiness for treatment and ways to deal with strong and unhelpful client emotions.

These chapters help clinicians understand the effect of emotions on the treatment process, facilitate the appropriate expression of emotions, and, if indicated, help clients modify harmful emotions. As in the previous chapters, the modified version of Bloom's taxonomy will be used to facilitate an in-depth understanding of the emotional dimensions addressed in Chapters 4 and 5.

THE THERAPEUTIC ALLIANCE

The nature and quality of the therapeutic alliance has profound effects on the success of the treatment process. Research study after research study has found that the therapeutic relationship is the best predictor of therapeutic outcome (Orlinsky, Grawe, & Parks, 1994). Horvath and Symonds (1991), for example, conducted a meta-analysis of 24 studies "relating the quality of the working alliance to therapy outcome" (p. 139). They found a "moderate but reliable association" between outcome and therapeutic alliance that was not a function of the length or type of treatment. These researchers found that collaboration, along with negotiation of mutually agreeable goals and plans, were particularly important ingredients in enhancing the therapeutic alliance.

You may be surprised by the importance of the therapeutic alliance. Most graduate programs that train counselors, social workers, and psychologists devote much less time to helping clinicians learn to develop a positive therapeutic alliance than they do to helping them learn the important theories and strategies of treatment. Of course, the treatment approach also has a significant effect on outcome. Yet without a collaborative alliance that promotes client motivation and hopefulness, the most rigorous application of an established treatment approach and the most appropriate and detailed treatment plans are unlikely to succeed.

In this way, the connection between client and clinician resembles many other relationships. You will probably return to a restaurant that feels warm and welcoming and that pays attention to your needs, as long as the food is also satisfactory. Of the many people you meet at a party, you will probably remember and perhaps contact the ones who seemed interested in you and with whom you felt some rapport. In counseling and psychotherapy as well, the initial contact and the relationship that evolves usually are the primary determinants of the success of treatment and even of whether the client returns for subsequent appointments.

The Nature of the Therapeutic Alliance

Therapeutic alliances vary in terms of their nature, quality, and pattern of development. Bachelor (1995) surveyed clients on their perceptions of the therapeutic relationship and found three types of alliances:

- **Nurturant:** Of those surveyed, 46% described their clinicians as respectful, nonjudgmental, empathic, and having good listening skills. Support and reinforcement were emphasized. These clients had a trusting relationship with their clinicians and felt comfortable accepted, and at ease during the treatment process.
- **Insight-oriented:** Of those who responded, 39% described their treatment as focusing on improving self-understanding. Clinicians emphasized underlying causes and dynamics and used interpretation, exploration, and clarification to increase self-awareness.
- **Collaborative alliance:** Only 15% of clients surveyed reported that they were actively involved in the treatment process and described an alliance that emphasized mutuality as well as client commitment and responsibility.

The relatively low percentage of clients who reported a collaborative alliance is troubling. More recent research, such as Smith's (2006) writing on strength-based counseling, suggests that a therapeutic relationship that increases people's feelings of empowerment, raises their awareness of their assets and skills, and instills hope and motivation toward change is strongly associated with a positive treatment outcome. A collaborative alliance, in which clinicians and clients work together to help clients reach their goals seems more likely to fit the paradigm of strength-based treatment than alliances that rely heavily on either the clinician's interpretation of clients' difficulties or the clinician's caretaking of the client.

At the same time, some essential ingredients of a successful therapeutic alliance are encompassed by what Bachelor termed the "nurturant alliance." Clinicians who embody what Carl Rogers (1967) called the core conditions of effective treatment, including empathy, respect, and acceptance, and who demonstrate good listening skills, facilitate the development of a sound therapeutic alliance. In such a relationship, clients feel accepted, supported, and valued. They believe that their clinician cares about them and can be trusted, and they feel hopeful and comfortable in the presence of their clinician.

The most desirable therapeutic alliance, then, seems to embody characteristics of two of the three types of common alliances identified by Bachelor (1995). Combining these, the term *collaborative-nurturant* captures the essence of these two approaches. Keep this in mind as we present additional information on the nature and development of a successful therapeutic alliance.

Development of the Therapeutic Alliance

I have heard beginning clinicians speak of spending the first session or two building rapport and then moving into the treatment process. I think this reflects a misunderstanding of how to develop successful therapeutic alliances with clients. That process begins at the first moment of contact between client and clinician and does not end until the last contact with the client. Although initial interactions are especially important, as first impressions usually are, the development of the therapeutic alliance is intertwined with all aspects of the treatment process and evolves and changes over time.

Kivlighan and Shaughnessy's (2000) research focused on the development of the therapeutic alliance from a temporal perspective. In addition to affirming that the alliance was a strong predictor of therapeutic outcome, their research identified three common patterns that characterize the evolution of the therapeutic alliance over time. (Of course, some client-clinician relationships end rapidly and fit none of these patterns.)

- **Stable alliance:** The initial strength of the alliance remains constant throughout the treatment process. This may refer to both positive and negative alliances.
- **Linear growth:** The therapeutic alliance improves consistently over time.
- **Quadratic growth:** A strong alliance develops initially, then declines or is damaged during the middle phase of treatment, followed by a rebuilding in the concluding phase of treatment.

Particularly important is the finding that the therapeutic alliance does not always develop smoothly. Both in my own work as a therapist and in the work of the many novice and advanced clinicians I have supervised, I have often seen misunderstanding, tension, and even disagreements and conflicts develop between client and clinician. However, if these are addressed quickly and in healthy ways, they can be positive learning experiences, teaching clients how to address problems effectively, and they can lead to a strengthening of the therapeutic alliance. More will be said on this later in the chapter as well as in the next chapter, which discusses clinicians' own feelings and responses to their clients.

Regardless of the specific pattern of development of the therapeutic alliance, the literature suggests the importance of rapidly establishing a positive therapeutic alliance. Walborn (1996) concluded that a positive therapeutic alliance must be in place by the fifth session if treatment is to have a successful outcome. Kivlighan and Shaughnessy (2000) found that clinicians and clients could even develop the foundation for a strong working alliance by the end of the first session! Keep this in mind when you receive an initial telephone inquiry from a potential client, when a student asks if you are the school counselor or social worker and when he can meet with you, when a college student stops by the counseling center and asks you if counselors can help with roommate problems, and even when someone asks you for the name of the local community mental health center. All contacts between client and clinician contribute to the development of the important therapeutic alliance.

Characteristics of a Positive Therapeutic Alliance

We have already identified the collaborative-nurturant therapeutic alliance as the ideal client–clinician relationship. This, like all types of therapeutic alliances, is a synthesis of many elements, which we will examine here. The most important of these are the characteristics of the clinician, the characteristics of the client, and their interface. In addition, factors such as the treatment setting, the nature of the referral, the attitudes that significant people in the client's life have toward the treatment process, and even the weather and traffic at the time of the client's first appointment all contribute to the development of the therapeutic alliance. Clinicians can control only some of these factors, but they should keep the others in mind as potentially important variables. Having a vision of a positive therapeutic alliance can help clinicians build such an alliance with their clients.

A review of the literature suggests that a positive therapeutic alliance has the following characteristics:

- It provides a safe and protective environment for clients.
- It encourages collaboration, with both clients and clinicians playing an active role in the treatment process.
- It has mutuality or a feeling of shared warmth, caring, and respect.
- It is affirming, identifying, and building on clients' strengths and competence and promoting hope of positive change.
- It promotes client empowerment and resilience.
- Clients can identify with their clinicians, perhaps using them as role models.
- Client and clinician agree on goals and procedures; sessions are structured in such a way as to move clearly toward accomplishment of those goals.
- Client and clinician view themselves as engaged in a shared endeavor that seems likely to succeed.

Initiating and Developing a Positive Therapeutic Alliance

Clinicians can maximize the likelihood of developing a positive therapeutic alliance if they take steps to understand the essential ingredients of such a relationship and strive to include those ingredients in the treatment process. The research studies conducted by Bachelor and by Kivlighan and Shaughnessy demonstrate that sound therapeutic alliances can take many forms and develop in a variety of ways. However, strong and positive therapeutic alliances, and the clinicians who facilitate their development, typically share some key characteristics.

The literature suggests that the following 10 characteristics reflect the work of clinicians who are skilled at developing positive therapeutic alliances with their clients (Seligman, 2001). Review the following descriptions of these qualities and their associated strategies.

1. Empathy   "Empathy is the clinician's ability to see the world through the client's eyes and to communicate that understanding so that the client feels heard and validated" (Seligman, 2001, p. 18). This does not mean that clinicians participate in clients' feelings or feel pity for them; rather, clinicians let clients know that their emotions are neither strange nor distasteful but, rather, make sense in light their life experiences. According to Rogers (1980),

> It [empathy] means entering the private perceptual world of the other and becoming thoroughly at home in it. It involves being sensitive, moment by moment, to the changing felt meanings which flow in this other person, to the fear or rage or tenderness or confusion or whatever that he or she is experiencing. It means temporarily living in the other's life, moving about in it delicately without making judgments. (p. 142)

Empathy is an orientation toward people, a way of being with them, not just a technical skill.

Demonstrating Empathy: Reflection of feeling is a powerful tool for communicating empathy. This strategy is particularly effective when it not only reflects people's verbalized emotions but also acknowledges both covert and nonverbal emotions. Identifying core emotions or persistent feelings can be especially powerful and helpful. By letting people know clinicians are attuned to their deepest emotions, many of which may even be outside the clients' own awareness, clinicians truly let clients know that the clinicians understand them.

Use your own emotional reactions to help you tune into the client's affective world; if you are feeling confused and overwhelmed by the client's story, that may well be how the client is feeling too. Remember to communicate empathy frequently, even when the focus is on background, thoughts, or actions. Empathy is best conveyed when clinicians use their own words, rather than restating what the client has said, to deepen client self-awareness and demonstrate understanding. Clinicians should be tentative and allow the client ample opportunity to react to or revise empathic statements so that clients increase their self-awareness and clinicians really understand what that other person is feeling.

Let's look at the following client statement, followed by three clinician responses, so that you can better understand how to communicate empathy effectively.

> *Client:* I was sober for nearly two months and then I lost it. I was out the door as soon as my friend called me from the bar. I was feeling so lonely, I just couldn't stop myself.
> *Clinician 1:* So after nearly two months, you started to drink again.
> *Clinician 2:* What kept you from calling your AA sponsor or using your coping skills?
> *Clinician 3:* You sound pretty disappointed in yourself and even look discouraged. And yet I can hear your pride in those two months of sobriety.

Which of these most effectively communicates empathy? You probably had no difficulty identifying the third statement as the most empathic. Unlike Clinician 1, who simply restates the client's words, or Clinician 2, who sounds critical, Clinician 3 acknowledges the client's negative emotions, picks up on nonverbal communication, and yet also reminds the client of the two successful months of sobriety.

2. Good Listening Skills   Clinicians who listen carefully and deeply to their clients and communicate that listening and understanding serve as a mirror for their clients, helping them to hear and understand themselves better. Communicating empathy and demonstrating good listening skills are closely related. To succeed in both, clinicians must focus intently on the client and not allow themselves to be distracted by their own needs unless they are relevant to the therapeutic situation. They should listen for and acknowledge both overt and covert messages and recognize that silence and the absence of a response or an action are often important messages. If clinicians are listening closely but are not understanding, they may ask questions; perhaps the session has touched on an area that is conflicted or confusing to the client as well.

Demonstrating Good Listening: All of the fundamental skills you probably have already learned are important in demonstrating effective listening. Paraphrases and other encouragers let people know you have grasped the point of what they are saying. Open questions are important in clarifying confusing information. Reflections of feeling and meaning, as well as summarization, synthesize what has been said, identify themes, and recognize indirect communications. Remember that listening is an active, rather than a passive, process; clients only know that we are listening well if we demonstrate that to them in helpful ways.

3. Trustworthiness, Reliability, and Ethical Behavior   Many people enter treatment with a history of impoverished and unstable relationships. They may expect all their relationships to follow that pattern and may feel leery and mistrustful of the therapeutic relationship. Consequently, clinicians must facilitate and nurture clients' trust in them to counteract the clients' negative expectations.

According to Kottler and Brown (2000, p. 93), trust is crucial to productive treatment and includes "respect for the client's right to be his or her own person, warm regard for the client as a unique being, and genuineness, which means being honest and real." When clients trust their clinicians, they believe that the clinicians are on their side, that the clinicians will never hurt or shame them, that the clinicians will follow through on their commitments, and that they will always behave in ethical and professional ways.

Demonstrating Trustworthiness, Reliability, and Ethical Behavior: Clinicians must demonstrate to clients, through both words and actions, that they are not interested in exerting power over the clients or forcing them to change to meet clinician needs. Rather, the clinicians want to help clients be the best they can be and to meet both the clients' and the clinicians' needs in healthy ways.

To promote the clients' trust, clinicians must demonstrate and model reliability for their clients. For example, clinicians should be on time for appointments, remember important information about their clients, and return telephone calls in a timely way. If clinicians make a mistake, and all do that sometimes, they acknowledge that to the client and make amends as needed. For example, a clinician who inadvertently scheduled two clients at the same time did not charge the client for the appointment she had to reschedule for the next day. Clinicians are aware of the ethical standards of their profession and always behave ethically, never crossing boundaries inappropriately and always considering what will promote clients' healthy development.

Clients sometimes test the limits and create situations that raise boundary issues or challenge clinicians' efforts to be reliable and responsive. Clients may telephone clinicians many times a day; they may tell clinicians that if they really cared, they would meet them for lunch or lend the clients some money; they may cancel sessions frequently; or they may give an inappropriate gift. Situations such as these are difficult even for experienced clinicians. To address such situations effectively, clinicians should explain clearly to their clients the guidelines and limitations of the therapeutic relationship.

Rather than waiting for problems to arise, clinicians should provide clients with both written and verbal information on the appropriate nature of the therapeutic alliance. Reviewing this during the initial session, and then referring to it as needed, is critical to maintaining an atmosphere of acceptance, comfort, and safety during treatment. If clinicians find themselves having feelings or considering behaviors that conflict with the ethical and other guidelines of their profession, they should probably discuss this with a supervisor or trusted colleague to ensure that they do not compromise their professional roles. More is said on how therapists can deal effectively with their own reactions to clients in Chapter 5.

4. Caring and Concern   An angry adolescent once said to one of my colleagues, "If you weren't paid to see me, you wouldn't bother to talk to me. I'm just a 45-minute slot in your week." The role of the clinician is a complicated and often confusing one. Nearly all clinicians are paid for their work, and that is essential to their well-being, but finances are unlikely to be the primary reason that people chose to enter a mental health profession. They are mental health professionals because they care deeply about the welfare of others and believe that they can contribute to making people's lives better. Caring entails empowering clients, helping them in proactive ways, being interested in what is important to them, and consistently communicating support, empathy, and good listening.

Demonstrating Caring and Concern: Clinicians communicate caring when they teach clients the tools they need to feel more powerful and take charge of their lives, when they inquire about important milestones in clients' lives, when they do something out of the ordinary that demonstrates concern about a client, and when they let clients know that they are there to help them. Clinicians also demonstrate caring when they point out to clients the negative as well as the positive consequences of their actions, when they think about them in context and offer help to their communities and families, and when they accept, understand, and empathize with both their clients' joys and their disappointments. Caring usually is expressed in the context of the treatment sessions. However, moving slightly, but always ethically, away from the standard role of the clinician can be especially powerful in communicating caring and concern. Examples of this include calling a client who has just returned home after surgery, contacting a client's teacher to discuss his progress (of course, with the client's permission), sending a client an encouraging e-mail before a big event, and asking clients to bring in photos of their wedding or new baby.

5. Genuineness, Sincerity, and Congruence   Another way to build trust and counteract the exploitive and hurtful relationships experienced by so many clients is for clinicians to be genuine and sincere. This does not mean that they should be brutally honest with clients, but rather that they find sensitive and tactful ways to communicate clearly, accurately, and honestly. Being congruent is an important element in transmitting genuineness and sincerity. Clinicians' verbal and nonverbal messages must be consistent and compatible, providing clients with unambiguous messages.

Communicating Genuineness, Sincerity, and Congruence: Clinicians can best communicate these variables by being real people in their sessions, not just blank slates. They can laugh with their clients, feel sad with them when they hear bad news, and even become tearful when clients experience a great loss. As long as clinicians' interventions are intentional and have a helpful purpose, they can share their reactions with clients, provide encouragement, and let them know when the clinicians are concerned about the clients' potentially harmful choices. Of course, clinicians must respect clients' right to self-determination, unless they present a danger to themselves or others, but most clients can more easily form a positive working alliance with a real human being than with an anonymous and inexpressive one. Again, more information is provided in Chapter 5 on appropriate clinician self-disclosure.

6. Persuasiveness and Credibility   Clinicians who have credibility with their clients have what Kottler and Brown (2000) refer to as "benevolent power" or "interpersonal influence." In describing this dimension, they say, "Interpersonal influence is that dimension of counseling that involves the application of expertise, power, and attractiveness in such a way as to foster self-awareness and constructive change" (pp. 94–95). When clients perceive their clinicians as admirable and believable, the clients are more likely to view their clinicians as role models and to take reasonable risks to achieve goals. Clients' perception of some similarity between their clinicians and themselves enhances interpersonal influence; this connection can inspire clients and give them hope that they, too, can achieve personal and professional success. Clinician–client similarity can be particularly important for people who have had few positive role models, who have not yet become acculturated to this society, or who have had little exposure to mental health services. People such as these typically feel reassured by knowing that their clinicians have a cultural background, belief system, values, or experiences that are similar to their own.

Communicating Persuasiveness and Credibility: Although clinicians should not exaggerate the power differential between themselves and their clients, they do need to inform clients of their training and credentials. This can easily be done through a written consent-to-treatment form, given to clients before they begin treatment, or through a brief verbal description of the clinician's professional background. Information on clinicians' training, degrees, licenses, experience and other professional credentials all enhance credibility.

Interpersonal influence develops when clients see that their clinicians are competent, have a clear sense of direction, give structure to the sessions, and show understanding of their clients and their concerns. In addition, clinicians can enhance their influence by highlighting similarities between clients and themselves, being careful to remain professional. Some cautious sharing of common experiences or backgrounds can increase clinicians' credibility and let clients know that the clinicians' lives have been in some ways similar to those of the clients. This may involve no more than telling a client that the clinician, too, was an only child, or immigrated to the United States, or returned to college in midlife, or felt overwhelmed and scared when his or her first child was born.

7. Optimism When people seek counseling or psychotherapy, they often feel discouraged and sometimes even hopeless and suicidal. They may perceive treatment as their last resort, perhaps one that makes them feel inadequate and defective in some way. Understanding these feelings and countering them with hope and optimism can make a difference in treatment outcome. Clinicians can give their clients the message that treatment can improve their lives and help them achieve realistic goals. Balancing discussion of failures and disappointments with a focus on clients' strengths and accomplishments can further engender optimism.

Communicating Optimism: The communication of optimism generally will make a difference for people only if it is realistic and linked to their specific goals. Clinicians need to be honest with clients about the time and effort involved in effective treatment and the uncertainty of the outcome. However, they can also provide assurances. Consider the following illustrative and helpful clinician statements:

- Depression feels like it will never go away but, in reality, therapy is usually very successful in helping people feel less discouraged.
- I can see that you have already taken some important steps to help yourself stop drinking. I think we can find some ways to help you build on the gains you have made.

- I can hear that you felt terrified and embarrassed about the way you reacted when Todd made fun of you, but together I think we can come up with some ways for you to deal with him differently.

In addition, treatment should encourage, emphasize, reinforce, and celebrate successes. Establishing a series of small, readily achievable goals that build on each other can establish a pattern of successes.

8. Sense of Structure and Direction Mental health treatment is such a complex and ambiguous process that even experienced clinicians are sometimes unsure how to help someone. Although this feeling is understandable and although clinicians usually work collaboratively with their clients, clinicians must keep in mind that they are the experts on mental health treatment. People come to treatment for help and resources they have not been able to provide for themselves. Clinicians are responsible for giving structure and direction to the sessions, for developing sound treatment plans, for helping people formulate realistic goals, and for seeking consultation or making a referral if needed. Having a sense of structure and direction is important in helping clients move forward and in sustaining their hopefulness and optimism.

Communicating a Sense of Structure and Direction: Most clinicians today, especially those in mental health settings, keep written records that pave the way for treatment to move smoothly from one session to the next. The foundation for these records is generally a list of clear, achievable, and measurable goals, developed in collaboration with the client. Once goals have been agreed on, clinicians can develop a treatment plan based on their knowledge of the individual client, that person's concerns and diagnosis, and treatment approaches and strategies that have demonstrated success with similar clients and concerns. Many clinicians discuss their treatment plans with their clients so that they can be fine-tuned if necessary, as well as to obtain the client's understanding of and agreement to the work they will be doing together. When clients participate in the development of their treatment plans and view them as likely to be helpful, they usually are more motivated to accomplish their goals and more hopeful that treatment will help them. Keeping weekly progress notes, being sure to follow up on tasks that have been suggested to clients, reinforcing accomplishments made each week, setting an agenda at the start of each session, and summarizing and eliciting feedback at the end of each session are other ways that clinicians can give treatment direction and structure.

9. Support, Encouragement, Reassurance, and Affirmation Perhaps the most important shift in mental health treatment since the beginning of the 21st century is an emphasis on strengths, assets, and accomplishments, rather than on pathology and deficits. Part of the overall movement called *positive psychology* developed primarily by Martin Seligman, this change in treatment orientation has been associated with increased client motivation toward positive change (Smith, 2006).

However, promoting clients' empowerment and awareness of their strengths is not as easy as it may sound. One of the most challenging skills for clinicians is encouraging and reassuring clients without judging them. Saying to a client, "You did a good job of getting your work done on time," may seem benign and even helpful. However, once clinicians put themselves in the role of evaluating clients, they emphasize the power differential between clients and themselves. This can lead clients to place greater emphasis on pleasing the clinician than on pleasing themselves and can make them apprehensive that, if clinicians can judge them positively, they can also judge them negatively. Clinicians should find ways to enable clients to provide themselves the support, encouragement, reassurance, and affirmation they need, rather than looking to their clinicians for that help.

Communicating Support, Encouragement, Reassurance, and Affirmation: Many strategies are available to facilitate clinicians' efforts to help clients to become their own cheerleaders. Probably most important is directing clients' attention to their accomplishments and helping them to praise themselves. Clinicians might say, for example,

- "You must have been very proud of yourself when you turned in all your work on schedule this week."
- "It sounds to me like you achieved all your goals this week."
- "How did you feel when you got a positive response from your mother after you talked to her differently?"

Helping people identify the steps they took to achieve their successes can be particularly empowering and can reinforce their efforts and successes. A clinician might say,

- "What did you do differently this time?"
- "Let's review the steps you took so you can repeat them the next time."
- "What can you learn from this that you can use next time?"
- "How did you manage to make that happen?"
- "What strengths and resources helped you accomplish that?"

Acknowledging the effort clients expended to achieve their goals is yet another way to affirm and reinforce their efforts. Being specific and concrete when providing this affirmation helps clinicians avoid the pitfall of sounding judgmental. In other words, focus on the facts rather than making a value judgment. For example, a clinician might say, "Although you didn't get your desk organized as you had hoped, you did spend three hours on that project and have nearly reached your goal."

Helping clients develop their own *affirmations,* short meaningful slogans that they can repeat to themselves, is another way for them to give themselves support and reassurance. Typical affirmations include:

- "I know I can do this."
- "I have the skills I need to deal with my family successfully."
- "That is my depression talking, but I can talk back to it."
- "I'm doing the best I can and it's good enough."

Finally, helping people plan effective ways to deal with recurrent challenges provides an additional source of support and self-confidence. For example, the woman who fears her husband's violent behavior can develop a step-by-step plan to protect herself, whereas the man who is having difficulty maintaining his sobriety can list and rehearse new thoughts and actions to help him control his harmful impulses.

10. Ability to Address Problematic Client Behaviors and Attitudes   People are not always willing and cooperative clients. Many clients are mistrustful, unmotivated, or confused about how to make good use of treatment and help themselves. Whether fear, rage, or despair drives their reactions, they sometimes present challenging barriers to effective treatment. Nearly everyone wants to lead a happy and fulfilling life. Sometimes, however, this feeling is deeply buried or blocked by fear or hopelessness. To provide successful treatment, clinicians need strategies to circumvent or reduce barriers to treatment without shaming or attacking their clients. They need to help clients appreciate the potential benefits of treatment, create an environment that is conducive to change, and teach people the skills they need to engage productively in the treatment process.

Engaging People in Treatment: Resistant clients have been the subject of many clinical articles and discussions. Today, clinicians recognize that so-called resistance is usually a way for people to protect themselves and often is an understandable response to their difficulties and disappointments. Clinicians need to respect clients' caution rather than viewing reluctant clients as difficult or undesirable or personalizing their negative reactions to treatment. Through understanding and demonstrating empathy for the barriers that prevent people from forming a positive therapeutic alliance, clinicians can often begin to develop that alliance. They can further accelerate progress by matching treatment strategies to the client's level of readiness for change. Because this is such an important clinical issue, it is discussed further in Chapter 5 in the section on client reluctance and readiness for change.

Illustration of Ways to Develop a Positive Therapeutic Alliance

The following dialogue encompasses the important clinician characteristics and behaviors we have discussed. Notice that all 10 important clinician characteristics are illustrated in this brief interview.

Clinician: Alice, I know you were worried about Mother's Day. How did that go for you? (Trustworthiness, caring)
Alice: I guess I should talk about Mother's Day. Boy, I really lost it.
Clinician: Sounds like you feel badly about the way you handled it. (Empathy)
Alice: Yes. I don't know why I can't just get used to it. Every Mother's Day is a disaster for me. My son never called, my daughter called at midnight, my husband tossed a card at me as he ran off to play golf, and there I was making dinner for my mother. Well, it's over for another year. What's the point of dwelling on it?

Clinician: And yet I hear great sadness when you talk about it. (Empathy, good listening skills, caring and concern, genuineness)

Alice: Yes, you're right. I spent most of the day crying. But nobody knew. Whenever anyone was around, I just put on that happy face.

Clinician: Having to keep your sadness to yourself must have made it even harder. (Empathy, caring)

Alice: I guess so, but I'd feel really stupid if my family knew how badly I felt. Who am I to think that everybody should give up what they want to do and pay homage to me, just because it's Mother's Day?

Clinician: It sounds like you don't think you deserve anything special. And yet I know how committed you are to your family, how hard you are working now to plan for your daughter's wedding, to help your son pay for graduate school, and to help your husband launch his new business. (Good listening, genuineness, persuasiveness)

Alice: But I can't be doing enough or they would have done something special for me on Mother's Day.

Clinician: Am I hearing you say that you feel like a failure as a wife and mother because your family didn't do much for you on Mother's Day? (Empathy, good listening)

Alice: Yes, I guess that is the way I feel.

Clinician: That concerns me. You're devaluing yourself because of your family's behavior on one day rather than deciding for yourself the value of what you do for your family. (Caring and concern, genuineness and sincerity, affirmation)

Alice: I can see what you're saying, but how do I change how I feel?

Clinician: These feelings seem insurmountable to you. And yet I can think of several ways we can work together to perhaps make a shift in those feelings. One place to start is by identifying and checking out the thoughts you have that underlie those feelings of worthlessness. Another approach would be to talk about ways to communicate your thoughts and feelings to your family. Yet a third is to look at the strengths and abilities you use effectively in other situations and see if they can help you deal more effectively with this situation. Perhaps you have other ideas. (Persuasiveness and credibility, optimism, structure and direction, encouragement, ability to address problematic behaviors and attitudes)

Alice: Well, they all sound worth a try. I especially like that third one; that might really help me feel better about myself. Let's start with that one; it would be too hard for me to share my feelings with my family right now and I don't want to revisit those bad feelings I had on Mother's Day.

Clinician: All right. Let's begin by identifying a time when you felt really proud of how well you handled a challenging situation. (Structure and direction, addressing problematic behaviors and attitudes)

Many of the clinician statements, illustrating important strategies to build a successful therapeutic alliance while also advancing the treatment, are brief and deceptively simple. However, integrating into the therapeutic process these strategies to build a positive therapeutic alliance is an art that usually requires considerable practice. The Learning Opportunities at the end of this chapter will enable you to practice integrating interventions such as these into your own work.

CLIENT CHARACTERISTICS THAT ENHANCE TREATMENT

Thus far, this chapter has focused on the important characteristics, attitudes and interventions that clinicians contribute to the development of a positive therapeutic alliance, as well as on hallmarks of that alliance. Of course, clients also bring with them attitudes and traits that exert a strong influence over the quality and development of the therapeutic alliance.

Clinicians have two ways to help people develop and make use of those qualities that will assist them in engaging productively and collaboratively in the therapeutic alliance and process. Clinicians can identify those strengths that people bring with them into treatment, and they can try to teach, reinforce, and build up those qualities in their clients. The following client qualities have been linked to successful treatment:

- Maturity—being responsible, well informed, and reasonably well organized
- Capacity to trust others and form caring and stable relationships
- Ability to establish appropriate interpersonal boundaries, being neither too dependent on others nor too isolated from others
- Capacity for introspection and insight
- High frustration tolerance and ability to delay gratification
- Motivation toward accepting help and making positive changes
- Positive but realistic treatment expectations
- Good self-esteem and feelings of empowerment (Seligman, 2001, pp. 541–542)

Such a list can help clinicians identify those qualities the client already has and those that can readily be developed. By nurturing in clients those characteristics that will enable them to make good use of treatment, clinicians are likely to enhance the therapeutic alliance, increase the likelihood that treatment will be successful, and build strengths that clients can transfer to and use in other situations.

ROLE INDUCTION

Whether or not clients bring with them attitudes and traits that enhance the treatment process, clinicians can teach people how to be successful clients and how to engage productively in a collaborative therapeutic alliance. This process of orienting people to the treatment process is known as *role induction.* A study conducted by Acosta, Yamamoto, Evans, and Skilbeck (1983) found that people who received a pretreatment orientation to counseling or psychotherapy were more motivated and optimistic, had a better understanding of the treatment process, and were more willing to participate actively in treatment.

Although role induction is a learning process for the client, role induction should not be done in a didactic style; rather, it should be an interactive process—a dialogue. Clinicians not only transmit information, they also model those qualities that promote the development of a positive working alliance and elicit and explore client reactions to the information provided. Role induction typically occurs during the first session or two of the treatment process. In role induction, the clinician explores the client's preconceptions of the treatment process, clarifies the nature of that process, and helps the client develop realistic expectations and an accurate understanding of treatment, including both the role of the client and that of the clinician. This process is likely to engender hope in clients, increase their motivation to engage productively in treatment, and develop in them positive feelings toward both the clinician and the treatment. An initial session, including a role induction, might include the following 10 steps (Seligman, 2001, p. 29):

1. Initial exploration of presenting concerns

   - Immediate precipitant of client's seeking treatment
   - Nature, duration, and symptoms associated with presenting concerns

2. Discussion of client's expectations for treatment procedures and outcome
3. Explanation of how treatment promotes positive change and identification of client concerns that usually respond well to treatment
4. Description of the collaborative nature of treatment

   - The positive working alliance
   - Roles and responsibilities of the clinician
   - Roles and responsibilities of the client, including the importance of truthfulness and self-disclosure
   - Discussion of the client's reactions to and questions about the collaborative nature of treatment

5. Ethical aspects of the therapeutic relationship, especially confidentiality, boundaries
6. Practical information on treatment

   - Information on how to contact the clinician
   - Fees, appointment schedule, cancellation policy
   - Obtaining third-party payments

7. Further exploration of presenting concerns
8. Transition to gathering relevant background information (see section on intake interviews in Chapter 3 for details)
9. Linking of relevant background information to presenting concerns
10. Conclusion of session

    - Summarization of session
    - Suggestion of tasks for client to complete
    - Opportunity for client reactions and questions
    - Scheduling of next appointment

This may look like a great deal to accomplish in one session. Having some of the role induction information in written form can streamline the process. Suggesting that clients review the written information at home, after it has been explained in the session, can solidify understanding of the treatment process. In addition, only a preliminary exploration of presenting concerns and background usually occurs in the first session, paving the way for subsequent in-depth discussion of those areas in later sessions. At the same time, these 10 steps may well require more than one session. That is therapeutically sound, as long as they are included in the early stages of the treatment process.

CLINICIAN SELF-DISCLOSURE AND IMMEDIACY

Two of the most powerful ways to build a connection with another person are sharing information about ourselves and giving people helpful information. These strategies also can have a great influence on the treatment process and on the development of the therapeutic alliance.

Knox, Hess, Petersen, and Hill (1997) found that, although self-disclosure was infrequently used by clinicians, clients rated this intervention highly for its helpfulness and reported that clinician self-disclosure had a considerable effect on them. Edwards and Murdoch (1984) arrived at a similar conclusion: "Theory and research have suggested that counselor self-disclosure can be an effective technique if used for purposes that benefit the client" (p. 385).

Why, then, do clinicians make such limited use of an apparently helpful intervention? The answer is that clinician self-disclosure is a risky intervention that has both pros and cons (Simone, McCarthy, & Skay, 1998). Clinician self-disclosures can enhance the therapeutic process, create a sense of collaboration and immediacy, build rapport, make the clinicians seem more genuine and approachable, and introduce helpful new perspectives and reactions. On the other hand, clinician self-disclosure can blur the client–clinician boundaries, shift the focus from the client to the clinician, lead the client to feel judged and blamed, and exploit the client.

Although I believe that the great majority of clinicians act in ethical and professional ways and are dedicated to helping others, my clients have told me about the following:

- The psychologist who gave her client a running progress report on the clinician's own relationship with her partner and spent a session in tears when her partner ended their relationship
- The counselor who asked her client, a wedding planner, for advice on her daughter's wedding
- The social worker who asked his client, a personal trainer, to lend him weights and help him establish a weight-lifting program
- The therapist who invited himself to his client's home under the pretext of seeing her paintings and then initiated a sexual relationship with her

These examples may sound far-fetched to novice clinicians who are well versed in the ethics of social work, counseling, and psychology, but all are true.

Although you may never be tempted to engage in such boundary violations, even lesser instances of inappropriate clinician self-disclosure can damage the therapeutic alliance and lead to premature termination of treatment. Novice clinicians seem especially likely to overuse self-disclosure because of their eagerness to form a bond with their clients. The following guidelines for appropriate uses of self-disclosure can help clinicians make positive use of this powerful tool and avoid its pitfalls.

Guidelines for Beneficial Use of Clinician Self-Disclosure

Many have studied and written about the appropriate use of clinician self-disclosure. Knox et al. (1997), for example, found that the following types of clinician self-disclosure are particularly likely to be helpful:

- Self-disclosure that puts the client at ease and encourages client openness
- Self-disclosure that is normalizing and reassuring to the client
- Self-disclosure consisting of "a disclosure of personal nonimmediate information" (p. 274) about the clinician (e.g., "When I began college, I, too, had difficulty avoiding all the distractions and focusing on my studies. Many students experience that.")

Theory and research suggest the following guidelines to help clinicians make the best use of self-disclosure.

- Self-disclosures must be made for the primary purpose of helping the client. Clinicians should never share personal information in order to help themselves feel better or to use the client as a sounding board or source of information.
- Keeping the focus on the client rather than the clinician greatly increases the likelihood that the self-disclosure will help the client.
- Clinicians should have a therapeutic reason for making a self-disclosure and be able to articulate that reason; if they are unsure about the reason for or value of a self-disclosure, they should refrain from making the self-disclosure. Self-disclosures should not be made just to fill up time or make conversation, unless that is a valid therapeutic purpose.
- Clinician self-disclosures should be used sparingly and should be clear and concise; this minimizes the likelihood that they will distract the client or shift the treatment focus from the client to the clinician. Less is better in terms of clinician self-disclosures.
- Careful timing and wording of self-disclosures can ensure that they are well integrated into the treatment process. They should be relevant to the immediate discussion and should echo repeated phrases and key issues expressed by the client so that the relevance of the self-disclosure is evident.

- Using the present tense when making self-disclosures is likely to increase the relevance and immediacy of the statement.
- Self-disclosures should be relatively impersonal. Edwards and Murdock (1984) found that the most frequent topic for clinician self-disclosure was professional issues such as the credentials or experience of the clinician. The least common area of clinician self-disclosure was sexuality. This clearly reflects the continuum of self-disclosure, from the relatively benign, impersonal, and usually relevant topic of the clinician's professional background to the highly charged and usually inappropriate topic of the clinician's sexual attitudes and behaviors. Self-disclosures that are moderately personal rather than impersonal or very personal seem to be most meaningful to clients. This is illustrated by the following examples:

  ○ Impersonal/apppropriate—I have two sons and a daughter.
  ○ Moderately personal/usually appropriate—My son also had attention-deficit/hyperactivity disorder. I remember struggling, as you are, to find the best way to help him.
  ○ Very personal/usually inappropriate—My daughter was diagnosed with posttraumatic stress disorder after she was raped and I have never forgiven myself for leaving her alone with the neighbor who raped her.

- Be sure to incorporate the essential therapeutic conditions into all self-disclosures. Using empathy, as well as reflection of meaning, and highlighting the connection between the clinician's self-statement and the client's concerns, increase the relevance and meaningfulness of the self-disclosure. For example, the clinician might say, "I can hear how confused and anxious you are now that you have finished college and are unsure what to do next. I remember having some of those feelings when I graduated from college too."
- Self-disclosures should foster client self-determination, pride, awareness of strengths, and empowerment; they should not shame or attack clients or limit their options (unless those options present a danger). For example, the clinician might say, "I'm impressed by the way your motivation to support your family, your organizational skills, and your knowledge of technology all combined to help you identify and apply for over 25 jobs this week."
- Clinicians should be honest and authentic when offering self-disclosures. Credibility is an important component in successful self-disclosures. For example, in response to a client's request for feedback on his social skills, the clinician might say, "If I were to meet you socially, I think I would enjoy your sense of humor and the straightforward way in which you express yourself, but it might bother me that you are often late and sometimes even forget you have an appointment to meet a friend."
- Be aware that clinician self-disclosure is most likely to be effective with clients who have good ego strength (Simone et al., 1998). If clinicians are in doubt about the effect of a self-disclosure, they should wait until they are confident it will be helpful.

Objectives of Clinician Self-Disclosure

Clinician self-disclosure, following the previous guidelines, can accomplish many purposes. The following are some of the most important objectives of self-disclosure. An example illustrates each objective.

1. Providing clinically important information about the counselor or therapist.

    - Informing the client of the clinician's training, experience, theoretical orientation, and policies ("I have a doctorate in psychology and use primarily cognitive-behavioral approaches in the treatment I provide.")
    - Providing necessary information about the beliefs and biases of the clinician and the treatment setting ("This is a church-based agency and does not provide information on abortion as an option in dealing with an unwanted pregnancy.")

2. Building and deepening the therapeutic alliance.

    - Clinician self-disclosure can be helpful to clients whose backgrounds are different from those of the clinician, particularly when the client is from a traditionally oppressed or disenfranchised group. Clinician self-disclosure can highlight similarities in the face of apparently extreme differences and can enable clients to become more familiar and comfortable with the clinician. ("Our backgrounds are very different, and yet we have much in common. You know, I am also the parent of twins.")
    - Highlighting similarities when client and clinician have shared multicultural backgrounds also can build rapport and enhance treatment. ("Like you, I came to the United States as a teenager and had to deal with many changes and adjustments.")
    - Increasing clinician credibility, trustworthiness, and attractiveness ("Like you, I draw a great deal of strength from my spiritual beliefs and practices.")
    - Humanizing the clinician ("I was so upset when the terrorist attacks occurred that I had to stop my work for the day.")

3. Teaching and demonstrating new or alternative insights, emotions, thoughts, behaviors, and attitudes.

    - Modeling self-disclosure
    - Introducing new perspectives and reactions ("I think I would have been hurt if my best friend said that to me.")
    - Encouraging reality testing ("I know you are eager to attend that college, but I'm concerned that you have not paid enough attention to their admission requirements.")
    - Providing feedback ("You have worked very hard to resolve your difficulties through counseling.")

4. Empowering the client.

    - Normalizing a client's reactions ("You seem dismayed that you felt angry when your supervisor cursed at you, and yet I think I would have felt angry about that too.")

- Providing appropriate reassurance ("It sounds like you did everything you could to make the project a success.")
- Instilling hope ("I can hear that you feel pretty scared and hopeless when you have a panic attack, and yet I know from both the research and my work with other people that it is possible to learn to manage and even prevent these attacks.")
- Emphasizing client strengths and resources ("It sounds like your resourcefulness and quick thinking really made a difference when the caterer dropped the birthday cake.")

5. Promoting immediacy. Focusing on the current client–clinician interactions can have a beneficial effect on the treatment process when progress is stalled or when the client has strong feelings such as attraction, dependence, or mistrust toward the clinician. Discussion of ongoing and current interactions can promote client awareness and make feedback especially meaningful and useful.

- Promoting discussion of client–clinician interactions; these often mirror the client's interactions with people outside of treatment ("When you raise your voice and gesture like that, it makes me think that you are very angry even though you say you are not feeling anger.")
- Focusing on the treatment process ("You have come late for our last three sessions. I'm concerned that you are not really invested in our work together.")
- Addressing client feelings toward the clinician ("When you left our session last week, you gave me a note asking me to dinner. Although my professional guidelines require that we maintain a professional relationship, it sounds like you wish we could become closer. We have been working together for quite a while, and I can understand your developing some warm feelings for me. Let's talk about those feelings so we can understand them better and be sure that they do not get in the way of our work together.")

Examples of Clinician Self-Disclosure

Consider the following examples of self-disclosure. Each pair of examples illustrates one of the five major purposes or types of clinician self-disclosure. However, one follows the guidelines for appropriate self-disclosure while the other violates one or more of those guidelines; the assessment following each statement distinguishes the appropriate from the inappropriate self-disclosure statements. In the exercises at the end of this chapter, you will have the opportunity to identify the purposes of self-disclosure statements, to assess whether or not they follow the guidelines for helpful self-disclosures, and to develop some of your own self-disclosure statements.

Providing Clinically Important Information about the Counselor or Therapist

Clinician: I believe ending a marriage is a very serious matter and that we should do all we can to improve a marriage before deciding it should end.

Assessment: This clinician places great importance on the institution of marriage and communicates this attitude to clients. This statement is acceptable because it allows clients to seek a different clinician if they are not comfortable with this approach and to understand the clinician's point of view if they do continue treatment with this person. It does not shame, criticize, or blame clients but rather enables them to make an informed choice.

Clinician: You are putting your own needs in front of those of your children in deciding to end your marriage. Divorce is always devastating to children. Don't your children's feelings matter to you?

Assessment: This self-disclosure is countertherapeutic because it does blame and criticize the client. It misrepresents the research findings on the effect of divorce on children and does not allow the client to make choices.

Building and Deepening the Therapeutic Alliance

Clinician: You may be surprised to know that I, too, am a cancer survivor. It was one of the most difficult experiences I have ever had, as it probably is for you. What has it been like for you?

Assessment: Although this is a personal statement, it introduces an important similarity between the client and the clinician, increases the clinician's credibility, and can instill hope. It is concise, stated in the present tense, and keeps the focus on the client.

Clinician: You know, I, too, had cancer. Was that ever tough for me! I still think about the pain of the surgery, the nausea and vomiting from the chemotherapy, and the fear that I would die. You're lucky they have new drugs now that control the nausea; it shouldn't be so bad for you and you should have a better prognosis. I still worry that the cancer will catch up with me.

Assessment: Although this statement also identifies a similarity between the client and the clinician, it is too wordy and personal, and it shifts the focus from the client to the clinician. In addition, rather than communicating empathy, it minimizes the client's concerns.

Teaching and Demonstrating New or Alternative Insights, Emotions, Thoughts, Behaviors, and Attitudes

Clinician: I can hear you trying very hard to forgive your wife for her infidelities and her abuse of your children. I know that forgiveness is very important in your value system. However, from what you have said, she has never tried to change her behavior. If I were in your situation, I would probably put more energy into caring for my children and myself rather than focusing so much on my wife right now. What reactions do you have to that?

Assessment: This statement gives the client feedback and presents alternative thoughts and behaviors. The clinician is also trying to help the client become more concerned about the harm this situation may do to his children. It incorporates reflection of feeling and meaning, is authentic, and maintains a focus on the client, although it does give the client implicit advice.

Clinician: Week after week, you focus on your unsuccessful efforts to forgive your wife. And yet I think we're losing sight of who is really important here. I was abused as a child, and I know the life-long damage that can do. You need to face the fact that your wife is never going to change and do what a father is supposed to do, protect his children.

Assessment: Although this second statement has the same purposes as the first statement, it seems to be a harmful statement because it violates several guidelines. The clinician's reference to his own abuse is too personal and highly charged for this context. In addition, the statement shames and attacks the client and fails to incorporate the essential therapeutic conditions.

Empowering the Client

Clinician: You seem embarrassed about calling your physician last night when you had chest pains. If I'd had open-heart surgery recently, I would have been on the telephone to my physician as soon as I had pains like that. And I'm impressed that, even though you were scared, you used your deep breathing to relax, you made a list of your questions, and you talked calmly with your physician until you got the information you needed.

Assessment: This statement is designed to normalize the client's reactions and to provide appropriate reassurance. The statement also emphasizes client strengths and resources. Although the statement is lengthy, it does follow other important guidelines. It communicates empathy, keeps the focus on the client, and is honest and authentic.

Clinician: Why were you so reluctant to disturb your physician? Physicians expect emergency calls. Don't be like my brother, who was so afraid to bother anybody that he waited to get help until he had a heart attack that did permanent damage. Next time, get on that phone right away.

Assessment: Again, this self-disclosure is too personal. It takes the focus off the client and uses scare tactics and demands to try to change the client's behavior. Although the clinician is probably motivated by genuine concern for the client, these tactics detract from the client's power. In addition, the clinician fails to communicate empathy for the client.

Promoting Immediacy

Clinician: I'm feeling uncomfortable about our work together lately. You seem to be giving me all the credit for your progress, just as you did now when we discussed your good grades. You are ignoring the hard work you have done in treatment as well as at school. I wonder if you often devalue yourself in this way?

Assessment: This statement is intended to focus on the treatment process and promote discussion of the client's difficulty accepting credit for her accomplishments. This probably will raise her awareness of a pattern of behavior that she manifests in many settings. This statement also should contribute to her feelings of empowerment and can strengthen and build the therapeutic alliance. The statement is concise, uses the present tense, keeps the focus on the client, and is encouraging rather than shaming.

Clinician: I know you had planned to talk about your problems studying for finals, but I have something I want to bring up first. I noticed that you always tell me how wonderful I am and never say much about how great you are. Well, I think you are pretty wonderful, too, and I wish you could be more aware of it.

Assessment: This clinician is caring and supportive toward the client and is seeking to empower the client. However, the intervention is poorly timed, detracting from the topic the client has on her mind. It is vague and general rather than concise and clear, and it does not encourage dialogue about the immediate client–clinician interaction or about the client's patterns of behavior. In addition, the clinician sounds judgmental, a behavior to avoid even if the judgment is a positive one.

Client Requests for Clinician Self-Disclosure

Typically, clinician self-disclosures are initiated by the person providing treatment. However, sometimes clients ask clinicians to disclose information about their own values, beliefs, experiences, and lifestyle. In responding to such requests, clinicians should keep in mind the guidelines and purposes presented previously. Several additional considerations are also relevant under these circumstances.

- *Refusing to self-disclose can detract significantly from the trust and credibility inherent in the therapeutic alliance.* Even sidestepping client questions can be experienced as a rejection. For example, in response to a client's question about their marital status, some clinicians do not answer the question directly but instead ask, "What makes it important to you to know my marital status?" or "What leads you to ask this question?" or "What would it mean to you if I were married?" Although the answers to these questions may well be important, clinicians who respond to a question with a question run the risk of being perceived as manipulative and as emphasizing the power differential in the therapeutic relationship. This does not mean that clinicians must answer all client questions, but they do need to consider carefully the best way to respond.
- *Provide only as much information as is requested.* Just as young children who ask where babies come from do not generally want a lecture on biology, so do most clients want only minimal information. For example, if a client asks whether you are married or have children, a yes or no response usually is enough. Avoid providing details on the genders and ages of your children or the number of marriages you have had unless clients specifically request that information and you choose to disclose it.

- *Avoid making assumptions about what clients want to know.* Several years ago, I had to take time off from my practice for some surgery. I gave all clients the same minimal information: "I will be away from my practice for the next month in order to have surgery for a medical condition." (Of course, I also gave them the names of other therapists to contact in the event of an emergency, along with the opportunity to discuss my upcoming absence.) A few asked no questions and quickly resumed discussion of their own concerns. Most asked a few questions about my medical condition and treatment; once reassured that I was not in danger, they seemed satisfied. One expressed great concern about my health; after responding briefly to her questions, I helped her to recognize the link between her anxiety about my situation and the death of her mother from what was supposed to be minor surgery. People vary greatly in terms of what they want to know about their clinicians; let them tell you what they need.

- *Answer first, then explore.* Like the client who was reminded by my surgery of the unexpected death of her mother, people's questions typically reflect their own interests and concerns. Once clinicians have provided a brief response to clients' questions, the clinicians may well decide it would be therapeutic to explore the thoughts and emotions behind the questions. Clinicians can gently explore clients' motivations and reactions, as in the following example: "No, I don't have children. I know that parenting is one of your important concerns. What does it mean to you that I don't have children?"

- *Think carefully before responding to a client's questions.* Sometimes clients request information that may be harmful to them or that may undermine the therapeutic process. This might be the case with adolescent clients who ask, "Did you ever use drugs?" or "Didn't you have sex when you were my age?" Questions such as these may create a dilemma for the clinician who wants to be honest but also wants to serve as a positive role model for clients and discourage self-destructive choices. There is no formula for responding to questions such as these. However, this is a time for clinicians to draw on their in-depth understanding of the client. They should think about the meaning of the question for the client as well as the probable effect the response will have on the client and then craft a response that is most likely to have a positive effect.

  For example, to the question about the clinician's use of drugs, the clinician might reply, "Yes, like you, I wanted to be accepted by my friends and so I did smoke marijuana for a while. However, I felt it was getting in the way of my school work, so I got up my courage and told my friends that I didn't want to do drugs with them anymore. To my surprise, my decision didn't really hurt my friendships at all."

- *Remember that you have rights, too.* Sometimes clients ask clinicians questions that the clinician does not want to answer. Perhaps the question is personal and addresses information the clinician chooses not to provide. Perhaps the clinician believes that it would be countertherapeutic to respond to that particular question. Clinicians must still treat all clients with respect and acknowledge the legitimacy of their questions. They also usually should process with the client the decision not to provide requested information and explore the meaning this has for the client as well as the emotions it elicits. However, clinicians do not need to provide the answers. This is illustrated in the following examples:

Clinician: I don't want to color your decision about your pregnancy by telling you my beliefs about abortion. I hope you understand that I think it would be better to keep our focus on your choices. Whatever choice you make, I will continue to help you. How do you react to this?

Clinician: I realize you are very curious about me, but your questions are making it difficult for us to address your concerns. Remember, during our first session, I discussed with you your role as a client. I encourage you to shift your focus to your issues rather than to me so we can help you resolve your concerns.

Clinician: I'm glad to hear that you like my office, but I don't understand how it is relevant to our goals for me to tell you how much rent I pay here. If I am missing a connection, please help me understand it.

Clinician: I would rather not discuss my relationship with my partner. I prefer to keep my personal life and my professional life separate. How do you react to my decision not to answer your question?

The issue of clinician self-disclosure is a complex one. However, following the guidelines and models provided here should help you to deal effectively with this issue.

UNDERSTANDING CLINICIANS' OWN FEELINGS TOWARD THEIR CLIENTS

Just as clients have feelings and thoughts about their clinicians, so do clinicians have reactions to their clients. Clinicians' ability to identify their reactions and to deal with them in ways that benefit both themselves and their clients can make a difference in treatment outcome, in the therapeutic alliance, and in clinicians' self-awareness and feelings about themselves.

In determining how to make the best use of their reactions to clients, clinicians might ask themselves the following questions:

- "Are my reactions based on the reality of my interactions with the client, or do they have more to do with my own history and issues?" Chapter 3 discussed countertransference, reactions to clients that stem from clinicians' backgrounds. If clinicians' feelings reflect countertransference, they should deal with those emotions outside of the treatment room and perhaps seek help from a supervisor, a colleague, or their own therapist to help them understand and manage their feelings.
- "If my reactions are based on my interactions with the client, will it help the client if I share those reactions, and are they relevant to the client's treatment goals?" Although feedback on their feelings, thoughts, and actions

can be useful to clients, clinicians should keep in mind the importance of emphasizing client strengths and protecting clients from harmful embarrassment and discomfort. Clinicians should phrase feedback carefully, embedding it in a review of client strengths, and give clients specific and relevant information on how they might make positive changes.

- "Are my reactions hunches or intuitions?" Most clinicians are sensitive and intuitive and, as a result, often pick up information about people without knowing exactly how they acquired that information. Using hunches cautiously as a way to broaden discussion and help clients talk more openly can be useful, although clinicians need to guard against pressuring clients or insisting that the clinicians have the answers. The following is a constructive way to use intuition: "You've said very little about the uncle who lived with your family for several years. I have a hunch it is difficult for you to talk about him. What do you think about that?"

- Clinicians often hear stories that are painful for them, that may reawaken issues of their own, and that may lead them to doubt themselves and their abilities. Posttraumatic stress disorder occurs in police and firefighters who are exposed to violent and life-threatening situations. Therapists, too, can experience such reactions, as well as feelings of helplessness and of being overwhelmed in the face of their clients' difficulties. Although these reactions are normal and understandable, they can impair clinicians' functioning, lead to depression and to problems concentrating or sleeping, and even make clinicians think they are inadequate in their work and should change professions. Recognizing these reactions early and addressing them quickly are the keys to dealing with them effectively. I am often surprised to learn that a therapist or counselor is reluctant to seek help from another mental health professional, but many clinicians view it as a failure if they need help with their own emotional concerns. Think about the confusing messages inherent in this stance: Clinicians believe they can help others and yet many avoid seeking help themselves. In fact, personal therapy can be an excellent learning experience for mental health professionals, particularly when they are experiencing self-doubts and feelings of discouragement and burnout in relation to their work.

- Clinicians have rights too! They have the right to be treated respectfully by clients, to have agreements honored, to have their privacy and time respected by clients, and to be paid for their work. If clinicians feel that a client is violating their rights and is not treating them in a healthy way, they have the right to discuss this with the client and request a change in behavior. Of course, this must be handled with great care and in ways that show empathy for the client and emphasize the client's strengths. Clinicians might say, for example, "Mark, I noticed that you didn't pay for your session again this week and that you have a balance due of over $400. I'm concerned that this might undermine our work together and put you in an uncomfortable situation. I know that being responsible is an important value for you. I'd like to talk about this and see if we can come up with a payment plan that will work for both of us."

Although this section has reviewed a broad range of emotional reactions that clinicians might have to their clients and their work, clinicians may have reactions other than those discussed here. What is important is to recognize that clinicians have reactions to clients just as clients have reactions to clinicians, to be aware of those feelings and their sources, to understand and address them, and to be sure to use those feelings in ways that enhance the treatment process.

LEARNING OPPORTUNITIES

This chapter introduced an array of conceptual skills and strategies focused primarily on emotions, the second element in the BETA format. These skills help clinicians engender positive feelings in the treatment setting, develop a sound client–clinician relationship, work collaboratively with their clients, and deal productively with their own emotional reactions. This chapter included information on the following:

- Initiating and developing a positive therapeutic alliance
- Understanding the client and clinician characteristics that contribute to a strong therapeutic alliance
- Role induction
- Clinician self-disclosure
- Ways for clinicians to better understand and make therapeutic use of their own emotional reactions to clients and to the treatment process

The following exercises provide the opportunity to apply the conceptual skills presented in this chapter. This section includes written exercises, discussion questions, exercises and an assessment tool to use in your practice group, and topics to write about in your personal journal.

Written Exercises/Discussion Questions

1. Many modern clinicians and researchers believe that the treatment alliance between the client and the clinician is more important than the treatment plan that is used. Does this point of view surprise you? Why or why not? What evidence can you present that supports or refutes this position?
2. Beginning on page 98 is a list of 10 dimensions that characterize clinicians who are skilled in developing sound therapeutic alliances with their clients. For each of the following clients, identify two or three clinician qualities from that list that you believe will be especially conducive to the development of a positive working alliance with that client.
   a. A seven-year-old boy who has lived in several foster homes has recently been reunited with the parent who neglected him as an infant.
   b. A 56-year-old man who was recently fired from his job because of arguments with supervisors and co-workers. He believes he was fired because of his high salary.

    c. A 27-year-old woman with two young children who sought treatment because her husband recently left her when the woman with whom he was having an affair became pregnant. The client is depressed and humiliated.

3. Assume that you forgot a scheduled appointment with a client and were not in the office at the time of the appointment. How will you deal with this? Identify the characteristics you will model in an effort to maintain a positive therapeutic alliance with the client.

4. Ada has been a challenging client for you. Your first two sessions have largely been monologues by Ada, blaming her parents and friends for her difficulties and reiterating her hopeless feelings. At the end of the second session, Ada asks you whether you like her. How will you respond to her question, keeping in mind the importance of communicating both caring and genuineness to clients?

5. Discuss the probable benefits, drawbacks, and purposes of the following clinician self-disclosures.

    a. I also am a marathon runner. I find it helps me stay well, both physically and mentally.

    b. Alcohol can ruin families. It damaged my family just as it did yours.

    c. I have a perfume allergy and ask that you not wear strong perfume to our appointments.

    d. I'm impressed that you got here on time. The weather really slowed me down this morning.

    e. You really look terrific in that red outfit.

6. How would you respond to the following client requests for you to disclose information about yourself?

    a. Did you ever feel like killing yourself?

    b. I brought my wife to our last session so that I could get your feedback on her. What did you think of her?

    c. Because of her accident, my wife suffered brain damage and has become a quadriplegic. I'm only 28 years old and want to have a life. Would you divorce your wife if you were in my situation?

7. Clinicians seem to be increasingly aware of the importance of role induction in getting the treatment process off to a good start. What do you see as the advantages and disadvantages of role induction? For what types of clients do you view role induction as especially important? Under what circumstances are you likely to omit doing a role induction?

Practice Group Exercise: *Role Induction and the Therapeutic Alliance*

This practice group exercise provides the opportunity to practice your conceptual skills and further refine your fundamental skills. As usual, be sure to record (on audio or video tape) both the practice session and the subsequent discussion.

This practice group exercise involves the following skills:

- Initiating treatment
- Demonstrating characteristics that will build a sound therapeutic alliance
- Role induction
- Responding to clients' questions

Practice Group Exercise

As usual, in each role-play, one person will assume the role of clinician, another will assume the role of client, and the other one or two participants will serve as observers. This role-play should be viewed as an initial treatment session. Those in the client role may determine their specific concerns. During the course of the initial interview, they should ask the clinician at least two questions, one of which requests the disclosure of personal information.

Clinicians in this exercise have three major goals:

1. To demonstrate those characteristics that promote the development of a sound therapeutic alliance
2. To conduct a role induction in which the clinician informs the client about the nature of the treatment process and the desired roles of the client and the clinician
3. To deal effectively and therapeutically with the client's questions

Timing of Exercise

If possible, allow approximately two hours for this exercise, with each role-play and its processing taking about 30 minutes. If you do not have this much time, do only two role-plays, one for each dyad. Each person will then have the opportunity to be either client or clinician but will not experience both roles.

- Allow 20 minutes for each role-played interview.
- Allow about 10 minutes to provide feedback to the person in the clinician role. As you have done with other exercises in this book, begin the feedback process with the person in the clinician role, focus on strengths first, and offer concrete suggestions for improvement. Remember to make this a positive learning experience. Feedback should focus on the areas listed in the Assessment of Progress form that follows.

Assessment of Progress Form 4

1. a. What strategies and clinician characteristics were used to initiate the session and build a positive treatment alliance?

   _____

   _____

   _____

    b. Which of these seemed particularly successful? What made them effective?

_____

_____

_____

    c. What else might the clinician have done to further develop the treatment alliance?

_____

_____

_____

2. What is your overall assessment of how the clinician conducted the role induction? What were the strengths of this process? How might it have been improved?

_____

_____

_____

_____

3. How well did the clinician handle the client's questions? Were different strategies used to respond to personal questions than were used to address professional questions? What were the strengths of this process? How might it have been improved?

_____

_____

_____

_____

4. How successful was the clinician in integrating a variety of interventions into the interactions with the client? What strengths did you observe in the clinician's use of interventions? How might the clinician's use of a variety of interventions have been improved?

_____

_____

_____

_____

5. Summary of feedback

    a. Strengths:

_____

_____

    b. Areas needing improvement:

_____

Personal Journal Questions

1. Which of the 10 important clinician characteristics and skills (described beginning on page 98) do you believe you will be able to use well in developing positive therapeutic alliances with your clients? Which ones do you think will be the most challenging for you to use and why?

2. If you have been in therapy yourself, did your clinician conduct a role induction with you? If yes, was that helpful to you? If not, in what ways, if any, do you think that process would have been helpful to you?

3. List two questions that clients might ask you that you would find difficult to answer. Write an effective response to each of the two questions.

4. What sorts of clients or treatment situations seem most likely to raise feelings of inadequacy or other negative emotions for you? How might you deal effectively with such clients or situations so that you do not experience strong negative reactions?

SUMMARY

This chapter focused on ways to establish a positive therapeutic alliance, conduct a role induction, make helpful self-disclosures, and deal with clinicians' own emotional reactions to clients and to the treatment process. Chapter 5 focuses on dealing with strong client emotions, such as suicidal ideation and rage, and with variations in client readiness to engage productively in treatment.

Chapter 5

USING CONCEPTUAL SKILLS
TO MAKE POSITIVE USE OF
AND MODIFY EMOTIONS

ADDRESSING STRONG CLIENT EMOTIONS AND VARIATIONS IN CLIENT READINESS FOR TREATMENT

OVERVIEW

Chapter 4 began our discussion of applying conceptual skills to eliticing, exploring, and addressing emotions. That chapter focused on ways to develop and enhance the therapeutic alliance and presented information on role induction as well as on client and clinician characteristics and behaviors that can contribute positively to the client–clinician alliance. Chapter 4 also looked at the therapeutic use of clinician self-disclosure and provided guidelines, as well as examples, of ways in which clinicians can share their own feelings and perceptions of the client and the treatment process.

Chapter 5 continues our focus on using conceptual skills to address emotions. This chapter focuses on understanding and dealing with strong negative client emotions, including suicidal ideation, anger, and others. This chapter also looks at variations in people's readiness for treatment, especially their reluctance to engage in treatment, and suggests ways for clinicians to adapt treatment to the client's level of readiness for help.

DEALING WITH STRONG NEGATIVE CLIENT EMOTIONS

Clients often bring strong negative emotions with them into treatment—emotions such as rage, suicidal thinking, and despair. Often, these extreme reactions occur in response to a crisis or upsetting event. These emotions may feel as overwhelming to the clinician as they do to clients and those around them. In addition, these emotions may interfere with the development of a positive therapeutic alliance and with the role induction process. To provide successful treatment and safeguard clients and those who might be affected by their strong feelings, clinicians must find effective ways to address and modify these powerful emotions and help their clients deal with the crises that may have triggered these feelings.

The following sections of this chapter review ways to help people manage and change three types of strong emotions that are often seen in clinical settings: suicidal ideation; anxiety and upset associated with a crisis or critical incident; and strong anger. The models presented here can be adapted and used to help people deal with other strong and harmful emotions.

SUICIDAL IDEATION

Estimates suggest that approximately 25,000 to 35,000 people commit suicide each year in the United States. Not only is suicide the cause of many deaths, it has far-reaching negative effects; family members, friends, colleagues, neighbors, and fellow students of the person who has committed suicide may experience loss, guilt, self-blame, and other negative emotions.

Clinicians suffer, too, when a client commits suicide. Recently, in a class of 10 relatively new counselors, the topic turned to suicide and strong feelings began to emerge. Of the 10 people in the class, four had experienced the suicide of a client. According to Westefeld et al. (2000), 97% of psychology trainees reported working with suicidal clients, 29% had at least one client who attempted suicide, and 11% had a client commit suicide.

Suicidal thinking is far more common than completed suicides. All clinicians, even counselors in elementary schools, need to be on the alert for the presence of suicidal ideation. Whether or not clinicians believe a person is likely to act on the suicidal thoughts, the devastating effects of a suicide mandate that clinicians take suicidal thinking seriously and implement effective strategies to prevent self-injury.

Strategies for Addressing Suicidal Ideation

Working with a suicidal person can be frightening and confusing for clinicians. Having a conceptual model or plan for addressing suicidal thinking, such as the one that follows, can provide helpful reassurance to both client and clinician.

Step 1. Determine the Presence of Suicidal Ideation   Before clinicians can address suicidal ideation effectively, they need to determine whether such thoughts are indeed present and the level of risk to the person experiencing the suicidal thoughts. Although suicide attempts and completed suicides cannot be predicted with good accuracy, developing awareness of common indicators of suicide potential and becoming alert to the presence of those indicators in clients are important in sensitizing clinicians to the possibility that a client may be at risk of making a suicide attempt.

Risk Factors: The following factors, grouped in categories, have been associated with a higher-than-average risk of having suicidal ideation and attempting suicide (Carney & Hazler, 1998; Motto, Heilbron, & Juster, 1985; Westefeld et al., 2000):

Biological

- Age: Suicide is particularly common among adolescents and people over the age of 65.
- Changes in eating and sleeping patterns.
- Gender: Men are more likely to kill themselves than are women, although women are more likely to attempt suicide.
- Serious physical illness, especially a terminal illness.

Psychological

- Depression
- Flat affect
- External locus of control—being more strongly influenced by external signs of approval and disapproval than by inner values and self-assessment
- Psychotic disorders
- Feelings of hopelessness and helplessness
- Low self-esteem
- Questioning the meaning of life, one's own identity
- Social isolation, lack of support systems

Cognitive

- Extensive cognitive distortions
- Ideas of reference or persecution—having pervasive, unwarranted thoughts that people are criticizing, talking about, or seeking to harm the person
- Inflexibility in thinking
- Negative self-talk
- Self-centeredness
- Suicidal ideation (Of course, this is often present, either sporadically or consistently, before a suicide attempt.)
- Verbalizing thoughts of wanting to disappear or cease to exist
- Thoughts of invulnerability

Behavioral

- Giving away possessions (especially in adolescents)
- Negative outcome of previous efforts to obtain help
- Substance misuse
- Talking, writing, or drawing about suicide and death

Environmental/Contextual

- Availability of lethal weapons, especially guns
- Coming from a culture that is competitive and goal-directed, especially if that culture views suicide as honorable (suicide rates are especially high in the United States, Japan, and Sweden, and among Native Americans)
- Occupational problems, especially loss of position or prestige
- Living in an urban, metropolitan region

- Socioeconomic status that is middle-class or above—risk increases with financial resources
- Significant marital/partner/family conflict
- History of suicide, substance misuse, or depression in the family
- Unusual stress, loss, or threat of loss

Assessing Presence of Suicidal Ideation: More than 20 "recognized suicide prediction scales" have been identified in the literature (Cochrane-Brink, Lofchy, & Sakinofsky, 2000, p. 445). One of the simplest is the SAD PERSONS scale. Its validity and reliability have not yet been well established. Used cautiously, however, this scale affords clinicians a rapid and helpful way to assess the likelihood that someone will attempt suicide. The SAD PERSONS scale is an acronym, with each letter representing one of the important risk factors to consider when assessing for suicidal ideation. Developed by Patterson, Dohn, Bird, and Patterson (1983), this scale includes the following risk factors (Juhnke & Hovestadt, 1995, p. 32): sex, age, depression, previous suicide attempt, ethanol (alcohol) misuse, rational thinking loss, social supports lacking, organized suicide plan, no spouse, sickness.

When clinicians believe a person may have suicidal thoughts, particularly when at least two of the risk factors in the SAD PERSONS scale are present, they should inquire, matter of factly, about the presence of such thoughts. For instance, a clinician might say to a client, "Have you ever felt so bad, you thought about hurting or killing yourself?" Raising this question gives the client permission to express suicidal thoughts and is likely to reduce any shame associated with having such thoughts. Talking about suicide will almost always decrease, rather than increase, its likelihood.

Step 2. Determine the Level of Risk   Having suicidal thoughts is very common; the nature and intensity of these thoughts and the availability of means for killing oneself determine whether a person is in danger. Information on level of risk can be obtained by asking, "Do you have those thoughts now? When you have those thoughts, how likely do you think it is that you actually would harm yourself?"

Determine Whether the Person Has a Plan and the Means to Commit Suicide: The likelihood of an attempted or completed suicide is strongly related to the presence of a plan and the means to commit suicide. Clinicians might ask a client, "When you thought about killing yourself, how did you think you would go about doing it? Do you have those means available to you? Did you think about a particular day and time when you might kill yourself?"

Review the Client's History: People who have a history of suicide in their families or who have made prior suicide attempts are more likely to consider suicide as a solution to their problems. Ascertaining the presence of suicidal thinking and behavior in the client and in the family can provide further information about the level of risk. Questions that might provide this information include: "As far as you know, has anyone in your family thought about suicide, made suicide attempts, or even killed themselves? Have you had thoughts about killing yourself in the past?

How long/how often have you had those thoughts? Have you made suicide attempts or harmed yourself in the past? When, how, and under what circumstances?"

Step 3. Assess for Coping Mechanisms Determining the presence of coping mechanisms in people who are depressed and suicidal can be challenging. Clinicians should be sure to use empathy and provide support, reassurance, caring, concern, and optimism when exploring resources with people who have suicidal thoughts. If the clients view themselves as having few resources or coping mechanisms, they can become even more discouraged. A clinician might ask questions such as, "When you have suicidal thoughts, what do you do to help yourself? How does it work? What gives you a reason to stay alive and keep trying to feel better? When you have had other crises or been very upset in the past, what have you done to help yourself?" Clinicians should emphasize and reinforce successful coping skills, as well as the client's strengths, throughout this dialogue.

Step 4. Explore the Client's Concept of Suicide and Death People have a reason for considering suicide. That reason may not seem logical to others, but understanding the client's reasoning can be useful in preventing a suicide. Three common reasons for suicide are

1. Feelings of hopelessness and a wish to escape from pain ("If things get too bad, I'll kill myself.").
2. A desire to manipulate another person ("If you don't change or do what I want, I'll kill myself or scare you with a suicide attempt.").
3. Revenge ("I'll kill myself and then you'll be sorry for what you did to me.").

Asking clients about their concepts of suicide and death can be helpful. Clients may have been raised to think of suicide as honorable, or they may believe that, when they are dead, they will go to heaven and find peace. On the other hand, they may have been raised with religious beliefs that prohibit killing oneself, and they may view suicide as sacrilegious behavior. Understanding people's motives, as well as their images of suicide and death, can guide the development of effective preventive interventions.

Step 5. Process and Organize the Information Once clinicians have gathered information about a person's suicidal thinking, they can summarize that information by answering the following questions:

- What suicide risk factors are present?
- Is suicidal ideation present?
- What is the level of risk?
- What plan, if any, does the client have for committing suicide?
- What factors in the client's background or family history might predispose the person to a suicide attempt?
- What coping mechanisms has the client used successfully in the past? What coping mechanisms seem to be readily available to the client now?

- What seems to be the client's primary reason for considering suicide?
- What views does the client have of suicide, death, and the afterlife?

This information falls into two broad categories:

- What factors contribute to the likelihood that this person will commit suicide?
- What factors can protect this person from committing suicide?

Step 6. Analyze and Synthesize the Information Now that clinicians have obtained, thought about, and organized the information, they can take a deeper look at that information and consider its connections and implications. Particularly important is understanding the dynamics of the suicidal thinking. Answering the following questions can facilitate this process.

- Assuming that suicidal ideation is present, what patterns does it follow? Is it chronic or acute? How long has it been present? Is it worse at particular times of day or under certain circumstances? What life events, thoughts, or emotions seem to trigger suicidal ideation for this person?
- How are the risk factors linked to the suicidal ideation? For example, is a depressive disorder or chronic alcohol dependence creating feelings of hopelessness, are previous treatment failures making the person believe that nothing will help, or is an interpersonal rejection leading the person to crave both revenge and escape from pain?
- What is the meaning or the message of the suicide plan? For example, is the person contemplating shooting himself in the parking lot of the company from which he was fired? Is he considering taking an overdose of pills right before his parents are due home from work so that they will realize how unhappy he is? Plans such as these are intended to give a message.
- How do background factors contribute to the likelihood that a person will commit suicide? Perhaps a man whose mother committed suicide believes that her action condones his behavior. Perhaps previous suicide attempts brought the person sympathy, attention, and other secondary gains. What background factors need attention in treatment, not only to prevent them from contributing to the likelihood of a suicide attempt, but also to help the person identify and work through unresolved past concerns?
- What are the person's views of suicide, death, and the afterlife? Here is an opportunity for clinicians to use their multicultural competencies to understand the context of the suicidal thinking. The client's cultural and religious background may be compatible or incompatible with the concept of suicide. For example, a Japanese American man may view suicide as an honorable behavior after he has experienced a loss of face, and this may increase the likelihood that he will commit suicide. On the other hand, a depressed woman from a Roman Catholic background may be aware that suicide is antithetical to the tenets of her faith; this may reduce the

likelihood that she will make a suicide attempt. Ideas for helpful interventions will begin to emerge through understanding of a person's multicultural background.

Step 7. Make Sense of the Suicidal Ideation   Now clinicians should be ready to understand the underlying purpose and meaning that suicide has for the client, the last step before formulating treatment interventions. The basic question here is, "What makes suicide an acceptable and appealing alternative for this person?" The answer should reflect a deep understanding of this person as well as an integration of the information obtained about the dynamics of the suicidal ideation.

Step 8. Develop Interventions   Clinicians can now develop effective interventions to address and reduce a client's suicidal ideation and behavior and improve the person's coping skills. The following suggestions may help clinicians determine how best to accomplish these goals.

- The clinician has already identified factors that are important in determining the level of suicide risk. How might those factors be changed to reduce the level of risk? For example, helping the client recognize that both her family problems and her accompanying depression can be alleviated can promote hope and a reason to live.
- What might be done to interfere with any plans to commit suicide and to separate the person from the means? For example, an adolescent's parents might be notified that she has been taking their Valium and now has more than 50 pills hidden in her drawer. A person who owns guns might be encouraged to remove the ammunition and guns from the home and leave them with a trusted friend.
- Having determined whether the primary motivation for the suicidal ideation is escape, manipulation, revenge, or another purpose, in what better ways might the person accomplish the same purpose? For example, cognitive therapy might help alleviate emotional pain, while training in communication skills might help people find healthier ways to get attention, let others know what they need, or communicate anger and disappointment.
- What previously effective coping skills have been identified? What prevents the client from coping effectively at the present time? How can the clinician help the client make effective use of formerly successful coping skills? Perhaps the client turned to support systems in the past but now lives far away from family and friends. Perhaps the client views the current crisis to be of greater magnitude than any previously experienced. Developing interventions to help the person overcome these barriers to effective coping can avert a suicide attempt.
- What coping skills does the person seem likely to develop easily? Teaching coping skills that are appealing and acceptable to the client will, of course, make them more likely to be used successfully. For example, a person who is generally well organized might benefit from looking at the current situation step by step to figure out how to handle it best. A person who tends to

be quiet and private might benefit from reading about the current problem or learning meditation and relaxation strategies. Development of coping skills can emerge from information on the four elements in the BETA format: background, emotions, thoughts, and actions. The following provides information about approaches that clinicians frequently use to try to prevent suicide, grouped according to whether they focus primarily on emotions, thoughts, or actions.

Emotions

- Use reflections of feeling, open questions, and other helpful interventions to communicate caring, concern, and understanding.
- Make a referral for medication, particularly medication to reduce depression or psychotic thinking.
- Help the client to express feelings, but also teach ways to contain and control emotions.
- Become a support system for the client by scheduling follow-up telephone calls and future appointments.

Thoughts

- Dispute the client's motivation for committing suicide.
- Use statements such as the following to give people a different perspective:

  "Perhaps we can find other ways to lessen that great pain you are experiencing."

  "Perhaps your friends will feel sorry about making fun of you but, if you kill yourself, you won't be alive to enjoy that. While they are graduating from school and going onto college, you will be lying in your grave."

- Dispute cognitive distortions.
- Teach the client positive affirmations to solidify changes in thinking.
- Help the client find a reason to stay alive.
- Focus on the client's strengths and accomplishments to build self-esteem and clarify identity.
- Emphasize any religious, spiritual, or cultural beliefs that might discourage suicide.
- Help the client learn more effective ways to make decisions and solve problems.

Actions

- Develop a verbal or written safekeeping contract, agreed to (and signed, if written) by both client and clinician. An example is "I will not either accidentally or on purpose hurt or kill myself no matter how bad things might get and no matter how awful I feel." People who are highly suicidal may not agree to an open-ended contract but may be willing to agree to a time-limited contract of 24 or 48 hours, with a daily telephone call to renew the contract. This strategy inspires hope and reassures the client that the clinician is concerned and is trying to help.
- Teach the client improved communication skills.

- Collaborate with the client in the development of a list of coping strategies that can be used if suicidal thoughts or impulses arise. This should be a lengthy list, giving the client many options, and might include any or all of the following:

Go to the local emergency room or hospital.

Call a hot line.

Call your therapist.

Call a trusted friend or family member.

Go to a public place, such as a shopping mall, where you know you will not harm yourself.

Engage in relaxation or meditation.

Do something physically active (e.g., take a walk, work out, do sit-ups).

Do something to make yourself laugh (e.g., read a humor magazine, watch a funny movie or television program).

Remind yourself of the reasons you have to stay alive (e.g., look at photographs of your children, focus on the important role you play at work).

Plan a pleasurable trip or activity.

Make use of your improved communication skills to tell someone or write about your negative feelings.

Take steps to further develop your support systems (e.g., join a 12-step program, call an old friend, or suggest meeting a new friend for dinner).

Ask someone to stay with you until you believe you are safe.

Step 9. Monitor Progress Because of the immediate risk presented by suicidal ideation, ongoing evaluation of the client and the effectiveness of treatment are essential. If rapid progress is not evident, changes in the treatment plan may be indicated. Ongoing consultation with a colleague, supervisor, or psychiatrist, as well as documentation of all information and interventions, are important to protect both the client and the clinician.

Example: Addressing Suicidal Ideation

Sydney, a 62-year-old divorced man, has had a moderately successful dental practice for many years. However, he has struggled with depression and frequent suicidal thoughts for more than 40 years. Sydney's mother reportedly suffered from long-standing depression and eventually did take her own life. Sydney stated that his father was "alcoholic" until the father's death at age 63. Sydney has been diagnosed with a progressive neurological disease that is affecting his ability to perform his work. He has low self-esteem and few support systems, deriving his primary identity from his work. The anticipated loss of his dental practice feels devastating to him.

Sydney reports that he is currently at high risk of attempting suicide and has lethal drugs readily available. He views suicide as a way to escape from his emotional pain. On the other hand, Sydney has never attempted suicide, largely because of his concern about the effect it would have on his two sons, now ages 27 and 24. Sydney is still troubled by the effect on him of his mother's suicide and does not want his children to suffer as he did. In addition, he was deterred from suicide in the past because he did not want to tarnish his reputation in the community, nor did he want his ex-wife to view him as a failure.

Sydney coped with past stressors such as his divorce and downturns in his business by reading and consulting with experts, including lawyers and accountants. He has no strong spiritual beliefs, but he was raised in the Jewish religion. He thinks of suicide as "an end to all this pain and struggle."

The following interventions can be used to help reduce Sydney's depression and suicidal ideation.

Emotions

- Discuss the suicide of Sydney's mother and the effect it had on him; help him to finally come to terms with that loss.
- Emphasize his wish not to hurt his children in any way.
- Provide Sydney with support via frequent telephone calls and reinforcement of his efforts to help himself.

Thoughts

- Dispute Sydney's reasons for committing suicide and help him become aware of other ways to reduce his pain.
- Help Sydney find more reasons to stay alive.
- Focus on the many accomplishments he has made over the years.
- Help Sydney find solutions to the problems inherent in his diagnosis of a neurological condition.

Actions

- Develop a safekeeping contract with Sydney.
- Draw on previous coping strategies; suggest that Sydney read about career development in the later years and the effects of suicide on the survivors.
- Encourage regular exercise, as sanctioned by Sydney's physician.
- Facilitate development of Sydney's support system.
- Encourage Sydney to consult with specialists, such as his physician, his accountant, and a financial planner, so that he can more clearly understand his medical and financial situation.

Reviewing and Implementing the Conceptual Model

The conceptual model outlined here for dealing with suicidal ideation may seem long and cumbersome. However, clinicians can implement the first eight steps during a single session, and the follow-up can extend over as many subsequent sessions as are needed. In addition, this model can be applied to a broad range of other negative emotions and impulses, such as hopelessness, the wish to escape and avoid one's problems, self-injurious behavior, dysfunctional eating, and unwise sexual activity. Let's look at the model in skeleton form so you can easily see the steps involved.

1. Determine the presence of suicidal ideation.
2. Determine level of risk.
3. Assess for coping mechanisms.
4. Explore the client's concept of suicide and death.
5. Process and organize the information.
6. Analyze and synthesize the information.
7. Make sense of the suicidal ideation.
8. Develop interventions.
9. Monitor progress.

Now let's look at crisis intervention, another common and challenging situation that is often faced by clients and clinicians, as well as a conceptual framework for helping people in crisis.

CRISIS INTERVENTION

In addressing suicidal ideation, we drew on the BETA format (background, emotions, thoughts, actions) to facilitate the development of interventions. To illustrate another useful model, the modified version of Bloom's taxonomy (see Chapter 2) is used here to help clinicians deal with other strong client emotions.

People often enter treatment because of crises in their lives. Crises take many forms and can be viewed in terms of the following categories:

- An actual or threatened loss, such as a bereavement, a job loss, or a divorce
- An important decision point, such as whether to accept a marriage proposal, adopt a child, end a troubled relationship, make a career change, or move an elderly and ill parent into a nursing home
- A traumatic event, such as a rape, an automobile accident, a terrorist attack, or a hurricane or other natural disaster

Although these crises vary in terms of their nature and magnitude, a standard protocol can help clinicians treat nearly all people who are dealing with crises or critical incidents.

When helping people deal successfully with crises, clinicians generally focus their attention on the current situation and take a more active role than they might usually assume (Srebalus & Brown, 2001). They typically collaborate with clients in determining immediate plans to either minimize the negative consequences of a crisis or prevent a negative outcome, while helping the clients to regain equilibrium, make positive decisions, and move ahead with their implementation. In learning to cope successfully with a crisis, people commonly develop new strategies for handling problems and often become more empowered and self-confident than they had been.

The modified Bloom's taxonomy, along with the BETA format, illustrates the steps in the process of helping people cope with crises. There are many similarities between this format and the steps that were suggested previously for suicide prevention.

Modified Bloom's Taxonomy Applied to Crisis Intervention

Content (What are the facts?)

- Obtain a clear description of the crisis situation, including precipitants.
- What options does the client perceive as available to him or her?
- What decisions or actions does the client believe need to be taken immediately?
- What has the person already done in response to the crisis?

Process

Comprehension (What do I know and understand about the facts?)

- What is the true nature of the current crisis?
- What does the crisis mean to the person?
- What risk factors are present that may exacerbate the situation?
- What is the current level of danger?
- What has the person already tried to do to address the crisis, and how well have those solutions worked?
- What coping mechanisms has the person used effectively in the past to cope with crises?
- What coping mechanisms has the person used that have not been effective?

Organization (What principles, categories, and generalizations help me to understand this information?)

- What factors contribute to the difficulty the client is having in coping with this crisis?
- What factors are protecting or helping the person in this time of crisis?
- What immediate decisions and actions are needed?
- What are the viable alternatives?
- What are the available resources?
- What has worked and what has not worked in coping with crises of this nature, both for the client and for people in general?

Analysis/Synthesis (How are these facts related, and what inferences can I draw about their connections?)   Take a closer look at the information and consider its connections and implications. Begin to think about ways to empower the client and enable him or her to see options more clearly. Focus especially on the following:

- Ways to enable the client to make urgent decisions and take immediate steps
- The underlying significance of the crisis for the client
- Implications of the crisis for the client's life
- Links between the current crisis and the client's history, especially previous crises
- Options available for dealing with the crisis
- Coping skills, resources, and strengths available to the client

Interpretation (What does all of this mean, and what sense does all of this make?) The basic question to answer here is, "What has made handling this crisis particularly difficult for this person?" Perhaps the crisis is reminiscent of an earlier and very painful crisis, perhaps it is only one of a long series of crises, perhaps it is life-threatening, or perhaps it calls into question the meaning and value of the person's life. These and many other factors and patterns contribute to making a crisis feel insurmountable. Draw on all the information obtained about both the person and the crisis in determining the answer to this question. Once clinicians have figured out an answer to this question, they can move forward with interventions that are likely to help.

Application (What approaches seem most likely to be effective in helping the client cope with this crisis?) Once the clinician and the client have developed a clear picture of the nature of the crisis, the effect it has on the client, and sound strategies for coping with the crisis, the client and clinician are ready to address the crisis. Clinicians should be careful not to rush or pressure the client unnecessarily; that can compound the stress for an already fragile person. Typically, the process of helping someone cope with a crisis includes the following steps.

Background

- Help the client see the connection between the current crisis and that person's history, especially past crises.
- Develop a list of coping skills that the client has used effectively in the past.

Emotions

- Facilitate the client's awareness and expression of emotional reactions to the crisis.
- Help the client manage and change emotional reactions as needed.
- Provide support and resources to help the client cope with the crisis.

Thoughts

- Identify any distorted cognitions related to the crisis. Common examples include "I am unable to handle this," "I am powerless," "This is a hopeless situation," and "There is nothing I can do about this."
- Help the client modify distorted cognitions.

Actions

- Teach new coping skills if needed.
- Identify coping skills that the person used successfully in the past and facilitate their application to the present situation.

The following behavioral coping skills are especially likely to be useful to people in crisis.

- Relaxation
- Imagery, focusing on empowerment and success, as well as an image of a safe place
- Decision-making skills
- Clarifying priorities
- Dividing large tasks into manageable actions
- Developing and drawing on support systems
- Affirmations
- Thought stopping

Evaluation (How effective has my treatment been, how could I make it even more effective, and what can I learn from this experience?)   For several reasons evaluation is a crucial component of helping people cope with crises. The crises themselves may be long-lasting and may change or evolve over time, necessitating changes in coping skills. Examples include coping with chronic and life-threatening illnesses, going through a separation and divorce, and embarking on a new academic or occupational venture. In addition, the full emotional effect of a crisis may not be felt until the crisis is long past. Posttraumatic stress disorder, for example, may begin months or even years after the end of a crisis and may continue indefinitely, exacerbated by reminders of the crisis. Clinicians dealing with people in crisis need to include long-term follow-up, education on the warning signs of posttraumatic stress disorder, and prevention strategies in their treatment plans. Continual evaluation of treatment effectiveness is essential in helping people cope with crises.

Example: Helping Someone Cope with Crisis

The following example, using the case of Eileen Carter presented in Chapter 2, illustrates the application of this conceptual format for helping people cope with a crisis. As you review this case, think about what other questions and strategies you could incorporate into your work with this client.

1. *Content:*   Eileen Carter recently received a call from her older brother informing her that their mother had been hospitalized following a heart attack. This raised both practical and emotional issues for Eileen. She believed she had no one to care for her son if she went to visit her mother nearly 200 miles away. She was taking a college course and did not want to

fall behind or have to drop the class. In addition, she and her mother had a conflicted relationship. Eileen had taken no action thus far, but she believed that she must make decisions quickly in light of her mother's medical condition.

2. *Process*
   a. Comprehension

      Nature of the crisis: Eileen's mother had been hospitalized following a heart attack. Eileen felt torn between her loyalty to her family of origin and her current commitments to her son and her education.

      Meaning of the crisis: Her mother's heart attack brought home to Eileen the fact that she could not avoid dealing with her past indefinitely. She was fearful that this would be her last opportunity to resolve her differences with her mother and act in ways that reflected Eileen's efforts to overcome her difficult past. Now that she was a mother herself, Eileen felt greater empathy for her own mother. However, she was uncertain whether she wished to reconcile with her mother and perhaps bring up painful memories from the past. Eileen was also concerned about the welfare of her son and her progress in college and did not want to compromise those.

      Risk factors: This situation brought back to Eileen many painful memories of her childhood, the abuse she had experienced, her mother's failure to care for Eileen, and the rage she had felt at both parents. However, she also remembered the closeness she had felt to her mother and her father before his death. These strong and conflicted feelings might interfere with Eileen's ability to make a wise and healthy decision. Under stress, Eileen might relapse into feelings of self-hatred as well as dysfunctional behaviors such as misuse of drugs and alcohol and involvement in self-destructive relationships.

      Level of danger: Eileen was not in any physical danger. However, she had to address the crisis quickly because of her mother's tenuous health.

      Efforts to address the crisis: Eileen had not yet taken any steps to address the crisis, other than discussing the situation with her counselor.

      Past coping mechanisms: Until the birth of her son, Eileen coped via escape into drugs and unhealthy relationships. However, with her marriage and the birth of her son, she began to learn improved problem-solving and decision-making skills. She began to confide in other women and to use relaxation strategies. Prayer provided her another way to cope.

   b. *Organization*

      Factors contributing to the difficulty of the crisis: Eileen's conflict with her mother, her troubled and difficult childhood, her current commitment to doing well in college, and her reluctance to leave her son with his father or another caregiver all contributed to the difficulty she had in resolving this crisis.

      Factors that are helping and protecting the client: Eileen's recent realization of the importance to her of family and the mothering role, her acquisition of new coping skills, her spirituality, and her own intelligence were protective factors.

Immediate decision/action: The decisions included whether to visit her mother, whether to reconcile with her, whether to miss one or more college classes, and whether to leave her child with a caregiver.

Alternatives: Eileen could visit her mother or decide not to make that visit. In addition, her visit could take many forms, ranging from a brief casual visit to a lengthy reconciliation.

Resources: Eileen's husband's reassurance that he could take care of their son for a few days, the financial resources to allow her to visit her mother, a friend in class who could take notes for her, and a good relationship with her course instructor all constituted accessible resources.

Coping strategies likely to work in this situation: Potentially effective coping strategies included sound decision-making, information gathering, awareness of feelings, behavioral rehearsal, and identification and modification of cognitive distortions.

c. *Analysis/Synthesis*

Immediate effect of the crisis: Initially, Eileen felt overwhelmed by unhappy memories of her background and of the unanticipated pressure on her to reconcile with her mother.

Underlying significance of the crisis for the person: This experience called into question Eileen's feelings about her family of origin. She had distanced herself from her mother in anger and, although the two had resumed contact, Eileen had not planned on reconciliation yet. However, she now thought that this might be her last chance to reconnect with her mother before her death. Eileen's ambivalence about visiting her mother led her to view herself as a "bad and unloving person" and contributed to her already low self-esteem.

Implications of the crisis for the person's life: Eileen would have to make practical arrangements for her son and for obtaining notes from her class. Far more important was her recognition that if she reconciled with her mother and her mother survived her heart attack, this would affect Eileen's current family life. She wasn't sure whether she wanted to make space in her current life for her family of origin or whether she wanted her son to have contact with his grandmother.

Links between the current crisis and prior history: Since her marriage, Eileen had tried to shut out the pain of the years between the death of her father and the birth of her son. However, the call from her brother brought back to her all the difficulties of those years and the guilt and anger she felt.

Options available for dealing with the crisis: Eileen could refuse to see her mother at this time, perhaps precluding any opportunity for reconciliation. On the other hand, she could visit her mother. How much time she spent with her mother and how she interacted with her mother were unanswered questions that depended on both Eileen's and her mother's choices.

Coping skills available to the person: Although she tended to devalue her coping skills, Eileen had both internal and external resources. Her husband was supportive of whatever decision she made about visiting her mother, the presence of her son reminded her of the importance of family, and her contacts at school could help her avoid missing too much in her class. She was motivated to take care of herself for the sake of her son and had begun to develop improved self-esteem and problem-solving skills. Her faith had helped her through many difficult situations.

Ways to enable Eileen to make necessary decisions: Because of the urgency of this decision, short-term counseling, focused on the benefits and drawbacks of visiting her mother, seems most likely to help Eileen. In addition, reminding her of the strengths she has demonstrated, especially in recent years, could motivate Eileen to deal effectively with her current crisis.

d. *Interpretation:*   Many factors made handling this crisis particularly difficult for Eileen, including the potential urgency of the situation, her mother's neglectful behavior after the death of Eileen's father, Eileen's mistreatment by people she hod trusted, the unhealthy ways in which she had coped with the difficulties in her family of origin, her cutoff from that family, her strong commitment to her son and her education, and the value she placed on her current family. In addition, Eileen, now a mother herself, identified with her mother and recognized how painful it must be to cope with a life-threatening illness without the support of one of your children. Part of her believed that the right thing to do would be to visit her mother and attempt reconciliation. At the same time, Eileen feared that if she returned to her hometown, the pain and problems of her adolescence would overwhelm her once again and she would not be able to move forward with her life.

e. *Application (Interventions):*   Now that Eileen's inability to make a decision has been explored and understood, her clinician can identify interventions that are likely to help her move forward. The following are some that will probably be helpful.

Background

- Help Eileen recognize and understand the effect of the past on her reactions to this current crisis.
- Enable her to see that she has learned and grown from her past experiences and that she is able to make more mature choices now.
- Help her to develop a more balanced and sympathetic picture of her mother, encompassing both her strengths and her weaknesses.
- Facilitate Eileen's efforts to develop a list of the coping skills that she has used and can use successfully.

Emotions

- Help Eileen vent her fears and anxieties and learn ways to reduce and modify her strong emotions.
- Normalize Eileen's upset about this situation but help her see that the intensity of her emotions is getting in the way of her making a sound decision.

- Encourage Eileen to use prayer and her faith to counteract her hopelessness and help her find the best decision.
- Help her use her love for and dedication to her son to enable her to develop some empathy for her mother and perhaps even to forgive her.
- Enable Eileen to value her own needs and to care for herself as well.

Thoughts

- Help Eileen clearly identify her options for dealing with the current situation and then explore and evaluate each one to facilitate decision-making.
- Explore Eileen's cognitions regarding herself and her fear of falling back into her former self-destructive patterns; identify, dispute, and modify any distorted cognitions.
- Use meditation and imagery to enhance Eileen's efforts to make decisions.

Actions

- Encourage Eileen to find solutions to the practical problems presented by this situation, including child care and obtaining the notes for any missed classes.
- Teach Eileen communication skills that she might use with her mother and role-play her anticipated interactions with her mother.
- Encourage Eileen to use relaxation, affirmations, and thought stopping to help her cope more effectively with her current crisis.

f. *Evaluation:* Treatment should continue, either after Eileen visits her mother or while she comes to terms with her decision not to visit her mother. Eileen needs to deal with the long-term implications of her decision for herself and her current family, with the resurfacing of painful and guilt-ridden memories of her past, and with her doubts about herself as a daughter and a mother. Coping with this situation and getting her life back on track can be an experience that further empowers Eileen. It can help her clarify her priorities, improve her relationships, and value herself even more.

UNDERSTANDING AND ADDRESSING CLIENT RAGE, ANGER, AND VIOLENT IMPULSES

Anger is a universal emotion and can provide useful information and energy when it is understood and managed. On the other hand, clients with anger that is explosive, destructive to relationships, and even dangerous can present a challenge for clinicians. Anger can cause people both interpersonal and legal problems, particularly when it leads to violence. Anger directed toward the clinician also can elicit strong negative reactions; clinicians may respond to the anger with fear, discouragement, and reciprocal anger. Such responses on the part of a clinician can undermine the therapeutic relationship, reduce treatment effectiveness, and exacerbate rather than alleviate the client's anger and other difficulties. Clinicians need to identify the early signs of clients' anger; help them recognize, curtail, and modify their strong negative emotions; and channel them in positive directions.

Modified Bloom's Taxonomy Applied to Anger

The modified version of Bloom's taxonomy is used here to illustrate ways to help people learn anger management. This section presents both general information about the treatment of anger and the example of Henry, a 54-year-old Caucasian man who expresses his anger in harmful ways.

1. *Content:* Anger manifests itself in a wide variety of ways under a broad range of conditions. Anger may be a pervasive and enduring aspect of a person's personality, or it may flare up only in transient and stressful situations. The diverse ways in which anger is expressed can complicate diagnosis and treatment. As Tavris (1989) pointed out, "There are different angers, involving different processes and having different consequences to our mental and physical health. No single remedy fits all" (p. 22). Anger is not a mental disorder in itself but can be a symptom of many disorders (Deffenbacher & McKay, 2000). Identifying the components of an anger reaction is a good way to gather information about the manifestation of a specific person's anger.

Physiological

- *Identify the client's characteristic pattern of anger arousal.* Anger activates the sympathetic nervous system and releases epinephrine and norepinephrine into the bloodstream, producing a variety of physiological changes and sensations. Primary changes include accelerated heart rate, elevated blood pressure, increased blood sugar in the muscles, pupil dilation, changes in bodily functions such as digestion, blocking of physical pain, an urge to scream, and a rush of energy through the entire body. According to Stosny (1995), "Anger is the only emotion that activates every organ and muscle group of the body" (p. 56). Clinicians need information about what the client experiences when anger begins and what signals indicate that the anger is rising into out-of-control rage.

  Henry initially was unaware of any physical cues connected to his anger. However, after paying attention to his bodily sensations, he described a feeling of a rotating ball in the pit of his stomach as the first internal signal that something was distressing him. Next, he typically experienced tension in his forehead, an increase in his heart rate, and an urge to yell, which led to outbursts of rage he later regretted.

- *Determine whether any organic or physiological factor is creating or fueling the anger.* Although it has physiological manifestations, anger is not usually generated by a biological condition. However, some conditions, such as brain injury and epilepsy, have been connected to anger. Ascertain whether the client has experienced head trauma, hormonal fluctuations, or other medical conditions that might be generating or compounding factors.

- *Determine level of substance use.* Alcohol and other substances, notably stimulants, can worsen anger problems. Assess the client's level of substance use and identify any connection between substance use and angry outbursts.

Emotional

- *Assess the client's patterns of emotional experience.* "All emotions, including anger, have what amount to goals that [people] press hard to achieve" (Fein, 1993, p. 18). Understanding the goals of a person's anger can deepen understanding of that emotion. This can be accomplished by obtaining a clear picture of the client's experience of anger, including the timing, nature, frequency, duration, and intensity of that emotion.

  Henry's anger became most intense when his child or wife did not comply with his wishes. At the start of treatment, his anger toward his wife was almost constant, an ever-present rumble that periodically erupted. His anger toward his son, while similarly intense, was interspersed with warm feelings, usually when Henry was not in Johnny's presence.

- *Identify the problem signaled or suppressed by the emotional response.* Anger often reflects issues related to one's sense of self and one's personal boundaries. It can express frustration connected to these concerns and cover emotions that are more difficult to acknowledge and express such as shame, loneliness, sadness, and grief. Stosny (1995) described anger as "ice on a wound" (p. 59). Like ice, anger may numb pain temporarily, but eventually it becomes a source of pain itself. In identifying the problem signaled or covered by the anger, the clinician needs to pay attention to the client's sense of self and to the client's relationships with others.

  Henry's anger was a reaction to his perception of himself as unlovable and powerless. His anger gave him a false sense of control. It protected him from experiencing the pain connected to his longing for power, closeness, and acceptance and the hopelessness he felt about ever achieving what he wanted in his relationships.

- *Determine the level of motivation for change.* People present for treatment at various stages of readiness to work on an issue (more on this later in the chapter). DiGiuseppe (1996) found that many people with anger problems focus on changing others and have little motivation to change themselves.

  When Henry initiated treatment, he was not motivated to change his anger toward his wife. He believed that curtailing his anger toward her would condone and encourage what he perceived as her unacceptable behavior. However, he was distressed at seeing his son copying Henry and becoming enraged with his friends. Henry's recognition of the harm he was doing to his son was a strong motivator for him.

Cognitive

- *Identify the thought patterns underlying the client's anger.* Anger typically arises in response to how one interprets or thinks about an event. Usually, anger begins with a perception of pain or injury and a feeling of distress. Another person or group is often seen as the cause of the pain, and that becomes the target for the anger.

For example, Henry reported that his days frequently got off to a bad start because his eight-year-old son Johnny was disorganized and was rarely ready for school on time. This led Henry to become anxious and upset and to scold Johnny for his lateness. Even after he dropped Johnny off at school, Henry ruminated on the boy's actions and saw his son as having ruined Henry's day.

Anger is particularly likely to escalate when blame is combined with the perception that another person is acting out of malice or a deliberate intention to inflict pain, thereby prompting strong feelings of injustice (Beck, 1999). Henry fueled his anger by seeing Johnny as a "spoiled brat" who delighted in frustrating and irritating his father.

Behavioral

- *Determine the functions that anger serves.* The behavior of becoming angry attracts attention and changes people's interactions with others. According to Potter-Efron and Potter-Efron (1991), anger can provide communication, power and control, intimacy regulation (managing both distance and connection), status, self-defense, and problem solving.

  Henry's anger was a form of communication. It also served as a way of exerting power and control while regulating the intimacy between his wife and himself.

- *Determine the reinforcers.* Anger can have immediate payoffs. For example, Henry was able to remain in his marriage and maintain the illusion that he had power and control without having to risk emotional closeness with his wife. He was also able to coerce his son into complying with his commands.

- *Determine the costs.* Despite the short-term gains it may produce, anger can have a long-term negative effect on all areas of a person's life, including physical health, emotional well-being, relationships, occupational and economic success, and legal status. Henry had become aware of the negative effects of his anger on his son and their relationship.

Environmental/contextual

- *Review the client's history of experiencing and expressing anger in the family and community.* According to Beck (1999), "People continuously monitor and mimic one another's emotional reactions without realizing they are doing so" (p. 147). Many families experience multigenerational patterns of destructive anger.

2. *Process:* Once the clinician gathers information about a person's anger, that information can be processed as follows, continuing to use the example of Henry and the structure of the modified version of Bloom's taxonomy.

   a. *Comprehension/Organization:* The following questions can guide the organization of information on a person's anger.

Emotional

- What are the warning signs of anger for this client? What is the client's level of awareness of these signs?
- How does anger accelerate for this client? What successful and unsuccessful strategies has this person used to interrupt the anger arousal?
- What emotional needs underlie the anger? What boundary issues are involved in the anger? What emotional strengths does the person demonstrate?

Cognitive

- What thoughts and underlying beliefs fuel the anger? What level of insight does the client have into how thoughts affect the problem?
- What responsibility does this person accept for the problem?

Behavioral

- How does this person express and respond to anger?
- What is this person trying to accomplish through his or her expression of anger? Are there any rewards or beneficial effects of the anger? If so, what are they?
- What problems is the anger causing or aggravating? What potential exists for self-harm or harm to others? Is the anger related to substance use?
- How ready is the person to change?

Environmental/Contextual

- What experiences, especially in the family of origin, have shaped this person's understanding and use of anger?
- What environmental or contextual factors contribute to maintaining or inhibiting the person's anger?
- What positive experiences or models are available for learning new responses?

b. *Analysis/Synthesis:* After obtaining and organizing information on a person's anger, clinicians can develop an understanding of the client's anger-related concerns and how they fit into an overall picture of the person. Answering the following questions will facilitate development of a successful treatment approach for a client who has difficulty with anger management.

- *What is the pattern of anger escalation, and how clear is the person about the signs of initial and rising anger?* In other words, does this person go from 0 to 100 miles per hour in a second, or does the client experience a slow, prolonged buildup of anger, accompanied by rumination?
- *What self-perceptions contribute to the anger?* Understanding whether clients see themselves as wounded or inadequate helps clinicians to understand the clients' emotional pain and where healing needs to occur.

- *What cognitive strategies and perspectives does this person employ?* Perfectionism and demandingness often fuel anger. Many angry people rely on long lists of "shoulds" to direct their own behavior and judge others' behaviors. They often have conditional beliefs such as, "If he loved me, he would never disappoint me," or "If I were a responsible individual, I wouldn't have made that mistake" (Ellis, 1977).

- *What background and family-of-origin issues contribute to this person's current anger problem?* Consider the models and messages the client received about anger and how that person learned how to express and manage anger. Also, consider the effect of early experiences in shaping the client's self-image, understanding of relationships, and beliefs about anger. For example, if a client had a violent parent, does the client view the parent as admirable, or is the client determined not to be like the angry parent? Has the client accepted the parent's criticisms as valid, or has the person been able to create a more positive and valid self-image?

- *Does this client recognize the negative effects of the anger?* Often, what a person strives to achieve with anger becomes even more elusive, thus generating further anger unless the cycle can be clarified and interrupted. Awareness of the negative consequences of anger can increase motivation to change.

- *What are the person's overall levels of self-awareness and life skills?* When skill deficits contribute to the problem, appropriate training, such as in communication skills or parenting, can reduce anger.

- *What is motivating the client to change, and how can that motivation and interest in treatment be encouraged?*

- *Is the anger a deviation from the person's usual way of operating, or is the anger reflective of long-standing patterns of thoughts and actions?* If the anger reflects a change, understanding and addressing what led to this shift is essential. If, however, the anger is a long-standing pattern, a more comprehensive approach to treatment is probably indicated.

- *What risks to self or others are presented by the anger?* Does the clinician need to warn others of potential danger? Does the client's danger to the self need to be addressed immediately?

   c. *Interpretation:* Now that the clinician has developed a deep understanding of the anger and its connection to the person's view of self, others, and the world, the clinician can understand the meaning the anger has for the person.

Henry was an intelligent, self-employed, though unsuccessful, photographer, who had a long history of anger, anxiety, and depression. He described his father as an "angry alcoholic" and a "bully." Henry's mother was usually withdrawn and depressed but occasionally would rage at Henry and his three younger siblings. Henry reported that he was anxious and angry as a child and was a bully himself. He played contact sports and enjoyed the aggressive interactions. As a young adult, Henry abused drugs and alcohol. He described his wife as depressed and emotionally unavailable and reported that his son Johnny exhibited depression and periodic temper outbursts.

By bullying people, both as a child and as an adult, Henry experienced a sense of potency that helped him feel good about himself and see himself as better than others. This viewpoint led him to believe that others should welcome his direction and appreciate his great strengths and ideas. When others did not value and accept his frequent criticisms and reprimands, Henry became enraged and contemptuous.

At a deeper level, Henry's anger reflected his underlying self-doubts and his ambivalence about relationships. Henry craved the closeness denied him in childhood but also feared that closeness might allow others to see through his façade and recognize and confirm his negative view of himself. Henry's anger reflected this ambivalence, as did the emotional and physical cutoff that usually followed his angry outbursts. On the surface, Henry believed his behaviors would impress people, but, in reality, he was pushing them away and creating a wall around himself.

Because he was repeating long-standing multigenerational patterns of behavior and relationships, Henry did not recognize that his anger led others to engage in the very behaviors that were most frustrating to him: his wife's emotional withdrawal and his son's stubbornness. Henry lacked knowledge of healthy parenting and relationship strategies. However, his love and concern for his family provided the motivation for him to continue in treatment.

    d. *Application:* The following offers an array of treatment options.

Physiological

- Recommend referral for medication, physical examination, and substance use evaluation.

Emotional

- Empathy and respect can prevent an angry client from becoming entrenched in a hostile and defensive position.
- Provide self-esteem training. Helping people identify and value their strengths can counteract their resentment and jealousy of others.
- Provide compassion training. Stosny (1995) identified compassion as "an emotional regulator incompatible with contempt and anger" (p. 10). Learning to have compassion for others as well as for oneself can contribute to anger reduction.
- Teach emotional self-regulation. This can slow down the progression of anger and facilitate use of anger-management strategies.
- Enhance motivation to change, especially by building a positive therapeutic alliance with shared and meaningful goals.

Cognitive

- Keeping a journal of angry thoughts and events or a mood diary provides a basis for identifying and modifying cognitive distortions and monitoring progress.

- Use imagery in the session so that the client can reexperience a recent anger-provoking incident. This can provide access to cognitions as well as to physical signs of anger.
- Cognitive therapy is one of the most effective approaches for helping people identify and challenge the distorted thinking that underlies counterproductive anger. This also can help reduce any accompanying depression.
- Some people benefit from reading relevant self-help books such as *The Dance of Anger* (Lerner, 1985), *The Feeling Good Handbook* (Burns, 2007), *Angry All the Time* (Potter-Efron, 1994), and *Anger Kills* (Williams & Williams, 1993).
- Offer stress or anger inoculation training. Develop a hierarchy of anger-evoking situations and use cognitive skills to help the client become more tolerant of frustration and learn to formulate and use new and more effective responses. Practice these in treatment sessions.
- Help the client recognize the costs of anger and how it detracts from goal achievement.
- Model and teach effective problem solving so that the person does not need to use anger to gain power and control and can successfully resolve interpersonal and other problems.

Behavioral

- Incorporate training in assertiveness, communication, and parenting into treatment.
- Introduce behavioral experiments. Encouraging a client to try out a new and effective response can change perspectives and lead to new behaviors.
- Teach recognition of signs of rising anger. Potter-Efron (1994) suggests an anger thermometer as a metaphor for levels of anger.
- Teach relaxation strategies, such as progressive relaxation, imagery, meditation, and simple diaphragmatic breathing to interrupt rising anger.
- Teach the client to call a time-out when anger rises into the danger zone, doing so in a way that does not seem like abandonment of another person.
- Teach stress management. Anger and rumination accelerate under high stress. Living a balanced life with minimal stress and ample support facilitates anger management.
- Encourage regular exercise to promote stress management and alleviate any symptoms of depression related to anger.

Environmental/Contextual

- Enable the client to build healthy relationships and support systems.
- Consider referrals to relevant resources, such as Alcoholics Anonymous or other self-help and support groups.

e. *Evaluation:* Continued monitoring of progress and reevaluation of the treatment plan is necessary in helping people with anger-related concerns.

Relapse is common, and additional strategies may be needed to help people cope with backsliding. Continued follow-up helped ensure that Henry maintained the gains he had accomplished through treatment.

Example: Henry's Treatment

Determining which interventions to use depends on the individual client and the nature of that person's difficulty with anger. Because Henry's concerns dated back to his childhood and his family relationships and were a pervasive and enduring issue for him, his treatment was lengthy and involved interventions from most of the previous categories. The following outlines the interventions used with Henry:

Physiological

- Henry was referred for antidepressant medication, a physical examination, and substance use evaluation.

Emotional

- The clinician's empathy enhanced the therapeutic alliance, thereby increasing Henry's motivation to change. Seeing the benefits of empathy helped Henry develop and demonstrate more empathy for others.
- Self-esteem training was woven into the course of treatment, and Henry gradually became aware of his many strengths.
- Compassion training helped Henry to talk about his injuries from a vulnerable, rather than a morally righteous, viewpoint and to develop more compassion toward others.
- Emotional self-regulation was integrated into the entire treatment process.
- The development of the therapeutic alliance enhanced his motivation to make positive changes, as did an emphasis on how Henry's improved anger management might benefit his son.

Cognitive

- Henry wrote about his anger when it flared up.
- Henry became more successful in applying problem-solving strategies to issues in his life; this led to a sense of mastery and improved self-esteem.
- Henry responded well to learning problem-solving strategies, because he prided himself on his intelligence and clear thinking.
- Via cognitive therapy, Henry slowly learned to change his counterproductive thinking, which in turn led to an improvement in his mood.
- Teaching him to recognize signs of rising anger proved helpful.

Behavioral

- Assertiveness and communication training helped Henry become less aggressive and more able to find a middle ground in his interactions with others.
- Henry learned new ways of parenting, such as the use of natural and logical consequences.

- Henry did behavioral experiments in his interactions with his wife. He was surprised by the outcome of these experiments, which increased both his wife's responsiveness and his own warm feelings toward her.
- Imagery helped Henry become more aware of his thoughts and his physical experience of anger.
- Henry learned to use relaxation strategies, especially diaphragmatic breathing.
- Initially, Henry used angry withdrawal, but he was able to replace this behavior with constructive use of time-outs.
- Henry reduced the stress in his life in order to achieve greater balance.
- Henry started walking his dog daily.
- Henry put significant effort into stress inoculation training, creating and practicing new responses to provocations.

Environmental/Contextual

- Working with Henry to build healthy relationships and support systems was a central focus of treatment.
- Increasing the structure and consistency in his environment helped Henry to feel calmer and more in control of his life.

Henry and his clinician noted reductions in frequency, duration, and intensity of Henry's anger, both with his son and his wife. When Henry reported that his new, calmer responses were becoming automatic, a major part of his goals had been accomplished.

Henry's therapist made sure she had supervision and peer consultation to help her manage any negative feelings that she might develop toward Henry and to deal with times when his anger was directed at her. Henry eventually became able to express negative feelings toward his therapist in direct and calm ways; his success in that area was another sign of progress.

Thus far in this chapter, we have reviewed conceptual approaches to dealing with three strong emotions: suicidal ideation, distress in response to a crisis, and harmful anger. These conceptual models and illustrations can enhance clinicians' effectiveness in helping people deal with almost any harmful emotion.

VARIATIONS IN CLIENT READINESS FOR TREATMENT

Among the most difficult emotions for clinicians to address in treatment are clients' negative reactions to the treatment process itself. People may have little interest in changing, they may not recognize a need for change, they may resent those who suggested or required that they seek help, and they may be fearful of sharing and addressing aspects of themselves that they find shameful or fragile. This part of the chapter focuses on dealing with variations in client readiness for treatment and on clients who are reluctant to engage productively in treatment. We begin by looking at a model for assessing people's readiness for change and for matching treatment strategies to their level of readiness.

In many settings, a substantial percentage of clients are not initially eager for assistance. This is particularly likely in correctional settings, substance use treatment programs, and inpatient treatment programs. People who have been court-referred or strongly encouraged to seek help by a dissatisfied supervisor, a concerned teacher, or an unhappy family member also often are reluctant clients. Even among people who seek counseling or psychotherapy voluntarily, some will have little understanding of the treatment process and no interest in personal change.

Of course, clinicians do encounter many motivated and enthusiastic clients in all treatment settings. These people recognize that they have difficulties, take some responsibility for their problems, believe they would benefit from help in making changes, and are willing, at least initially, to engage in treatment.

Clearly, clinicians should not treat both groups of people in identical ways. Rather, social workers, counselors, and psychologists are more likely to succeed in developing a collaborative treatment alliance, establishing mutually agreed on goals, and getting the treatment process off to a positive start if they can meet clients where they are and build rapport and involvement in treatment. Assessing a person's stage of readiness for treatment and matching intervention strategies to that stage is essential to effective treatment (Miller & Rollnick, 1991).

Assessment of Readiness for Change

An array of factors should be considered when assessing a person's readiness for change via counseling or psychotherapy. These include:

- The referral source (self or other).
- The presenting concerns (symptoms and precipitants).
- The multiaxial assessment according to the *Diagnostic and Statistical Manual of Mental Disorders* (*DSM-IV-TR*, American Psychiatric Association, 2000).
- The severity of the symptoms and their effect on the person's life.
- The person's expressed level of distress and motivation to change.
- The person's support systems and lifestyle.
- Current stressors and crises in the person's life.
- The person's strengths and coping skills.
- The person's level of insight, self-awareness, and empathy.

In general, people with a high level of readiness for change are those who are self-referred, have an identifiable cause or precipitant for their difficulties, a mild to moderately severe emotional disorder that is affecting their personal and professional functioning, and strengths that include a capacity for insight, self-awareness, and empathy. On the other hand, people who are mandated or pressured into seeking treatment, who have long-standing difficulties with no apparent precipitant or stressor, whose lifestyle is unstable and very stressful, who have either very mild or very severe difficulties, and who have little capacity for insight into themselves or others are far more likely to have a low level of readiness for change.

Stages of Change Model

Prochaska and Norcross (1999) delineated six levels of readiness for change in a model known as the *stages of change model* (SOC) or the *transtheoretical model of change* (TTM). They described the following six levels of readiness for change and suggested accompanying interventions that are likely to be successful.

1. *Precontemplation:* People in this stage do not recognize a need for change and consequently have no intention of making changes in their emotions, thoughts, or actions in the foreseeable future. They will probably be reluctant to disclose personal information about themselves and are unlikely to engage in realistic goal setting.

Strategies: Clients must recognize their need for change before they can be engaged in the treatment process. Strategies should focus on raising doubts about the effectiveness of their current behaviors. Looking at the results of their choices and whether their actions are meeting their needs is a good place to begin discussion.

2. *Contemplation:* People in this stage recognize that they have some difficulties, and they have some preliminary awareness of their need for personal change. However, they have not yet decided whether to invest themselves in the process of changing. They may be dubious about their ability to change successfully, they may not know effective ways to make changes, or they may not even be aware of alternatives to their current emotions, thoughts, and actions.

Strategies: As with people in the precontemplation stage of change, clinicians can promote motivation by helping clients see the drawbacks and risks of continuing their current behaviors and choices. In addition, helping people become more hopeful about the prospects of change also can facilitate progress. Clinicians can accomplish this by making people aware of the availability of effective procedures for change, strengthening their optimism and confidence in their ability to make positive changes, and educating them about better choices they might make.

3. *Preparation:* People in this stage of change not only recognize the importance of making some changes in their lives, they are even planning on making some changes within the next month. They may not know exactly how or what they want to change, but they are ready to move forward.

Strategies: Clinicians can build on the commitment these people have already made to change. Helping them to develop specific, achievable, and meaningful goals; identifying the best routes to change; and formulating an action plan, including a timeline and initial steps toward successful change, can propel these clients forward in their efforts to change.

4. *Action:* People in this stage are ready to make some positive changes; in fact, they have already taken steps to change their environment, emotions,

thoughts, or actions. However, they are still struggling to find the most effective ways to change. They may have established unrealistic goals, may not know how to tackle even sound goals, or may expect too much of themselves.

Strategies: Congratulating people in this stage for moving forward and helping them develop positive feelings about their progress can solidify the gains they have already made. Additional strategies that build on those gains include: developing realistic and meaningful goals; breaking down goals into manageable pieces; identifying steps toward change that are small, specific, and achievable; teaching coping, communication, and other relevant skills; and giving a logical sequence to clients' steps toward change. Encouraging continued progress via rewards, reinforcements, and other methods can prevent loss of momentum and backsliding.

5. *Maintenance:* In this stage, people have already made many positive changes and have achieved most or all of their objectives. They have developed a repertoire of new emotions, thoughts, and actions that are healthy and growth-promoting. They see gratifying changes in their lifestyles. However, relapse continues to be a risk, and signs of relapse may even be present.

Strategies: Solidifying gains is the most important process in this stage. People may lack confidence that they can persist in the changes they have made, may not yet have encountered challenges to their newfound successes, or may have difficulty coping with the challenges they have encountered. Identifying and addressing risk factors, alerting people to the signs of relapse, and helping them develop the coping skills they need to ward off threats to progress can strengthen their resolve and ability to maintain positive change and give them confidence that they can stay on track. Developing both intrinsic and extrinsic sources of support and motivation can further enhance the likelihood that gains will be maintained.

6. *Termination:* In this final stage, people have satisfactorily attained their goals, made positive changes, and learned new attitudes and skills that can maintain and perhaps even build on progress already made. Clients in this stage typically are confident that they can cope more effectively with life's challenges and know how to find help if they feel overwhelmed or begin to revert to their former unhealthy behaviors and attitudes. Treatment is a success for both client and clinician.

Strategies: More will be said about the termination process later in this book (see Chapter 9). In general, treatment for people in this last stage of change emphasizes identification, consolidation, and reinforcement of gains. In addition, clients and clinicians may look to the future to help clients establish goals they are now likely to achieve on their own, using the knowledge and skills they have acquired through their treatment.

Of course, treatment does not always have such a positive ending. Miller and Rollnick (1991), applying the stages of change model to people with addictive behaviors, suggested that the final stage is sometimes *relapse* rather than termination. If that is the case, helpful strategies include strengthening clients' motivation, reinforcing their ability to change, helping them to reinstitute the successful coping skills they learned, and bolstering their morale.

Example: Matching Treatment to Stage of Change

The following three clients represent three different levels in the stages of change model. Notice how the planned interventions address the stage each is in when he or she seeks treatment. The Learning Opportunities at the end of this chapter provide you the opportunity to identify the appropriate stage of change for several clients and suggest interventions that match their level of readiness for treatment.

Client 1   Lita was court-mandated to a treatment program to provide help with anger management because she frequently engaged in explosive and aggressive behavior. One night, when her partner returned home later than promised, Lita pelted her with dishes and shoes. A neighbor called the police, who took Lita into custody. She explained her behavior by stating that she believed her partner had been with her former girlfriend. Lita viewed her behavior as justified in light of her suspicions and her partner's late arrival. Lita is in the *precontemplation* stage of change.

Strategies: Lita's therapist encouraged her to examine her long history of explosive behavior, along with the consequences of that behavior, to determine whether her behavior was meeting her needs. Her actions had cost her several important relationships, she had been beaten on more than one occasion when someone retaliated, and she was now threatened with imprisonment.

Client 2   Roberto, age 9, had been diagnosed with mild mental retardation and an attention-deficit/hyperactivity disorder. Since he began school, he had had noticeable difficulty paying attention, often interrupted his classmates to blurt out answers, and broke or lost items of importance. Although he was in a program to address his special needs, Roberto did poorly in school and had difficulty forming friendships. He recognized that he needed to make some changes and, with the help of his parents and teachers, had developed a list of changes he needed to make. However, Roberto felt overwhelmed by the long list and was discouraged by the process of change. Roberto is in the *preparation* stage of change.

Strategies: Roberto and his counselor reviewed the list of desired changes, shortened the list, and identified the two most important goals: completing his homework and waiting to be called on before speaking up in class. They then agreed on two small steps Roberto could take with the help of his family and teachers to initiate the change process. These steps, which included checking with his teacher at the end of each day to ensure that he had written down his assignments correctly and drawing a hand on the outside of his notebook to remind him to raise his hand when he had something to say in class, were specific, meaningful, and readily attainable.

Client 3   Khorn, a Cambodian woman who had immigrated to the United States, had worked hard in treatment to deal with the terrible experiences she had in her native land and to adjust to life in the United States. She was much less anxious, was sleeping better, had found employment, and had begun to form some friendships outside her immediate family. However, her difficult background and the enormous changes she had experienced left her feeling uncertain that she would be able to maintain her gains. Khorn was in the *maintenance* stage of change.

Strategies: Khorn's social worker helped her to identify support groups and community resources that would promote Khorn's efforts to maintain her gains. In addition, her therapist worked with Khorn to list her gains and coping skills. They discussed hypothetical situations that might cause her to resume her unhealthy thoughts and behaviors and identified ways she might cope successfully with those challenges. In addition, her therapist helped her identify warning signs of relapse, along with ways she might seek help to prevent a full relapse. This process was done in a way that would further empower Khorn, reinforce the many gains she had made, and consolidate them to make them readily accessible to her.

CLIENT RELUCTANCE

Despite the use of helpful and appropriate strategies to foster clients' involvement in treatment, people are not always willing or able to participate fully in the treatment process. Their reluctance to talk openly about themselves and take constructive steps to resolve their concerns can impede the therapeutic process and prove frustrating and discouraging to clinicians. This dynamic has been known by many terms over the years, including *defensiveness, resistance, reluctance, reactance,* and *noncompliance.* These clients might also be viewed as people in the *precontemplation stage.* Some clinicians perceive these clients as difficult, oppositional, unmotivated, or challenging. I will use the term *reluctance* because it is a relatively neutral term and does not imply criticism of clients for having difficulty engaging in treatment.

Clinicians identified client reluctance and its potentially negative effects on the treatment process more than 100 years ago. Freud wrote about resistance, manifested by the client's opposition to bringing unconscious material into awareness, and believed it reflected "the client's innate protection against emotional pain" (Cowan & Presbury, 2000, p. 411). Reluctance also has been viewed as reflecting a negative transference to the clinician, stemming from impairment in early childhood attachment to caregivers. For many years, client reluctance has been seen as undesirable.

However, attitudes toward this process and even the terminology used to describe it have changed considerably over the years. Today, reluctance is viewed as a common and understandable aspect of treatment. Although most clinicians probably still wish they did not need to contend with client reluctance, they seem to have more empathy for this reaction and also to take more responsibility for helping people get past their reluctance and engage productively in the treatment process.

Reluctance is particularly prevalent in people who are involuntary clients or those who are in treatment primarily to please someone else. Reluctance is also common in people who are mistrustful, shy and fearful, or dubious about the value of treatment. Reluctance is common and understandable, too, in people whose cultural backgrounds do not encourage counseling and psychotherapy and who believe they have little in common with their clinicians. Strong reluctance also can be found in people who are invested in proving that someone else is to blame for their problems, in demonstrating that they are incorrigible, in defeating the clinician, or in proving others wrong.

Conceptualizing Reluctance

In teaching both novice and experienced clinicians to understand and cope with reluctance in clients, I encourage them to take an optimistic but realistic attitude. Assume that all people have strengths they can use to help themselves, want to feel better, and desire more rewarding lives, but they have not yet found a way to make needed changes. Of course, clinicians are not successful in helping and joining with all of their clients, but taking an optimistic but realistic stance seems most likely to motivate clients to engage productively in treatment. Looking at reluctance through the lens of the modified version of Bloom's taxonomy can promote understanding of effective ways to work with reluctant clients.

Conceptual Analysis of a Reluctant Client

The treatment of Delaney, a 14-year-old Japanese American, female, illustrates the application of the taxonomy to client reluctance. Delaney had been referred for counseling because of her declining grades and withdrawn behavior. She was the youngest of three children born to a Japanese mother and an American father who met while the father was working in Japan. Delaney and her two brothers were born in Japan but moved to the United States when Delaney was 7. Delaney's father was emotionally and physically abusive toward her mother and frequently behaved in an inappropriately sexual way toward Delaney. On several occasions, Delaney had observed her mother talking to a man Delaney did not know and acting in secretive ways.

Delaney's reluctance is processed in the following example, according to an abbreviated version of Bloom's taxonomy. Understanding a person's reluctance to engage in treatment and make personal changes typically leads to identification of successful ways to address the reluctance.

Content   Reluctance is the process of acting in ways that seem to obstruct the progress of treatment. Reluctance can take many forms. The following are some of the most common.

Violating Rules

- Arriving late for sessions or failing to attend scheduled sessions
- Failing to pay for treatment in a timely way
- Not completing agreed-on tasks and activities
- Making excessive demands on the clinician (e.g., telephone calls, extra time)

Withholding Communication/Restricting Content

- Focusing the session on extraneous material such as the weather, the traffic, humorous anecdotes, the problems of a friend, or anything else not related to the treatment goals
- Talking excessively about facts and ideas
- Avoiding discussion of important experiences, emotions, thoughts, and behaviors
- Overtalking, so that the clinician has little opportunity to intervene; ignoring what the clinician does say
- Evading questions, responding with "I don't know" or "I don't remember" to the clinician's questions
- Dwelling on past concerns and avoiding discussion of the present as well as exploration of the relationship of past to present concerns
- Talking about the same topics or issues again and again, without attempting to make any changes
- Silence or withdrawal
- Asking many questions that are not germane to the treatment process

Hostility and Manipulation

- Verbal attacks or constant criticisms of the clinician and the treatment process
- Discounting the value of whatever the clinician says or suggests
- Seductive behavior toward the clinician
- Being angry, belligerent, argumentative, or defiant
- Threatening harm to oneself or another person
- Externalizing blame for one's difficulties

These and many other client behaviors and attitudes can impede the therapeutic process.

Delaney avoided discussing personal information in counseling. When her counselor asked her direct questions, she replied with, "I don't know" or "I don't remember." When she did talk, it was typically about singers or actors she admired. She failed to complete the few simple tasks the counselor had suggested to her and often asked how much longer she had to meet with the counselor.

Process

Comprehension/Organization: Just as all people have defenses, all clients probably have mixed feelings about beginning counseling or psychotherapy. Change is difficult, and even if current ways of coping are ineffective or painful, giving them up for the unknown can be frightening. The question is not whether a client is reluctant about participating in the treatment process but how strong that reluctance is, how it can affect the treatment process, and whether the reluctance is greater than the motivation to make positive changes. Also important is noting times when the reluctance is particularly strong; this is typically a sign that treatment is focusing on important and highly charged issues that need attention. Once clinicians have identified signs of reluctance (listed previously), they can determine whether the client's behavior in treatment is impeding the treatment process. If so, then they probably should address the reluctance.

Understanding the motivation behind the reluctance is important in determining the best way to address it. Following are some common reasons for reluctance.

Negative Thoughts or Feelings about the Clinician and the Treatment Process

- Lack of trust
- Lack of understanding of counseling or psychotherapy
- Belief that the clinician will not understand or accept the client
- A view of treatment as a punishment or source of shame
- Fear of change
- Disinterest in change; comfort with the known and familiar
- Discomfort with self-disclosure and expression of emotion

Feelings and Thoughts about the Self

- Shame or guilt about own behavior or situation
- Wish to gain power or control over another
- Need to assert independence or separateness
- Fear of success
- Need to protect the client's own view of reality
- Need to prove that the client is hopeless and beyond help

Feelings or Thoughts about Others

- Wish to protect another person
- Desire to prove another person wrong by ensuring that treatment is ineffective

Important in understanding a client's reluctance is looking at the clinician's reactions to the client as well as the interactions between the clinician and the client. Reluctance can be challenging and disturbing to hard-working clinicians, who are doing their best to help others. The clinician's feelings of anger and irritation can inadvertently manifest themselves during treatment. The clinician may appear short-tempered or impatient with a client. Empathy may diminish while questions and harsh confrontation increase in an effort to compel the client to change. Needless to say, this will probably exacerbate the client's reluctance and create a vicious cycle in which client reluctance leads the clinician to have negative reactions that, in turn, exacerbate the reluctance. Clinicians need to recognize any ways in which they are contributing to the reluctance and take steps to modify their own behaviors and attitudes.

Delaney's reluctance primarily took the form of withholding communication and restricting content. Her noncompliant behaviors were passive rather than active; she was not hostile or overtly negative. She complied, at least superficially, with the treatment process, but she did not really engage in that process.

Reasons for Delaney's reluctance to engage in treatment included all three areas listed previously:

- **Feelings and Thoughts about Treatment:** Delaney did not believe that counseling could help her. She also mistrusted her clinician and feared that he would not maintain her confidentiality and would tell her parents about the content of her sessions.
- **Feelings and Thoughts about Herself:** Delaney was uncomfortable with self-disclosure and expression of emotion, and she felt threatened and ashamed when encouraged to talk about herself.
- **Feelings and Thoughts about Others:** Delaney believed she was protecting her family by refusing to discuss her parents, their interactions with each other, and their relationships with her. The only comments she made about her family focused on how wonderful her mother was and how entertaining her brothers were.

Analysis/Synthesis: In analyzing and making sense of Delaney's reluctance, the counselor considered a range of factors:

- The nature of Delaney's reluctant behavior (withholding/restricting content):
  - Providing only superficial positive information about her family
  - Avoiding any mention of her father and the interactions within her family
- The probable reasons for her reluctance:
  - Delaney's cultural background which might, at least in part, explain her need for privacy and lead her to withhold information that might reflect badly on her family
  - The great change Delaney experienced when relocating from Japan to the United States, where she felt out of place and different from her peers
  - The decline in Delaney's grades, several years after the family's relocation to the United States, suggesting an additional problem that had developed fairly recently

Interpretation: Interpretation of reluctance is the process of making sense of that behavior, based primarily on clinicians analysis and synthesis of the material they have gathered on the nature and dynamics of the client's reluctance. The basic question to be answered is, "What purpose does the reluctance serve for this person?"

Delaney's self-doubts and feelings of differentness, cultural messages about family honor and privacy, as well as family behaviors she perceived as potentially shameful, seemed to be the primary causes of her reluctance. Multicultural factors certainly played a part in her attitude toward counseling, as did her family's relocation. Her lack of knowledge about counseling and her mistrust of that process were additional factors in her reluctance. In addition, more recent family issues, not yet fully disclosed, also seemed to contribute to Delaney's reluctance. All this information suggested that the motivation behind Delaney's reluctance was protection of herself, as well as her family, from experiencing additional humiliation and pain.

Application: Many strategies have been suggested for addressing and reducing client reluctance. Following are some of the more common ones.

Increasing Client Comfort with the Treatment Process

- Establishing mutually agreed-on goals
- Increasing use of empathy
- Providing information on the nature and purposes of treatment (role induction)
- Using relaxation and other strategies to reduce anxiety
- Giving the client more control over the treatment process
- Enhancing and strengthening the therapeutic alliance
- Focusing on the positive
- Teaching the client useful skills and strategies such as assertiveness and other communication skills
- Finding motivations or incentives for the client to engage productively in treatment

Normalizing the Reluctance

- Helping clients recognize that ambivalence about and discomfort with treatment is common and understandable
- Giving clients permission to talk about their conflicted feelings
- Viewing the reluctance as an important source of information

Using Indirect Treatment Strategies

- Paradoxical intention ("I'd encourage you to sit quietly until words come to you that want to be spoken.")
- Imagery
- Bibliotherapy (e.g., suggesting reading about the value of counseling)
- Doing something unexpected, such as going for a walk or playing a card game with a client during the time of the session
- Modeling appropriate self-disclosure
- Focusing on nonverbal cues
- Suggesting that clients review tapes of sessions
- Using humor
- Using metaphors or reframing ("I can see by your silence that you have a great deal to think about.")
- Becoming more silent
- Piquing client's curiosity, especially about what that person might learn through treatment
- Suggesting that positive change will happen ("When you are ready, you will be able to talk about this more freely.")
- Discussing the benefits of avoiding change

Challenging the Reluctance Directly

- Providing data to substantiate the presence of client reluctance ("Were you aware that you have been late five out of six sessions?")

- Using challenge or confrontation to point out the self-destructive nature of the reluctance ("You say that you want to get along better with people and yet you have not followed through on the between-session social activities you agreed to do. I don't know what to make of that.")
- Setting limits ("I cannot schedule any more sessions until you establish a schedule for paying what you owe for your treatment.")
- Interpreting the reluctance to the client to reduce blocks to progress ("I wonder if your reluctance to talk about your family is a way to protect them.")
- Disputing the client's negative perceptions of treatment ("You tell me that treatment has been a waste of your time. That surprises me since your grades have improved, you have stopped purging, and you have made a new friend.")
- Raising client anxiety and awareness of the need to make changes

Many types of helpful interventions are available to clinicians who are trying to reduce client reluctance. However, clinicians should generally guard against using the following potentially harmful interventions:

Unhelpful Interventions

- Letting reluctance go on and on without addressing it
- Personalizing the reluctance ("I want you to stop harassing me with your constant telephone calls.")
- Engaging in a power struggle with the client
- Allowing oneself to be abused or manipulated by a client
- Blaming and attacking the client
- Giving the client full control of the treatment process
- Greatly reducing expectations of what can be accomplished by the treatment process
- Quickly referring the client to another clinician or terminating the treatment process

In light of the analysis and interpretation of Delaney's reluctance, directly challenging the reluctance seemed to be the least desirable approach. This intervention probably would increase her mistrust, fear, and sense of shame; exacerbate her already low self-esteem; and make her even more reluctant to engage in treatment.

Normalizing the reluctance and using indirect treatment strategies might be helpful after Delaney had developed some trust in the clinician and in the treatment process. However, even those approaches run the risk of making Delaney feel manipulated, uncomfortable, and under pressure to comply with the clinician's requests.

Interventions that seem most likely to reduce Delaney's feelings of mistrust fear, and shame are those that increase her comfort with the treatment process and build her self-esteem and self-confidence. Consequently, her clinician increased the use of empathy in treatment, making sure not to be intrusive or overly personal.

The clinician gave Delaney greater control over the treatment process, letting her set the agenda for each session after educating her on appropriate issues for discussion. Her clinician focused on Delaney's strengths and accomplishments, such as her academic success in the first few years after the family's move to the United States. In addition, her counselor taught Delaney some study skills and communication skills that helped her perform better at school and engage more successfully in group projects. This helped Delaney see that her counselor did have caring and concern for her and was unlikely to humiliate or pressure her.

Subsequent interventions normalized Delaney's reluctance and encouraged her to discuss her ambivalence about getting help and talking openly about herself and her family. The counselor then emphasized indirect interventions such as suggesting that positive change was possible and using stories, metaphors, humor, and bibliotherapy. This combination of interventions eventually enabled Delaney to share with the counselor the problems in her family and to participate actively and productively in treatment.

Following a step-by-step process to understand client reluctance using the modified Bloom's taxonomy can help clinicians not only reduce client reluctance but even use it as an important source of information about a person and the way the person deals with new and challenging situations. The exercises in the following Learning Opportunities section include those that afford practice in applying the taxonomy to examples of client reluctance.

LEARNING OPPORTUNITIES

This chapter, like Chapter 4, presented concepts and interventions intended to help clinicians deal with strong emotions in treatment. The primary topics in this chapter included:

- Dealing with strong emotions in clients
  - Suicidal ideation
  - Crisis reactions
  - Anger and violence
- Variations in client readiness for treatment; stages of change
- Addressing client reluctance

Written Exercises/Discussion Questions

1. Your client is Nathan, a 17-year-old African American male. He was recently diagnosed with a sexually transmitted disease, although he had been sexually involved only with his girlfriend, age 15, who is Caucasian. When he confronted her about this, she acknowledged that she had been sexually involved with many of his friends. Nathan went home and consumed a bottle of aspirin along with a quart of vodka. Although he survived this suicide attempt, he continues to wish he were dead. Nathan's father, with whom he lives, is

unemployed. Nathan's parents are separated, and he sees his mother about once a month. Nathan has few friends, except for his girlfriend, and has never been a strong student. He had been involved in sports but was dropped from the team because of his many absences. Develop your understanding of Nathan's suicidal ideation by applying the modified Bloom's taxonomy to the information you have on Nathan. Then formulate a plan that seems likely to reduce the risk that Nathan will again attempt to commit suicide. In what stage of change is Nathan? How will that affect your treatment plans?

2. Beverly, a 76-year-old woman, has always lived with her twin sister, Valerie. Valerie recently had a stroke and is on life-support. The doctors say it is unlikely that she will recover and have encouraged Beverly to request that life-support be removed. Valerie did not have a living will but spoke often of not wanting to live unless she had dignity and quality of life. Beverly is devastated by Valerie's stroke and feels unable to make a decision. Following the modified Bloom's taxonomy applied to dealing with crises on pages 136–138, analyze the nature of Beverly's crisis and develop a plan to help her cope with this situation. In what stage of change is Beverly? How will that affect your treatment plans?

3. A common negative client emotion that was not addressed in this chapter is fear, particularly the terror, avoidance, and reexperiencing that often follows a traumatic experience. Create a client who has such a reaction to a trauma. Use the modified Bloom's taxonomy to improve your understanding of this person, and develop a treatment approach that seems likely to be effective.

4. Clinicians now view client reluctance differently than they did 10 or 15 years ago. Then it was called resistance and generally was seen as a negative emotion that needed to be eliminated so that treatment could progress smoothly. Now reluctance and variations in people's readiness for treatment generally are accepted as an important client variable, a source of information, and a message that can inform the treatment process. What are your reactions to this shift in perception? How do you think conceptions of people's readiness for change will continue to evolve?

5. Considering the types of clients you expect to work with, what sort of client reluctance do you think you are most likely to encounter? What do you think will be the three or four approaches you will be most likely to use to address reluctance?

Practice Group Exercise: *Dealing with Strong Client Emotions While Building the Therapeutic Alliance*

In this chapter, as in previous ones, you have the opportunity to refine and practice both your fundamental and your conceptual skills. As usual, record both the practice session and the subsequent discussion.

In this chapter you learned skills that will help you deal with your clients' strong feelings and assist them in expressing, understanding, and modifying their emotions. In this practice group exercise, you will build on what you learned in this chapter as well as in Chapter 4, where you learned ways to develop a positive client–clinician alliance.

Clinicians in this exercise have four major goals:

- To demonstrate those characteristics that promote the development of a sound therapeutic alliance (presented in Chapter 4)
- To enhance client motivation toward change
- To explore and begin to address effectively the unhealthy emotions and issues presented by the role-played client
- To demonstrate a broad range of effective fundamental skills and interventions

Your role-play will probably enhanced by sound use of the following fundamental skills:

- Ability to make good use of encouragers (restatement, paraphrase, summarization)
- Ability to make accurate and helpful reflections of feeling
- Ability to identify and make good use of nonverbal communication

Practice Group Exercise

In each dyad, one person will assume the role of clinician and the other will assume the role of client. This interaction should be viewed as an initial treatment session. Those in the client role may determine their specific concerns, as long as their presentation reflects one of the following types of clients discussed in this chapter:

- A client in crisis
- A suicidal client
- An angry or potentially violent client
- A highly reluctant client

Those of you in the clinician role may discover that you have some strong emotional reactions to this role-play. You may feel frustrated or irritated, and you may even feel some anger toward your partner for being such a difficult client. Keep in mind that this is a role-play, not a genuine interaction between the two of you, and try to make the most of what may be a challenging learning experience.

Timing of Exercise

If possible, allow at least 2 hours for this exercise. If you do not have this much time, do only two role-plays, one for each dyad. Each person will then have the opportunity to be either client or clinician but will not be able to experience both roles.

Alternatively, you can shorten the time required for this exercise by eliminating the discussion of client issues described in the following section.

- Allow approximately 15 minutes for each role-played interview.
- Take about 5–10 minutes to provide feedback to the person in the clinician role. As you have done with other exercises in this book, begin the feedback

process with the person in the clinician role, focus on strengths first, and offer concrete suggestions for improvement. Remember to make this a positive learning experience. Feedback should focus on the areas listed in the accompanying Assessment of Progress form.

- After you have given the clinician feedback, take about 5 minutes to discuss the issues presented by the client according to the information presented earlier in this chapter. Identify those treatment strategies that are most likely to be helpful in dealing with the client's strong emotions.

Assessment of Progress Form 5

1. What interventions and strategies were used to initiate the session, increase client motivation toward treatment, and build a positive treatment alliance?

   _____

   _____

   _____

   a. Which of these seemed particularly successful? What made them effective?

   _____

   _____

   b. What else might the clinician have done to further develop the treatment alliance?

   _____

   _____

   _____

2. Which of the clinician's interventions (e.g., encouragers, open questions, reflection of feelings) seemed particularly successful overall?

   _____

   _____

   _____

3. How might the clinician have improved on his or her interventions?

   _____

   _____

   _____

4. What was the clinician's strategy in dealing with the client's strong emotions?

   _____

   _____

   _____

   a. What interventions were especially effective in helping the client understand and modify his or her unhelpful emotions?

_____

_____

_____

b. How might the clinician have dealt even more effectively with this client's strong emotions?

_____

_____

_____

5. Summary of feedback

_____

_____

_____

a. Strengths:

_____

_____

b. Areas needing improvement:

_____

_____

Personal Journal Questions

1. What do you think it would be like for you to work with a suicidal client? What do you think would be the most difficult aspect of that process for you? What skills do you have that would help you work with that client?
2. What do you think it would be like for you to work with an angry and potentially violent client? What do you think would be the most difficult aspect of that process for you? What skills do you have that would help you deal with that client?
3. Listen to the recording of the role-played interview in which you were in the client role as part of this chapter. Respond to the following questions about that recording:
   a. How did you feel about working with a challenging client? Did your feelings interfere with your ability to provide effective treatment?
   b. What do you view as your greatest accomplishment during this role-play?
   c. What progress did you make toward improving your clinical skills?
   d. What goals do you have for your next role-play?
4. Client reluctance to engage in treatment is manifested in many ways as described in this chapter. What sort of reluctance would be particularly difficult and uncomfortable for you? What sort of reluctance is most understandable to you? What sense do you make of your reactions?
5. What is the most important thing you learned from this chapter and its exercises?

SUMMARY

This chapter focused on conceptual skills associated with addressing challenging client emotions and reactions to treatment, including suicidal ideation, responses to crises, anger, and reluctance to engage in treatment. This chapter also presented information on variations in people's readiness to change and ways to assess and address their stages of change. Continued use was made of the modified Bloom's taxonomy to promote learning of the skills presented in this chapter.

Chapters 6 and 7 focus on conceptual skills associated with thoughts. Included in those chapters is information on assessment, defining people's central concerns, diagnosis, and treatment planning.

Chapter 6

USING CONCEPTUAL SKILLS TO ENHANCE THOUGHTS

ASSESSMENT, MENTAL STATUS EXAMINATION, DEFINING MEMORIES, AND CASE CONCEPTUALIZATION

OVERVIEW

Most of the chapters in this book focus primarily on the client, helping clinicians to better understand and more effectively address clients' concerns. Chapter 5, for example, focused on changing strong and self-destructive client emotions as well as on identifying and increasing clients' readiness for change.

Chapters 6 and 7 take a somewhat different slant on the treatment process. These chapters focus on *thoughts,* the third element in the BETA format (background, emotions, thoughts, and actions). However, rather than focusing primarily on the clients' thoughts, most topics in these two chapters focus on a combination of the clinicians' thoughts and the clients' characteristics and concerns. These chapters are designed to help clinicians clarify and develop their own thoughts about their clients and then to use those thoughts to further the treatment process. Information in Chapters 6 and 7, as well as the Learning Opportunities at the end of each of these chapters, incorporate these new skills into what you have already learned. This will help you progress in your ability to provide effective treatment to your clients.

Chapter 6 includes information on the following topics:

- **Assessment:** Chapter 4 provided considerable information about client assessment. That chapter presented the steps in an intake interview and analyzed the information obtained according to the modified Bloom's taxonomy. Although the intake interview is usually the most important tool in the assessment process, sometimes it does not yield all the information the clinician needs to understand a person well enough to develop a sound plan for helping that person. This chapter discusses the nature and importance of assessment further, as well as tools to facilitate that process.
- **Mental Status Examination:** This chapter presents and illustrates the mental status examination, a tool that seems to be growing in use and usefulness.

- **Tests, Inventories, and Structured Observations:** This chapter discusses the appropriate use of these tools to facilitate the assessment process.
- **Defining Memories:** Many people have memories of important incidents that give shape and direction to their lives and their views of themselves. Identifying and understanding the significance of these memories is an important aspect of the assessment process and facilitates treatment planning.
- **Case Conceptualization:** Once clinicians have completed the assessment process, they should be ready to develop a comprehensive understanding of their clients. Several formats, including the modified Bloom's taxonomy, illustrate the process of case conceptualization.

ASSESSMENT

Assessment involves building a comprehensive picture of a person's background, personality, emotions, thoughts, and behavior patterns from a broad perspective, sampling pertinent sources of information (Kottler & Brown, 2000). This typically entails using a variety of tools to gather information. Assessment almost always includes an intake interview, often includes a mental status examination as well as tests and inventories, and sometimes includes structured observations. Assessment is a comprehensive and integrative process, combining information gleaned from multiple sources into a meaningful whole.

The intake interview, described earlier in Chapter 3, is usually the first step in the assessment process. The mental status examination, described in the following section, is often incorporated into the intake interview.

MENTAL STATUS EXAMINATION

The mental status examination has become an important tool for clinicians. Although some specific questions may be used to clarify aspects of a person's mental status, the term *examination* is misleading. In reality, most of the information for a mental status examination is inferred from the clinician's observations of and interactions with the client, rather than obtained from a formal evaluation. Few specific procedures are required of the clinician when conducting a mental status examination; the clinician needs only to listen and observe carefully the client's presentation, keeping in mind the categories encompassed by a mental status examination.

Benefits of a Mental Status Examination

The mental status examination is important in many ways:

- It deepens clinicians' understanding of their clients.
- It enables clinicians to systematically assess clients' areas of strength and difficulty.

- It facilitates the process of diagnosis.
- It enables clinicians to develop individualized treatment plans that are likely to be effective.
- It allows clinicians to assess their clients' progress by tracking changes in mental status.
- Its categories offer a semistandardized format for synthesizing important information about people's functioning and documenting that information in the client's file as well as on assessment reports and insurance forms. Mental health agencies, as well as managed care organizations, are increasingly asking clinicians to provide mental status information in order to assess clients' needs for services and the appropriateness of the services that are provided.

Categories in a Mental Status Examination

Information derived from mental status examinations is generally presented on a checklist or in a few descriptive paragraphs. Categories included in a mental status examination vary but typically include some or all of the following (Seligman, 2004).

1. Appearance

   - Overall appearance
   - Nature and appropriateness of clothing in light of the weather and the context
   - Cleanliness and grooming
   - Distinguishing physical characteristics

2. Behavior

   - Eye contact
   - Habits or mannerisms such as restlessness, nail biting, gum chewing, or blinking
   - Movement retardation, agitation, or difficulties in walking or other physical activities
   - Sensory difficulties such as problems in vision or hearing

3. Speech

   - Clarity of articulation and communication
   - Rate of speech (pressured, slowed, or normal)
   - Unusual or idiosyncratic speech or word usage
   - Speech reflective of cultural or ethnic background

4. Emotions and overall affect

   - Nature of observable emotions, both immediate and underlying
   - Range and lability (amount of change) of emotions
   - Appropriateness of emotional responses to content
   - Quality of emotions (e.g., flat and blunted, intense, flamboyant)

5. Orientation to reality

   - Awareness of time (hour, day, month, year)
   - Awareness of place (where interview is being conducted)
   - Awareness of persons (who client and clinician are)
   - Awareness of situation (what is happening, purpose of session)

6. Concentration and attention

   - Alertness (responsive, lethargic, or distracted)
   - Ability to sustain attention
   - Ability to follow a train of thought and maintain focus on a topic
   - Ability to provide clear and relevant responses

7. Thought processes

   - Capacity for abstract thinking
   - Clarity of thoughts (coherent and logical or reflecting confusion, tangential thinking, and loose associations)
   - Repetitions and perseverations
   - Responses rapid or delayed

8. Thought content

   - Suicidal ideation
   - Thoughts of violence, aggression, or rage
   - Obsessions and compulsions
   - Intrusive recollections of traumatic or other upsetting experiences
   - Other prominent thoughts, especially those that are recurrent

9. Perceptions

   - Hallucinations (auditory, visual, olfactory, gustatory tactile, other)
   - Bizarre or nonbizarre (within the realm of possibility) delusions
   - Ideas of suspicion, persecution, or reference
   - Other unusual beliefs or perceptions

10. Memory

   - Adequacy of immediate memory (less than a minute)
   - Adequacy of short-term memory (e.g., information provided at the beginning of the interview)
   - Adequacy of medium-term memory (e.g., client's activities a week ago)
   - Adequacy of long-term memory (e.g., childhood experiences, educational/occupational history, important world events during the client's lifetime)

11. Intelligence

   - Educational level
   - Adequacy of fund of information

- Level of vocabulary
- Overall intelligence

12. Judgment and insight

- Decision-making ability
- Problem-solving ability
- Awareness of and insight into self; recognition of strengths and difficulties
- Ability to accept appropriate responsibility for reported concerns
- Capacity for deferring action and controlling impulsivity

The Mini-Mental Status Examination

A variation of the mental status examination is the mini-mental status examination. This is usually used to assess people who show signs of severe cognitive difficulties such as loss of contact with reality, dementia, and other forms of cognitive impairment. The mini-mental status examination is similar to a general mental status examination but is more structured and is designed specifically to assess cognitive functioning. Psychiatric nurses and psychiatrists are more likely to use the mini-mental status examination than are counselors, social workers, psychologists, and other nonmedical clinicians.

A typical mini-mental status examination includes the following categories, illustrated by the sort of exercises or questions that might be used to assess each category of functioning.

- **Orientation:** What is the day/month/year/season?
- **Registration:** The clinician names three common objects such as "shoe, hat, dog" and then asks the client to immediately repeat the list of three items.
- **Attention and Concentration:** The clinician might ask the client to spell a word backwards or to count backwards from 100 by 7s.
- **Recall:** Midway through the session, the clinician might ask the client to name the three objects that were presented at the beginning of the session (see Registration, listed previously).
- **Language:** The client is asked to provide the names for common objects such as a chair and a pencil, to repeat a sentence, or to follow a three-stage command such as "Open the cabinet, take out a pad of paper, and put it on the desk."

Other exercises typically incorporated into a mini-mental status examination include writing a sentence and copying a design.

Example of a Mental Status Examination

Following is a mental status examination, describing Eileen Carter, discussed previously in several chapters of this book, when she first sought treatment. Brevity, conciseness, and of course accuracy are the hallmarks of a sound mental status examination.

- **Appearance:**   Eileen Carter is a tall, slender African American woman. She was casually and appropriately dressed and appeared well groomed. She has no distinguishing physical characteristics.
- **Behavior:**   Eileen initially had some difficulty making eye contact, but her eye contact improved as the interview continued. Some mannerisms, such as clasping and unclasping her hands and chewing on her fingernails, suggested anxiety. Agitation also was noted in her movements. Otherwise, no unusual mannerisms or sensory difficulties were evident.
- **Speech:** Eileen spoke rapidly but clearly. Although she occasionally mispronounced words, she made herself understood without difficulty.
- **Emotions/Affect:** Sadness and tearfulness generally characterized Eileen's presentation, except when she was talking about her son. A dysphoric mood seems to have been present for many years, exacerbated by current disappointments. Eileen also presented with some guilt and anger. Eileen's affect was fairly stable and was appropriate to the content of the session.
- **Orientation to Reality:** Eileen was oriented to time, place, person, and situation (oriented $\times$ 4).
- **Concentration and Attention:** Eileen had no difficulty following the direction of the interview. She was alert and responsive, provided relevant responses, and maintained attention.
- **Thought Processes:** Eileen was capable of thinking in a logical and coherent way and seems to have a sound capacity for abstraction. However, she sometimes responded to questions too rapidly; her answers seemed driven more by anxiety than by careful thought.
- **Thought Content:** Eileen repeated many times the importance to her of her son and her education. She expressed considerable anger toward her husband and described her own strong feelings of guilt. She did not seem to present a danger to herself or anyone else.
- **Perceptions:** No indications of hallucinations, delusions, or other unusual perceptions were evident during the interview with Eileen.
- **Intelligence:** Eileen completed her GED after leaving high school at age 17. She has begun to take college courses. Her fund of information and vocabulary reflect her limited education. However, her depth of thought and interest in learning suggest that she is of above-average intelligence.
- **Judgment and Insight:** Eileen has good awareness of her difficulties and accepts responsibility for the part she has played in her problems. She is trying to change past patterns of impulsivity and poor judgment but needs help in learning problem-solving and decision-making skills.

Now that you have read the previous mental status examination, notice how it organized and clarified information about Eileen. You can probably imagine how you could use this information, along with information from an intake interview with Eileen, to determine effective ways to help her. Later chapters of this book discuss the processes of formulating diagnoses and developing treatment plans. A diagnosis and treatment plan draw on information from an intake interview and mental status examination to determine effective ways to help clients.

Although the mental status examination is a powerful and useful tool, it does entail clinicians' making judgments about clients' levels of functioning and empasizing strengths. Clinicians should be cautious during this process and be sure that they are making good use of multicultural competencies, as discussed in Chapter 2. Using tentative language and factoring in information on clients' cultural backgrounds will help clinicians avoid premature and inaccurate conclusions.

USING TESTS AND INVENTORIES AS PART OF THE ASSESSMENT PROCESS

Incorporating tests and inventories into the assessment process requires careful thought, decision making, and planning on the part of the clinician. Both clients and clinicians probably bring with them some preconceptions about the use of tests and inventories. These may be positive, or negative, or a mixture of the two. Some people view standardized inventories as an objective, reliable, and helpful source of information, whereas others are apprehensive about such tools, believing that they stereotype, limit, and judge people. Both of these viewpoints are valid; standardized inventories can enhance treatment by providing new information, increasing client self-awareness, and promoting useful discussion. At the same time, these tools can indeed provide an inaccurate and incomplete picture of a person and can increase that person's self-doubts and mistrust of the clinician and the treatment process.

To emphasize the benefits and minimize the drawbacks of the assessment process, clinicians should be clear about what they hope to accomplish via testing and should be aware of their own reactions to incorporating tests and inventories into the treatment process. They also should discuss the prospect of testing and its pros and cons with their clients.

Maximizing the Benefits of Testing

Asking themselves the following seven questions will help clinicians determine whether testing can enhance their work with a particular person and what types of tests and inventories are most likely to be useful (Seligman, 1994):

1. What knowledge, insight, or information am I seeking?
2. Have I first reviewed available sources of information, such as intake interviews, mental status examinations, psychological and academic records, and previous tests and inventories administered to this client, to determine whether they can provide the needed information?
3. Does it seem likely that additional tests and inventories can provide important knowledge that is not available from other sources?
4. How is the client likely to benefit from and react to the use of tests and inventories?
5. How will the treatment process and the therapeutic alliance be affected by the use of tests and inventories?
6. What tests and inventories are most likely to yield the desired information? The selection process should take account of the client's multicultural,

socioeconomic, and educational background to maximize the likelihood of selecting instruments that yield valid, reliable, and meaningful information. The process should include identifying and obtaining information on strengths, although assessment also may be useful for determining whether and what mental disorders are present and what barriers and challenges may be hampering the client's progress.

7. How should tests and inventories be integrated into the treatment process?

Types of Tests and Inventories

Clinicians should be familiar with the array of tests and inventories available to them, so that they can choose instruments that are likely to provide the information they are seeking. Reference books, such as *Tests in Print* published by the Buros Institute of Mental Measurements, *Test Critiques* published by the Test Corporation of America, and the *Mental Measurements Yearbook* published by the Buros Institute, as well as catalogs issued by test publishers, can help clinicians identify appropriate tests for their purposes.

Five broad categories of assessment tools are available (Seligman, 1994). A brief description of these follows. However, reference books and test catalogs should be consulted for additional information about specific tests and inventories.

- **Measures of ability** include tests of achievement, aptitude, and intelligence. These are used primarily in school settings for academic purposes. School psychologists, school counselors, and career counselors most often administer these tests. Individual intelligence tests, such as the Stanford-Binet Intelligence Scale, the Wechsler Intelligence Scale for Children, and the Wechsler Adult Intelligence Scale, are also used by clinical and counseling psychologists to assess intellectual functioning, work habits, and personality. Ability tests that you have probably taken include the Scholastic Aptitude Test and the Graduate Record Examination.

- **Interest inventories** are widely used by counselors and psychologists, particularly those engaged in career counseling. The results of these inventories are typically combined with expressed interests (what people say their interests are) and manifest interests (what interests are reflected in people's activities) to develop an integrated and comprehensive picture of people's likes and dislikes. This information can help people to better understand their academic and occupational interests, to make wise choices of academic programs and occupations, and to develop their awareness of unexplored interests. These inventories also can provide information on leisure activities that might be of interest to a client. The Self-Directed Search and the Strong Interest Inventory are widely used interest inventories.

- **Personality inventories** include comprehensive measures of people's personalities, inventories of self-esteem and values, and measures of specific aspects of personality such as depression, dissociation, anxiety, social skills, and resilience. These inventories are helpful in promoting client self-awareness, in identifying emotional strengths and difficulties, in characterizing personality style, and in tracking changes in a particular variable such as de-pression or anxiety. Well-known comprehensive personality inventories in-clude the Minnesota Multiphasic Personality Inventory (MMPI), the Millon Clinical Multiaxial Inventory (MCMI), and the Myers-Briggs Type Indicator (MBTI). More narrowly focused inventories such as the Beck Depression Inventory and the Beck Anxiety Inventory are particularly useful to clini-cians in mental health settings who want to determine the nature and sever-ity of people's affective symptoms and assess the progress of treatment.

- **Measures of career development** assess such variables as decisiveness, work-related attitudes, and knowledge of careers. These assessment tools are often incorporated into computer-based assessment and information programs de-signed to facilitate career development. Computer-based programs typically also include interest inventories and career information systems and may also include inventories to assess abilities. These assessment tools are most likely to be available at high schools and colleges and at career counseling programs.
- **Nonstandardized approaches** to assessment also are sometimes used by cli-nicians. These are generally checklists and informal questionnaires that do not have proven validity and reliability. They are used primarily to promote thought and discussion rather than for assessment purposes.

Conceptualizing the Assessment Process for Eileen Carter

Eileen Carter will be used here to illustrate how clinicians might decide whether to use tests and inventories with a particular client and how to select the specific in-struments to use with that person. Although considerable information about Eileen is already available in the summary of her history presented in Chapter 2 and the mental status examination included in this chapter, there are significant gaps in the information Eileen has been able to provide about herself. Consequently, her clini-cian is considering whether tests and inventories might provide useful information for both the client and the clinician.

Let's look at the answers to the questions presented on pages 175–176 as they pertain to Eileen.

1. *What knowledge, insight, or information are you seeking?*

Eileen spoke openly about her background and present life situation. How-ever, her years of involvement with drugs and alcohol, as well as her limited work ex-perience and education, made it difficult for her to clarify her interests and develop sound future goals. Because Eileen wanted to continue her education, tests and in-ventories should help Eileen determine and clarify her areas of strength and inter-est. Exploring these could give more direction to her college coursework and increase her motivation and sense of accomplishment.

Just as Eileen has little sense of her interests and abilities, so also does she have little sense of her personality. Her background provides evidence of much strength. However, Eileen tends to denigrate herself and has little awareness of her assets. Personality inventories might present an objective view of those assets and give her language she can use to think of herself in more positive terms.

2. *Have available sources of information, such as the intake interview, the mental status examination, psychological and academic records, and previous tests and inventories administered to this client been reviewed first to determine whether they can provide the needed information?*

An intake interview and a mental status examination have already been conducted with Eileen; both were fruitful sources of information. However, no other tests or records are available that are relevant to Eileen as an adult. High school grades, tests, and inventories probably have little validity because of the difficulties Eileen was experiencing at that time. Eileen today is very different than she was as an adolescent.

3. *Does it seem likely that tests and inventories can provide important knowledge that is not available from other sources?*

Based on the answers to the previous questions, tests and inventories do seem likely to provide useful information on Eileen that cannot be obtained from other sources. However, care must be taken in both the selection and the interpretation of the inventories because of Eileen's cultural background, her limited interest in education as an adolescent, and her low self-esteem.

4. *How is the client likely to benefit from and react to the use of tests and inventories?*

Because of her recent interest in education and her self-referral for counseling, Eileen probably will have considerable interest in inventories and their results. The use of tests and inventories seems likely to enhance her self-awareness and self-esteem. On the other hand, the clinician should keep in mind the possibility that the use of these tools will reawaken negative reactions that Eileen had to testing as an adolescent. She may feel judged and categorized by the inventories, as well as by the clinician. Because of her hunger for learning and her self-doubts, Eileen also might overemphasize the importance of the test results and take them too literally.

5. *How will the treatment process and the therapeutic alliance be affected by the use of tests and inventories?*

The use of assessment tools with Eileen can enhance or detract from the therapeutic alliance. However, steps can be taken to maximize the benefits to Eileen and the treatment process and to safeguard the therapeutic alliance. Inventory results should be used primarily to promote discussion; identify strengths, abilities, and interests; and suggest new avenues for exploration. They should not be used to provide definitive answers and direction.

6. *What tests and inventories are most likely to yield the desired information?*

Because the goal of Eileen's assessment is promoting discussion and self-esteem, instruments should be selected, at least initially, that do not have right and wrong answers but instead encourage self-awareness and exploration. Two well-established inventories that meet these criteria are the Myers-Briggs Type Indicator, a personality inventory that focuses on the normal rather than the pathological personality, and the Strong Interest Inventory, a broad-based interest inventory.

7. *How should those tests and inventories be integrated into the treatment process?*

Time should be taken to develop a positive therapeutic alliance with Eileen before suggesting that she complete any inventories. In addition, Eileen needs to make a rapid decision about remaining in college; progress should be made toward resolving the current crisis before inventories are used. When the clinician presents to Eileen the possibility of taking personality and interest inventories, she should be given ample information about these tools and their benefits and potential drawbacks so that she can play an active and informed role in deciding whether to complete the inventories. Similarly, Eileen should play an active role in discussing the results of the inventories. Empowering Eileen is important, and that should be emphasized in her treatment. In addition, information already provided by Eileen on her interests and personality style should be reviewed and integrated into the discussion of the inventories. This should enable her to view the results of the inventories as enhancing the information she already has about herself rather than superseding her knowledge of herself.

Results of Eileen Carter's Inventories

Eileen's Myers-Briggs Type Indicator (MBTI) profile showed that her preferences were ISFJ, reflecting the following personality styles:

- **I/Introversion:** Eileen focuses on her inner world and prefers being alone or with a small number of close friends or family members to being with a large group. This was a high score.
- **S/Sensing:** People with a sensing preference on the MBTI typically focus on facts and information and tend to be practical. However, this score was low. Eileen also frequently uses intuition and sometimes experiences conflicts between her practical side and her intuitive side.
- **F/Feeling:** This was another high score, suggesting that Eileen is understanding and supportive, values relationships, and tends to make decisions subjectively, based primarily on her values and on the welfare of others, rather than on objective evidence and impartial analysis.
- **J/Judging:** This was a relatively low score. Eileen tends to prefer her life to be clear, structured, and well organized. However, she can be spontaneous and sometimes has difficulty meeting deadlines and following through on plans, especially when her need for structure conflicts with her wish to please and be close to others.

Eileen's overall MBTI type is ISFJ. According to Kroeger and Thuesen (1988), people with this personality type emphasize duty and responsibility and focus their energy outward, in the service of others. They are matter-of-fact, serious, and thorough in their activities and diligently pursue their goals. They take parenting seriously, are loyal to their partners and friends, but sometimes allow others to take advantage of them. As students, they prefer courses that are organized and practical.

This profile is consistent with and provides some clarification of what is already known about Eileen. She is dedicated to her family and is a caring and responsible parent. She has a small circle of friends and feels most comfortable with people she knows well. She currently is torn between two strong feelings: her love for her son and the joy she has discovered through attending college. She is eager to satisfy her J side and make a decision, but she has difficulty making an objective assessment of her options and determining a sound plan because of this emotional conflict.

On the Strong Interest Inventory (SII), Eileen manifested very high interest in the Social (S) theme and moderately high interest in the Artistic (A) and Conventional (C) areas. Occupations that reflect both her MBTI personality type (ISFJ) and her SII code (SAC) include librarian, preschool teacher, medical technician, dental hygienist, and licensed practical nurse. A clear pattern of interests emerges from these scores. Eileen would probably most enjoy working in a helping capacity, perhaps with children and in an educational or medical setting. This information, too, is compatible with what is already known about Eileen; these scores reflect her enthusiasm for education and for helping others and her enjoyment of children. Discussion of these personality and interest inventory results are likely to help Eileen develop a clearer picture of herself and identify occupations that are likely to be rewarding to her.

The Use of Observation as an Assessment Tool

Clinicians use informal observations of their clients throughout the treatment process, beginning with their first telephone contact. They observe clients' tone of voice, their style of dress, their physical mannerisms and movements, their greeting, and much more. However, sometimes clinicians find it helpful to conduct a formal and structured observation of clients in addition to their informal observations. Particularly useful is the opportunity to observe nonverbal behaviors without interacting with the client. Social workers, counselors, and psychologists who work in schools, as well as other mental health professionals who treat children, are most likely to conduct structured observations.

Structured observations are particularly useful when clients meet the following criteria.

- They do not disclose verbally very much information about themselves because of their age, their reluctance, their limited self-awareness, or the level of their intelligence and communication skills.
- They present with behavioral difficulties such as hyperactivity, aggressiveness, or social withdrawal.
- They are in a classroom or other setting in which they can readily be observed.
- Their parents or guardians, as well as their teachers, understand the potential benefits of an observation and consent to that process. Depending on age and abilities, children might also be involved in discussing and planning an observation.

Usually, the clinician prepares for an observation by developing a list of behavioral categories that will focus the assessment. For example, observation of a child suspected of having an attention-deficit/hyperactivity disorder might include the following categories:

- The number of times the child gets up from a seat without permission
- The number of times the child speaks out in class without being called on
- The number of times the child engages in inappropriate conversation or physical interaction with another child
- The approximate number of minutes or percent of class time that the child remains on task

Observational information such as this can promote understanding of a child, especially when discrepancies such as low grades and high inventoried ability are seen in available information.

CONCEPTUALIZING THE MEANING OF DEFINING MEMORIES

Yet another approach to assessment is the use of *defining memories.* Alfred Adler (1931), an early psychoanalyst, wrote about the importance of earliest memories. According to Adler, those memories that stood out in people's minds as their earliest memories were usually reflective of their lifestyles, their views of themselves, and their interactions with others. Adler emphasized that what mattered was not the reality of the memories, but rather the way they were preserved in people's minds.

Although early memories have special significance, people have other memories that shape their self-images, their views of the world, and the way they lead their lives. Important memories often are preserved in people's minds in an almost photographic way; some elements of the memory stand out sharply and clearly, while others are lost in the background. This has been described as a *frozen moment.* Probably all of us have such memories that come to us often and reflect a turning point in our lives. Visualize memories that are important to you to have a better sense of the defining moments in your life.

Memories of defining moments or critical incidents come in many forms.

- They may reflect *traumatic experiences.* Alonzo, for example, remembers being severely beaten by an older boy in his neighborhood. Ben, who is allergic to nuts, remembers the near-fatal reaction he had the first time he ate peanut butter. Carlena will never forget the car accident in which she was seriously injured and her companion was killed.
- They may be *peak experiences* that leave an indelible impression. Jenna vividly recalls winning the academic achievement award when she graduated from fifth grade, whereas Denuta remembers her excitement and apprehension when her family left Poland for the United States. For Russ, his parents' 50th wedding anniversary celebration, in which they reaffirmed their vows, was a peak experience.
- Defining memories also may reflect experiences that seem *insignificant to others but are very meaningful to us.* Lulu remembers the first day her parents

let her go to the playground alone and how independent and brave she felt, climbing on the play equipment without supervision. Gerard remembers the day his father accidentally ran over a squirrel that had run into the road. April often thinks back to the first time someone in her office invited her for coffee and how good that made her feel.

Application of Modified Bloom's Taxonomy

Once again, the modified Bloom's taxonomy can be helpful in determining the significance that particular memories have for a person. That information can then be used to promote self-awareness and to guide the treatment process.

Content

The first step is eliciting one or more memories that stand out in a person's mind. Using two or three memories typically provides a clearer and more reliable picture. Clinicians can ask people to simply recall and describe these important memories, or they can suggest that people visualize or imagine themselves in the memory and then report what they are seeing, feeling, thinking, and doing. Several meaningful memories provided by Eileen Carter, the client who has been highlighted throughout this book, illustrate how the use of memories can enhance the treatment process.

Eileen presented three memories that stood out in her mind.

1. She recalled a time when, as an adolescent, she had been involved with a man who had a motorcycle. Both of them had been using drugs and alcohol that evening when the man took her for a ride on his motorcycle. Along the way, they stopped to get gas for the motorcycle. They noticed that a woman had left her purse in the car while she paid for her gas. Eileen's boyfriend grabbed the purse and the two of them sped off on the motorcycle. Eileen vividly recalled this incident and her mixture of feelings: exhilaration at their successful crime but also shame that she had participated in such an experience.

2. Eileen remembered the first day of her first class at college. She felt a strong mixture of anticipation and anxiety. Because she had trouble finding a parking place, she had no time to purchase her books before class. When the teacher referred to the book and other students pulled out their books to follow along, Eileen felt ashamed that she did not have the book. However, when the student sitting next to her moved closer to Eileen so they could share a book, Eileen thought that perhaps college could be a positive experience after all.

3. Of course, for Eileen, the birth of her son was a defining moment. However, even during that experience, her reactions were mixed. She felt great joy and a sense of belonging and purpose in her life because of the birth of her son. At the same time, she remembers thinking, "Now I must stay with my husband; I can never be free again."

Process

Comprehension: Clarifying the emotions, thoughts, and actions associated with each memory can facilitate comprehension of these defining moments. For

Eileen, the emotions, thoughts, and actions associated with each memory include the following.

Memory 1: Theft of purse
Emotions: Exhilaration, shame
Thoughts: "I must be a terrible person to enjoy committing a crime."
Actions: Fled the scene of the crime, did not report the crime.
Memory 2: First day at college
Emotions: Fear, shame, and hope
Thoughts: "I don't belong here, I don't think I can succeed at college, but I really want to and perhaps people will help me enough so that I can succeed."
Actions: Continued college, with recognition of her need to be better prepared and to ask others for help.
Memory 3: Birth of son
Emotions: Joy, but also a sense of being trapped, self-doubts
Thoughts: "Now my life has meaning; I have someone to love who loves me, but I have lost my freedom in the process. Why can't I be contented with what I have?"
Actions: Eileen made a commitment to be the best mother she could be for her son, and resolved to stay with her husband.

Organization: The information obtained from the content and the comprehension of the memories can be organized according to themes. Eileen's memories reflect the following themes.

- **Conflicting emotions:** Joy is mitigated by guilt, shame, self-doubts, and regret.
- **Conflicting choices:** Part of Eileen is drawn toward socially acceptable behavior (obeying the law, becoming a wife and mother), but another part of her longs to break free and defy social conventions (the motorcycle incident).
- **Low self-esteem:** A confused and damaged sense of self.
- **Other-directedness:** Concern with how she is perceived by others.

Analysis/Synthesis: The conflicts in Eileen's memories reflect the split in her life. During her adolescence and early adulthood, she made some self-destructive choices: she misused drugs and alcohol, she became dependent on men who abused her, she had two unwanted pregnancies and two abortions, she rejected her family, and she even engaged in criminal behavior. However, all that changed with her marriage and the birth of her son. According to Eileen, "I became a totally different person." In reality, however, external influences have always greatly influenced Eileen's life. In her youth she molded herself in the image of her peer group, behaving in socially unacceptable ways even though they felt shameful to her. Now she has molded herself into the image of the middle-class wife and mother, dressing and acting the part as much as possible. Never has she clearly figured out who she wants to be, nor has she been able to integrate the two sides of her personality into a rewarding whole.

Interpretation: Eileen's conflicted views of herself and her goals seem to be at the root of her current difficulties. She believes that she should be the perfect wife and mother, never deviating from her perception of that role, but locking herself into unrealistic standards. Not only is Eileen driven by a desire to be well regarded by others and achieve a socially acceptable role for herself, she is also driven to counteract her own painful childhood experiences. She wants her son to have the good parenting and stable home she missed. However, the side of Eileen that longs for independence and achievement has found college to be a great source of gratification. Although college appears to be a healthy and growth-promoting choice for Eileen, the side of her that adheres rigidly to her prototype of the perfect wife and mother is uneasy about her decision to attend college. Reconciling her wish to attend college with her view of herself as a perfect wife and mother became especially difficult for Eileen when her husband expressed disapproval of her college attendance. Also difficult for her was the realization that, because of her husband's limited cooperation, Eileen would occasionally need child care for her son while she attended college. Eileen's self-doubts, her sense of shame, her reliance on others to tell her how to lead her life, and her lack of healthy role models in childhood all make it challenging for her to integrate the two sides of herself and find a healthy and rewarding balance of roles in her life.

Application (Intervention): Analysis of the defining memories in Eileen's life provides important insights that inform the treatment process. In her treatment, Eileen needs help in the following areas.

- Understanding and accepting both sides of her personality
- Integrating the two sides of her personality into a healthy self-image
- Developing emotions, thoughts, and actions that reflect her positive and integrated self-image
- Making choices that are rewarding to her, that take account of both societal norms and the needs and values of her loved ones, and that also reflect her own creation of her life rather than an unfulfilling effort to fit into a stereotype.

As you can probably see, eliciting and analyzing defining memories can be a fruitful source of information and can contribute greatly to treatment planning. The Learning Opportunities at the end of this chapter will enable you to identify and analyze your own important memories and to apply the modified Bloom's taxonomy to clusters of important memories presented by others.

The next section of this chapter focuses on using conceptual frameworks to obtain an in-depth understanding of people and their strengths and concerns. Having learned to analyze defining memories will make it easier to learn the skills in this next section and to work collaboratively with clients to understand them more fully.

Jean, a 37-year-old woman in crisis, sought help because of her diagnosis of ovarian cancer a month earlier and the effect this had on both Jean and her family. Jean is married and has two sons, ages 10 and 12. Jean is understandably upset about her diagnosis and is having difficulty making treatment decisions. In addition, she reports that her children, both previously diagnosed with oppositional defiant disorder, have become disruptive and almost uncontrollable in the classroom. Jean's husband, who has a history of accessing pornography on the Internet, spends most of his time at his computer and is often withdrawn and uncommunicative. In addition, Jean is apprehensive about informing her mother about Jean's cancer diagnosis; her mother, who is in her 70s, has a heart condition and is not in good health. Jean's father died of prostate cancer 12 years ago.

Jean believes in the value of psychotherapy and, as a result, has seen many mental health professionals to help her deal with her current crisis. She met with the school counselor and psychologist to discuss her sons' behavior, social workers at the continuing care facility where her mother lives, a family therapist, and a specialist in helping people cope with cancer. By now, Jean is overwhelmed, not only by the many stressors in her life but also by the conflicting interactions she had with all these mental health professionals. Apparently, each one viewed Jean's situation from the perspective of his or her own mental health specialization. This is not surprising, because Jean presented her concerns differently to each one.

In counseling and psychotherapy, more is often not better. More problems, more clinicians, more interventions, and sometimes even more sessions can exacerbate a person's difficulties rather than ameliorate them. What is necessary is to develop a clear conceptualization of the person's areas of concern, symptoms, difficulties, strengths, and resources. Once these have been clearly described and the case holistically conceptualized, appropriate interventions can more easily be identified. According to Mayfield, Kardash, and Kivlighan (1999, p. 504), "Client conceptualization is an important skill. . . . In forming a client conceptualization, counselors take in a vast array of client data (symptoms, familial background, etc.) and organize this information into a model of the client." According to Loganbill and Stoltenberg (1983, p. 235), "Case conceptualization involves the integration of cognitive, behavioral, emotional, and interpersonal aspects of the client, which can be synthesized into a comprehensive understanding of his or her current functioning." Case conceptualization entails understanding a person's story, making sense of that person's life, and formulating a central issue. In case conceptualization, clinicians seek to answer core questions such as "What might cause this person to feel/think/act as he or she is?" and "What treatment approach is most likely to be helpful to this person?"

Research suggests that beginning clinicians often have difficulty with case conceptualization, and I suspect this is a challenge for many experienced clinicians as well. Pfeiffer, Whelan, and Martin (2000) looked at how doctoral students in psychology made decisions about the nature of their clients' difficulties. Early in treatment, the doctoral students formulated a hypothesis as to their clients' central concerns. This can be a helpful starting point if clinicians then consider both confirming and disconfirming information. However, confirmatory bias led these clinicians to focus on information that supported their hypotheses and to overlook discrepant information. Schwitzer (1996, p. 259) agreed with this finding and concluded, "Novice clinicians, especially, typically lack the conceptual structures and extensive general knowledge of counseling required for making effective decisions." Keep in mind that you might find the skill of case conceptualization to be a challenging one. However, the work you have already done on understanding background and context (Chapters 2 and 3) and on clients' strong emotions (Chapter 5) should facilitate the development of your case conceptualization skills.

Information Needed for Case Conceptualization

Before clinicians can accurately and clearly conceptualize a case, they must gather information on the client and on that person's context. Intake interviews, a mental status examination, tests and inventories, observations, and previous client records all provide information that contributes to a useful case conceptualization.

Many models have been developed to facilitate the process of case conceptualization (Eells, 2007). Some of these will be discussed in the next section. First, however, we review the essential ingredients of all case conceptualizations. The following information should be obtained about a person before moving forward to develop a case conceptualization:

- Overt and presenting concerns
- Covert and unacknowledged difficulties
- Current lifestyle
- Relevant background information
- Nature, intensity, and effect of characteristic emotional responses
- Helpful and dysfunctional thoughts, especially those that are recurrent or pervasive
- Constructive and self-destructive actions, especially habits, impulsive behaviors, and violent and self-injurious behavior
- Context of person and problems
- Support systems and resources
- Multicultural considerations
- Barriers to change, including reluctance, transference, secondary gains of symptoms, fear of change, lack of information, or misunderstanding of the treatment process
- Other factors that worsen symptoms or block progress
- Client's accomplishments, strengths, and assets
- Other factors that enhance functioning or promote progress

Models of Case Conceptualization

The primary purpose of case conceptualizations is to "guide and shape the therapist's decision making" (Eells, 2007, p. 421.) Clinicians also may share case conceptualization information with clients, being sure to present the information clearly and gradually so that it is helpful and provides direction rather than overwhelming clients.

Although models of case conceptualization differ depending on clinicians' theoretical orientations and the steps in the conceptualization process, most focus heavily on understanding a person's interpersonal experiences and relationships (Eells, 2007). In addition, most involve three broad steps:

1. Obtaining and describing clinical information
2. Interpreting and organizing that information
3. Developing hypotheses or formulations that make sense of a person's difficulties and suggest effective treatment goals and strategies

Several models of case conceptualization are presented here, along with illustrative examples. In working with clients, you can use one of the following models, another model described in the literature, or a model of your own creation. Models that are helpful in facilitating case conceptualization typically meet the following three criteria:

1. They organize a great deal of client information into a small number of categories.
2. They present a concise understanding of the client.
3. They facilitate the processes of diagnosis and treatment planning (discussed in Chapter 7).

The Learning Opportunities at the end of this chapter offer experience in case conceptualization through application of one or more of the following models.

Concept Mapping

Concept mapping is a way of organizing many salient client statements into a small number of categories and then identifying the connections and patterns among those categories (Mayfield et al., 1999). This process begins with a listing of important client statements. Information elicited from Jean, the woman diagnosed with ovarian cancer, illustrates this process. The categories of information needed for case conceptualization, listed on page 186, are used as a framework to organize Jean's important statements as follows.

Overt and Presenting Concerns

1. I'm having great difficulty coping with my diagnosis of ovarian cancer.
2. I'm feeling depressed and anxious.
3. My family is not helping me but is actually making my situation worse.

Covert and Unacknowledged Difficulties

4. My husband and I sleep in separate bedrooms and rarely spend time together.
5. Our house is always in chaos.
6. I know that alcohol is bad for me, but I need something to help me relax.

7. At least I have some time off from work; I couldn't deal with that pressure, too.
8. I usually feel like I'm swimming against a strong current and just managing to hold my own.

Current Lifestyle

9. We live in a three-bedroom apartment on the outskirts of town.
10. The house is much too small for us and is always a mess.
11. My husband works at home.
12. I'm employed as a teacher's aide in an elementary school.
13. Every day it's just get up, get the kids off to school, go to work, come home, make dinner, get everybody to bed.
14. We manage, but I don't see the light at the end of the tunnel.

Relevant Background Information

15. My father, two of my mother's sisters, and a close friend all died of cancer.
16. My mother and I have never been close.
17. My mother has been treated for depression for many years.
18. My father doted on me. I was devastated when he died.
19. My mother always told me I didn't have much going for me so I'd better get married as soon as I had the chance.
20. My parents worked really hard to make ends meet; I wanted a different life for myself but I don't have it.

Nature, Intensity, and Effect of Characteristic Emotional Responses

21. I'm a lot like my mother; I may even have inherited her depression.
22. I've always had trouble making decisions. Now I have a life-or-death decision to make and I just can't figure out the right thing to do. I feel overwhelmed.
23. I've been crying at least two or three times a day.
24. I've even thought about killing myself, but that seems stupid when I'm working so hard to survive cancer. Maybe I should just let the cancer kill me.
25. I almost never get angry, but every once in a while I really explode.

Helpful and Dysfunctional Thoughts, Especially Those That Are Recurrent or Pervasive

26. I always thought something awful would happen to me; I'm just an unlucky person.
27. I'm a strong person, but I'm feeling like I can't handle any more.
28. I must have done something pretty bad to deserve this.
29. If I die, it will destroy everyone—my husband, my children, and my mother.
30. I often wish this would all just end.

Constructive and Self-Destructive Actions, Especially Habits, Impulsive Behaviors, and Violent and Self-Injurious Behavior

31. A few drinks are the only thing that gets me through the day.
32. I just live from moment to moment, never really looking down the road.

33. Sometimes my children are so difficult, I really lose my temper and hit them so hard they can't breathe.
34. I avoid my husband as much as possible.

Context of Person and Problems

35. Other than a few people I see at work, I don't talk much to anyone, not even my family.
36. I do have confidence in my physicians, but when they disagree about my treatment, I feel lost.
37. I do my job all right, but I sometimes feel like I'm just going through the motions, and that's not fair to the kids I work with.
38. At least money for my medical care isn't a problem; we do have good health insurance and sick leave at work.
39. It's taking care of my family that worries me.

Support Systems and Resources

40. I really haven't had any close friends and associates since I lost my father and my friend Josie.
41. I have a younger brother, but he's pretty useless, always after some wealthy woman or some get-rich-quick scheme.
42. My mother can't even take care of herself, let alone help me.
43. My husband acts like he's the one with cancer, not me, always complaining about how badly life has treated him and staying glued to the computer.
44. My husband should be taking care of me instead of vice versa.
45. I've tried to get my kids to help out around the house, but it's more trouble than it's worth.

Multicultural Considerations

46. I was raised Jewish but haven't been to synagogue since my father died.
47. I know that gynecological cancers are more common among Jewish women, and my aunts both died of breast cancer. Could this be hereditary? Does that mean I'm destined to die of this disease, too?
48. My parents were always very concerned about prejudice against Jews, but of course they grew up during the Second World War
49. There aren't any other Jewish families in our neighborhood. I tell my children not to talk about their religion so they won't be discriminated against. We even celebrate Christmas like everyone else in the neighborhood. That really feels hypocritical.

Barriers to Change, Including Reluctance, Transference, Secondary Gain, of Symptoms, Fear of Change, Lack of Information, or Misunderstanding of the Treatment Process

50. I think that counseling is a place where people tell you the right things to do.
51. I've talked to lots of therapists, but they all tell me something different; how do I know who to listen to?

52. I don't like to sit around and talk about things; I want to get moving.
53. My doctors say I should have decided about my treatment two weeks ago.
54. I don't have a lot of time, so I hope this counseling thing isn't going to take too long.

Other Factors That Worsen Symptoms or Block Progress

55. I was barely hanging on before my diagnosis; I don't know how I can handle one more thing.
56. I wish someone would just make the right decision for me.
57. My husband and children are driving me crazy; I feel like running away from home.

Client's Accomplishments, Strengths, and Assets

58. Even though my mother treated me badly all my life, I never cut her off and I'm still helping her.
59. My children may drive me crazy, but I love them and I'd do anything for them.
60. I'm the teacher's aide in the toughest class in the school, but somehow I do all right and the teacher really seems to appreciate me.
61. I was a pretty good student all through school.
62. I am a strong person and have coped with a great deal.
63. I'll do whatever I can for my family and myself. I just need some help.

Other Factors That Enhance Functioning or Promote Progress

64. My prognosis is pretty good.
65. My job is stable.
66. My husband and I may have our differences, but we're going to stay together.

Further organization of these statements into a concept map with only four categories yields the following syntheses of the information Jean provided and concludes with a case conceptualization.

> **Family of Origin/Family Dynamics/Background (items 3, 15, 16, 17, 18, 20, 21, 41, 42, 43, 46, 48, 58, 59):** Jean came from a hard-working Jewish family. She describes her father as loving and helpful, her mother as critical and demanding, and her brother as self-centered. She believes she may have inherited both cancer and depression from her family. Current family includes two active sons and a distant husband who may still be involved with Internet pornography. Jean seems to be the mainstay in her current family, just as she was the good child in her family of origin.
>
> **Current Stressors (items 1, 7, 22, 29, 36, 37, 39, 44, 53, 54, 57):** The primary stressors in Jean's life are her diagnosis with ovarian cancer, her need to make a rapid decision regarding her treatment, and her fear of death as a result of cancer. She also experiences stress as a result of her children's

behavior, her husband's withdrawal and overinvolvement with the Internet, the demands of her job, and her mother's condition and attitude toward Jean.

Factors Exacerbating Difficulties (items 2, 4, 5, 6, 8, 9, 10, 11, 19, 25, 26, 27, 28, 30, 34, 35, 40, 45, 47, 49, 51, 55): Becouse of cancer, Jean lost both her father and a good friend, apparently the strongest members of her support system. At present, she seems to have no helpful support systems, she lives in a chaotic environment, she has little free time, and she views herself as having primary responsibility for her family. She is not involved with her religion and, in fact, conceals her religion from others. She is experiencing depression and anxiety, contributing to her difficulty in making important decisions.

Strengths, Coping Strategies, and Other Relevant Behaviors (items 7, 12, 14, 23, 24, 31, 32, 33, 38, 50, 52, 56, 60, 61, 62, 63, 64, 65, 66): Jean is an intelligent person who is hard-working and action-oriented. Although she wishes she could escape from her difficult situation, she is willing to do all she can to help herself and her family. She has consulted many specialists to figure out how to help herself. At the same time, she is not introspective, looks to others to give her answers, becomes impatient and angry, and uses alcohol to relieve her anxiety.

Interrelationships of Concept Map: Jean's recent diagnosis with cancer and issues related to that diagnosis are the core of Jean's concerns. However, these stressors have been worsened by the underlying problems in her family of origin and current family, as well as by the secondary stressors she is experiencing, including her work situation, her limited support system, and her depression and anxiety. Her typical efforts to help herself have been moderately effective but may not be up to the challenge of coping with cancer.

Case Conceptualization: Jean is coping with many difficulties, including the immediate stressor of cancer and long-term stressors from both her current family and her family of origin. In many ways, Jean's current life replicates patterns in her family of origin; she is the responsible one, she seeks to please the other family members, and she is coping with cancer and depression. As in her family of origin, she has limited resources and support systems. However, in her family of origin, she was rewarded with the love of her father. Her husband apparently has not shown her caring in the same way, and Jean seems angry and resentful about this. Nevertheless, she often pushes her needs aside, is committed to her family, and keeps trying. Unfortunately, the added stress of cancer has been almost too much for her, and her already tenuous coping skills are letting her down, allowing her depression and anxiety to surface and leaving her immobilized and searching frantically for answers.

The process of organizing a broad array of diverse client statements into broad categories, then into narrower categories, and finally into a case conceptualization is one approach to deepening understanding of a client and moving toward a diagnosis and treatment plan. Clinical factor analysis is another approach.

Clinical Factor Analysis

Emmerson and Thackwray-Emmerson (1992) developed an approach to case conceptualization that involves an analysis of clients' statements. Their model "attempts to translate the principles of statistical factor analysis into an applicable clinical process of identifying factors or themes in therapy to assist in case conceptualization" (p. 404). This approach is structured and entails considerable listing and rating of statements. Such an approach might appeal to clinicians who enjoy and value research but may seem cumbersome to more intuitive clinicians.

The clinical factor analysis consists of the following steps.

1. Construct a list of the client's emotional statements over the course of at least one session. The client's voice quality, body language, and statement content are all criteria used to identify emotional statements.
2. Rate the level of emotional intensity and reactivity of each statement, using the symbols L for low, M for medium, and H for high. These symbols equate to numbers: L = 1, M = 2, H = 3.
3. Group statements that have a common theme.
4. Analyze and name each theme as succinctly and clearly as possible. Each theme will be viewed as a factor, representing the statements it includes.
5. Average the emotional intensity ratings for each factor.
6. Rank the factors according to their emotional intensity ratings and use this ranking to develop a case conceptualization and to identify and prioritize client needs.

An application of clinical factor analysis to a session with Jean, the client in the previous example, yielded the following rank-ordered factors, listed along with their average emotional intensity ratings:

- Cancer and related treatment issues—3.0
- Feeling overwhelmed by my life—2.77
- Concern about my children's welfare—2.65
- My relationship with my husband—2.53
- Limited support systems—2.23
- Job-related stress—2.03

This list clarifies treatment priorities and facilitates development of a sound treatment plan.

The Inverted Pyramid Heuristic

Yet another approach to case conceptualization is Schwitzer's (1996) inverted pyramid heuristic. This model provides a stepwise method for understanding and narrowing the description of people's concerns. Applied to Jean, this model looks like the following.

Step 1. Problem Identification and List of Client Concerns and Characteristics

- **Medical:** diagnosis with ovarian cancer; need to make treatment decisions; fear of dying
- **Emotions, thoughts, actions:** depression; anxiety; self-doubts; difficulty with problem solving and insight; concern about children's future; pessimism; some abuse of alcohol; weak coping; does see self as a strong person; willing to work hard to help self and family
- **Interpersonal:** overactive children; ailing mother; stressful job; husband withdrawn and overinvolved with the Internet; limited support systems; tendency to look to others for answers

Step 2. Organization of Concerns into Logical Thematic Groupings or Constellations

- Medical concerns
- Family stressors and lack of family support and closeness
- Emotional dysfunction
- Coping with many demands

Step 3. Theoretical Views of Thematic Groupings

- Self-doubts and other-directedness (humanistic perspective)
- Impaired attachment, poor role models (psychodynamic perspective)
- Overreliance on nonproductive and somewhat impulsive behaviors (behavioral perspective)
- Seeking perfection in self and others, as well as in her choices (cognitive perspective)

Step 4. Narrowed Inferences: Underlying Difficulties

- Limited sense of self and own wants; focus is on pleasing others
- Lack of support and validation, sharpened by cancer diagnosis

This approach to case conceptualization is a complex one, requiring knowledge of theoretical models and considerable insight. However, it, too, facilitates efforts to hone in on central client concerns.

Stevens and Morris's Format for Case Conceptualization

Stevens and Morris (1995) developed the next format for case conceptualization presented in this chapter. It consists of 14 components, reminiscent of a mental status examination. However, these components are carefully sequenced, moving from the observational to the inferential. This enables clinicians to gradually deepen their understanding of a person. The 14 components are as follows.

1. Relevant background information (e.g., age, physical appearance, living arrangements, education, medical history, family background, cultural and spiritual background)

2. Nature and severity of presenting concerns and current stressors
3. Content of sessions, especially important themes
4. Verbal style (e.g., tone of voice, fluency, quantity and rate of verbalization)
5. Nonverbal behavior (e.g., eye contact, facial expressions, body movements, posture)
6. Nature, intensity, duration, and range of client's emotions and their relationship to verbal content
7. Clinician's experience of and reactions to client
8. Client–clinician interactions and roles in treatment process
9. Results of tests and inventories, mental status examination, behavioral assessments, records, creative products
10. Multiaxial diagnosis according to the *Diagnostic and Statistical Manual of Mental Disorders* (DSM-IV-TR, American Psychiatric Association, 2000)
11. Inferences and assumptions, including a working model of the client's difficulties and factors that contributed to their development
12. Short- and long-term treatment goals, growing out of a clinical understanding of client's difficulties
13. Identification of interventions that will lead to accomplishment of goals
14. Evaluation of outcomes

This model will not be illustrated here because it repeats much of the material that already has been presented. However, you might draw on what you know about Jean to develop your own illustration of this model.

Modified Bloom's Taxonomy

The now-familiar Bloom's taxonomy can also be used as a structure to facilitate the development of a case conceptualization. The Learning Opportunities will enable you to prepare case conceptualizations according to the modified Bloom's taxonomy and several of the other models presented here.

LEARNING OPPORTUNITIES

This chapter focused on some of the thinking skills and conceptual frameworks that clinicians need to understand, clearly and accurately, the nature and dynamics of their clients' concerns. These skills and frameworks pave the way for clinicians to make accurate diagnoses and effective treatment plans, skills that are presented in the next chapter. The conceptual skills included in Chapter 6 are

- Appropriate use of assessment
  - Mental status examination
  - Selection and use of tests and inventories
  - Client observation

- Identification and therapeutic use of defining memories
- Case conceptualization and problem definition
  - Concept mapping

- ○ Clinical factor analysis
- ○ Inverted pyramid heuristic
- ○ Stevens and Morris format for case conceptualization

The following exercises, like those in previous chapters, provide opportunities to apply the conceptual skills presented in this chapter. This section includes written exercises, discussion questions, exercises and an assessment tool to use in your practice groups, and questions to address in your journal.

Discussion Questions

1. The term *mental status examination* is misleading because it does not require an actual examination. What would be a better term for this process of gathering information to formulate a picture of a person's overall functioning?
2. Clinicians often disagree on the value of incorporating tests and inventories into the treatment process. Discuss the pros and cons of using these tools as part of the assessment and treatment process. What can clinicians do to maximize the benefits and reduce the drawbacks of using these tools with clients?
3. What categories of tests and inventories seem most useful to you and why? Least useful and why?
4. Discuss the benefits and disadvantages of the following four approaches to case conceptualization presented in this chapter. Which seems to have the most overall usefulness to clinicians and why?
   - Concept mapping
   - Clinical factor analysis
   - Inverted-pyramid heuristic
   - Stevens and Morris format

Written Exercises/Discussion Questions

The following exercises and questions are based on the case of Zane, age 13.

Presenting Concerns

Zane's school counselors suggested that Zane needed some special help with his emotional and behavioral difficulties. Zane's school performance has been satisfactory, but recently he has been in verbal and physical fights with several of the other boys in his class. Zane will not talk with the school counselor about these conflicts, so the counselor has encouraged Zane's parents to take him to a therapist in private practice.

Zane is active in sports at school and excels particularly at soccer. He tends to keep to himself at school, appears to have only one friend, and does not make any effort to develop new friendships or engage in group activities other than sports. Zane is somewhat stocky and is above average in height. He has dark curly hair and a medium complexion. He dresses in age-appropriate ways and always looks neat and well groomed.

Background

Zane was adopted when he was three years old by Alan and JT, who have been in a committed relationship for 16 years. Alan is a Caucasian male from a middle-class Protestant background and is employed as a journalist. JT is an African American male, also from a middle-class Protestant background, and is employed as a lawyer. Zane is their only child. Zane's biological parentage is unclear; his mother, who gave him up for adoption, was Caucasian, and she reported that his father was African American. This mixed-race background appealed to Alan and JT because it reflected both of their races.

JT and Alan have a strong and positive relationship with considerable involvement with Alan's family, including his parents and his sisters. JT's family does not live in the area and have not been as accepting of JT and Alan's relationship, although they do visit once a year and call occasionally.

JT and Alan seem to love and appreciate Zane. They take turns helping him with his homework, attend his soccer games, and try to maintain open communication in their home.

Client Statements

In the course of his first two sessions with a clinical social worker, Zane made the following statements:

1. I guess I'm here because I don't get along well with the other kids.
2. The other guys have been teasing me about having two fathers, and they say that I'm probably gay too.
3. Maybe I am gay. I like girls, but I haven't dated or anything like that yet. Some of the other guys have girlfriends, and one even said he had sex with his girlfriend.
4. I love my Dads and I know they love me, but I never know what to say to people when they ask questions. My Dads always come to my games, but I almost wish they wouldn't. Somebody always asks me, "Who are those two men cheering for you?" or "How come your mother never comes to a game?" I guess by now most everybody knows what the story is.
5. I'm not big on academics. I do ok, but that's probably just because my Dads give me so much help. They both have graduate degrees and are real smart. I know they want me to do well so I try my best.
6. I wish I had a brother or sister. That would make it easier.
7. None of the other kids at school have two Dads like I do. There's this one guy, he has a bio Dad and a step-dad so he has two fathers, too, but it's not the same. He also has a biological mother who sees him often. He and I have become friends. He really struggles with his step-dad, who sounds like a jerk.
8. The only time I really feel good is when I'm playing soccer. I'm pretty good at it, and people cheer when I do well. That feels great. Sometimes I imagine I could really succeed in sports.
9. I have a dog who's real special to me. He's a mixed breed, part German shepherd and part I don't know what. He was abandoned when he was a puppy, and we adopted him at the animal shelter. I guess he's like me in lots of ways.

10. I don't really know anything about my mother or my biological father. My Dads said they thought my mother had a problem with drugs and couldn't take care of me so she gave me up for adoption. She's Caucasian and she said my father was African American, but I really don't know much about my background. I wish I did.

11. My two Dads usually get along really well, but a few nights ago they had a fight. I don't know what it was about, but it really scared me. What would happen to me if they split up?

12. We have a system at home. Usually, JT gets me off to school; Alan has to start work earlier. Then they take turns getting home in time to help me with my school work and make dinner. I help with dinner too.

13. My Dads told me about a cruise for other families with two Dads or two Moms. They asked me how I would like that. I don't know. At least I wouldn't feel so different. But it seems weird to think people would want to be together just because they're gay or lesbian. I didn't really say anything about the cruise.

14. I don't know if my Dads understand how different I feel. They tried to talk to me when I had the fights at school, but I didn't say anything. I didn't want them to feel bad about being my Dads. I just made up some other explanation for the fights.

15. JT is much older than Alan; he's almost 60. Lately he's been taking lots of pills every day. I asked about it and he just said not to worry, that it was for high blood pressure and was no big deal. I hope he was telling me the truth.

16. Sometimes I feel like my Dads still think I'm a little kid. Just a couple of years and I'll be driving. But they still try to buy my clothes for me and worry about what I'm eating and how much sleep I get.

17. I don't have much free time. Between soccer practice and school work, my time is pretty full. I watch some television before I go to bed, but I don't do much else. Usually, if I don't have a game on the weekend, my Dads and I will do something, go to the beach or to an amusement park or to a movie.

18. I think my Dads would like it if I became a lawyer. I just don't think I have what it takes to get all that education. I'll be lucky if I get a degree from a community college.

19. My Dads said I could go to a really good college after high school and then spend a year in Europe after I finish college, but I don't like school much.

20. I did like a few things we did in school this year; we saw the movie *Romeo and Juliet* and we read a book called *Of Mice and Men*. They're both about love and friendship and how much people need those things. I know I do.

21. We acted out part of *Romeo and Juliet* at school. I tried to get the part of Romeo, but the teacher just put me in a crowd scene.

22. My Dads gave me some books about growing up and dealing with adolescence. The books made it sound like other kids my age are confused about who they are and what they want to do with their lives too. That surprised me, but it was helpful.

23. My Dads go to this church that makes a point of welcoming everyone. They have a sign with a rainbow out front. I feel pretty comfortable there, but I haven't really connected with anyone or gotten involved with any of the task forces.

24. My Dad JT is real quiet and studious; my Dad Alan is more outgoing. I wish I could be more like Alan, but usually I'm quiet like JT.

25. We live in a big house. My room is full of all sorts of electronic equipment. I'm pretty good at figuring out how to use all that stuff. I even showed my Dads some things on their cell phones and computers. Our garage has space for three cars, even though we only have two cars.

26. I'll never forget the day of the fight with Sebastian. I was just walking by him, and he says, real low, "You're a fag, just like your whole family." I turned around and looked at him, and he said it again. I just lost control and tried to punch him in the face. He grabbed my arm and twisted it and so I kicked him. By them, somebody had called the school security guard and he was pulling us apart and taking us to the office. Lots of kids were just standing around, trying to figure out what was going on. I felt so ashamed of myself, but then not all that sorry that I had tried to hit Sebastian.

27. I think I can remember the day I was adopted. My Dads say I probably can't remember that far back, but I think I can. I had been in what I guess was an orphanage with lots of kids. Then these two men came into the room and picked me up. They were so gentle. They had a toy for me, a stuffed monkey. I still have it somewhere. Then they put me in a car seat and took me home. They had cookies for me there.

Questions

In responding to the following questions, you may provide additional details about Zane, as long as that information is consistent with the information you already have about him. Some of the questions are challenging and call for the use of new skills and ways of thinking. Unless you already have clinical experience, I recommend that these questions be discussed in class or in a study group rather than being completed individually.

1. Prepare a mental status examination for Zane.

2. What types of tests or inventories, if any, would you incorporate into your treatment of Zane? Discuss your responses to the questions on pages 195–196. as they pertain to Zane to help you answer this question.

3. Do you think it would be fruitful to observe Zane in class or playing soccer? If so, what categories of information would you include in your observation?

4. Select one of the critical incidents or defining memories presented by Zane. Analyze it according to the modified Bloom's taxonomy. What important information does that provide about Zane and your plans for working with him?

5. Develop a case conceptualization for Zane using one of the following models:
   - Bloom's taxonomy
   - Concept mapping
   - Clinical factor analysis
   - Inverted pyramid heuristic
   - Stevens and Morris's format

Practice Group Exercise: Defining Memories and Case Conceptualization

Divide into your practice groups. In this exercise, you have the opportunity both to practice your conceptual skills and to further refine your fundamental clinical skills. As usual, record both the practice session and the subsequent discussion.

This exercise encompasses the following skills:

Conceptual Skills

- Identification and analysis of defining memories
- Case conceptualization

Fundamental Skills

- Reflection of meaning
- Open questions, used especially to elicit cognitions

As usual, in each dyad, one person will assume the role of the clinician and the other will assume the role of the client. The focus of this role-play should be a critical incident or defining memory of an event in the life of the client. The person in the client role may present an actual incident in his or her life or may role-play another person (real or imaginary). Presenting an actual incident in your life may have personal benefits for you and is likely to lead to a more powerful dialogue. However, this has risks, and you should think about what and how much you are willing to disclose and be sure to take care of yourself.

Clinicians have the following major goals for this exercise:

- To continue to use interventions that promote a sound therapeutic alliance
- To use reflection of meaning and other interventions to elicit and explore a defining memory

Observers play a particularly important role in this exercise. They should take careful notes on key client statements so that they can take an active part in the discussion of the case conceptualization following the role-play. This discussion will afford participants the opportunity to apply some of the skills presented in this chapter.

Timing of Exercise

Ideally, this role-play should extend over a 2-hour period. However, the exercise can easily be modified so that it requires only half that time. What determines the amount of time this exercise requires is how many role-plays are completed and whether the discussion of the case conceptualization is included in the exercise. Regardless of whether group members have the opportunity to assume client or clinician roles, they will play an active part in this exercise.

Each role-play should follow this schedule:

- Allow 15 to 20 minutes for each role-played interview, eliciting and exploring the important memory.

- Take about 10 minutes to provide feedback to the person in the clinician role. As always, begin the feedback with the person in the clinician role, focus on strengths first, and offer concrete suggestions for improvement. Remember to make this a positive learning experience. Feedback should focus on the areas listed in the accompanying Assessment of Progress form.
- At the conclusion of the role-played interview, if time allows, take about 20 minutes in your small group to develop a conceptualization of the role-played client according to one of the models presented in this chapter.

Assessment of Progress Form 6

1. What strategies were used effectively to enhance the therapeutic alliance and conduct a productive session?

   _____

   _____

   _____

2. Describe ways in which the clinician elicited and explored the defining memory.

   _____

   _____

   _____

3. Which interventions seemed particularly successful?

   _____

   _____

   _____

4. How might the clinician have improved on the use of these interventions?

   _____

   _____

   _____

5. Summary of feedback
a. Strengths:

   _____

   _____

b. Areas needing improvement:

   _____

   _____

Personal Journal Questions

1. List three critical incidents or defining memories that have had an important effect on your life. Briefly analyze the meaning one of them has for you according to the modified Bloom's taxonomy.
2. If you could create the perfect test or inventory for assessment of yourself, what would that instrument be like and what information would it provide?
3. Write a mental status examination on yourself.
4. What is the most important thing you learned from this chapter and its exercises?

SUMMARY

This chapter focused on conceptual skills associated with thinking. Particular attention was paid to conducting a mental status examination, making appropriate use of tests and inventories, understanding and analyzing important memories, and conceptualizing a case. The chapter presented an array of models to facilitate use of each of these skills.

Chapter 7 continues to focus on conceptual skills that help clinicians think more clearly and with greater clinical acumen about their clients. That chapter emphasizes the importance of developing accurate diagnoses and effective treatment plans and presents both of those skills.

Chapter 7

USING CONCEPTUAL SKILLS TO FACILITATE DIAGNOSIS AND TREATMENT PLANNING

OVERVIEW

Chapter 6 considered a range of conceptual skills and approaches, including the mental status examination and case conceptualization, that can help clinicians better understand their clients and find effective ways to help them. Chapter 7 focuses on two additional tools to facilitate those goals: diagnosis using the *Diagnostic and Statistical Manual of Mental Disorders* (*DSM-IV-TR*, American Psychiatric Association, 2000) and a systematic approach to treatment planning. Diagnosis and treatment planning are two of the most important clinical skills. Although some clinicians make more frequent and more formal use of these skills than do other clinicians, nearly all mental health professionals in all settings use and recognize the importance of diagnosis and treatment planning.

DIAGNOSIS

According to Hinkle (1994, p. 174), "At the foundation of effective mental health care is the establishment of a valid psychodiagnosis." An accurate diagnosis, derived from a careful and valid case conceptualization, contributes to the treatment process in many ways (Seligman, 2004). Diagnosis of mental disorders, based on the latest edition of the *Diagnostic and Statistical Manual of Mental Disorders* (*DSM*), is an essential clinical skill, for the following reasons:

- Diagnosis of a mental disorder provides important information about the symptoms associated with that disorder as well as the probable course of the disorder.
- Information presented about a diagnosis in the *DSM* can deepen the clinician's knowledge and understanding of age, gender, familial, ethnic, cultural, and other factors related to that diagnosis.

- Helping people to recognize that they have a mental disorder can reduce their guilt and self-blame, promote greater self-awareness, provide reassurance that they are not alone in their difficulties, and increase both their hopefulness and their engagement in the treatment process.
- Diagnostic terminology is a common language that enables clinicians from all specializations and theoretical orientations to communicate with each other and with insurance companies providing payment for their services.
- Records of diagnosis, treatment plans, and treatment outcomes provide a way for clinicians to demonstrate accountability, determine their areas of effectiveness and weakness, improve their work, and protect themselves in the event of malpractice lawsuits.
- With knowledge of a client's diagnosis, clinicians can make good use of the extensive research literature on treatment effectiveness to determine those treatment approaches and strategies that are most likely to ameliorate a particular mental disorder.

Clearly, knowledge of diagnosis and the *DSM* can be very beneficial to clients and clinicians. At the same time, the information, use, validity, and reliability of the *DSM* still needs improvement. Imprecisely defined disorders, clinician subjectivity and lack of knowledge of the *DSM*, and the frequent need to make rapid diagnoses to satisfy mental health agencies and insurance companies can lead to erroneous diagnoses. Clinicians should be sure they have the information, training, and supervision they need to make accurate diagnoses.

Although a detailed presentation of the current edition of the *DSM* is beyond the scope of this book, an overview of that volume is provided here to introduce readers to the skill of diagnosis and the range of mental disorders. A more detailed discussion of the *DSM* is provided in other readings (Seligman, 2004; Seligman and Reichenberg, 2007).

Multiaxial Assessment

The *Diagnostic and Statistical Manual of Mental Disorders* provides a multiaxial format for diagnoses. This format consists of the following five axes or perspectives, which help clinicians think about clients holistically rather than focusing exclusively on pathology.

Axis I: Clinical Disorders and Other Conditions That May Be a Focus of Clinical Attention—Nearly all of the mental disorders are listed on Axis I, including some of the most common diagnoses such as mood disorders, anxiety disorders, adjustment disorders, and substance-related disorders.

Axis II: Personality Disorders and Mental Retardation—As indicated by the title of this axis, only two categories of disorder are included on Axis II, personality disorders and mental retardation (along with borderline intellectual functioning, also reflecting impairment in intellectual abilities). Axis II encompasses disorders that, by definition, are long-standing, often life-long. Axis I, on the other hand, includes disorders that tend to be time-limited, although many of them persist for many years.

Axis III: General Medical Conditions—Axis III includes medically verified physical conditions as well as physical signs and symptoms that may be related to or affect people's emotional functioning, such as frequent headaches and loss of appetite.

Axis IV: Psychosocial and Environmental Problems—Axis IV is where clinicians list the stressors in people's lives. This axis may include

- Recent and circumscribed stressors, such as a relocation or job loss.
- Enduring stressors, such as coping with a chronic illness, poverty, or an abusive partner.
- Stressors that occurred many years ago but that are still relevant to a client's mental condition, such as a combat experience that led to prolonged posttraumatic stress disorder.

Axis V: Global Assessment of Functioning (GAF) Scale—On Axis V, clinicians rate a person's current level of functioning on a scale from 1 to 100. The higher the number, the better is the functioning. This axis is useful in assessing the severity of people's difficulties, determining the nature and level of treatment they require, and measuring their progress during treatment.

Following is the multiaxial assessment for Eileen Carter, the client who has been presented throughout this book.

Axis I

309.28: Adjustment Disorder with Mixed Anxiety and Depressed Mood
300.04: Dysthymic Disorder, Moderate
304.80: Polysubstance Dependence, Prior History

Axis II

Dependent Personality Traits

Axis III

424.0: Mitral Valve Prolapse

Axis IV

Problems with primary support group: conflict with husband
Educational problems: barriers related to continuing education

Axis V

GAF = 63 (current)

In this multiaxial assessment, Axis I reflects Eileen's recent anxiety and discouragement in response to her husband's efforts to stop her from attending college (adjustment disorder), her long-standing moderately severe depression (dysthymic disorder), and her prior history of misusing multiple drugs and alcohol. Her tendency to be other-directed, to defer to the men in her life, and to involve herself in unhealthy relationships is reflected on Axis II as dependent personality traits. Axis III alerts the clinician to the presence of a medical problem, mitral valve prolapse, which can produce symptoms resembling an anxiety attack. Axis IV identifies the current stressors in Eileen's life. Finally, Axis V, indicating that Eileen has a Global Assessment of Functioning Score of 63, suggests that she has some mild-to-moderate symptoms but is functioning fairly well overall.

Determining the Presence of a Mental Disorder

Although nearly everyone who presents for counseling or psychotherapy has problems or difficulties, not everyone has a mental disorder. Determining whether a mental disorder is present and, if it is, identifying the nature and severity of that disorder, is essential to effective treatment. *DSM-IV-TR* (American Psychiatric Association, 2000) defines a mental disorder in the following way:

> In *DSM-IV-TR*, each of the mental disorders is conceptualized as a clinically significant behavioral or psychological syndrome or pattern that occurs in an individual and that is associated with present distress (e.g., a painful symptom) or disability (i.e., impairment in one or more important areas of functioning) or with a significantly increased risk of suffering death, pain, disability, or an important loss of freedom. (p. xxxi)

This definition suggests the following series of questions that can help clinicians determine whether a mental disorder is present.

- Does the person manifest "clinically significant symptoms" such as depression, anxiety, impulsive and harmful behaviors, or loss of contact with reality?
- Have the duration and severity of the symptoms been such that the person meets the criteria for one of the mental disorders listed in the *DSM-IV-TR*? Although several of the disorders in the *DSM-IV-TR*, such as major depressive disorder, brief psychotic disorder, and adjustment disorder, have a minimum duration of days or weeks, the most common minimum duration for mental disorders is six months. In addition, although some people with mental disorders have Axis V GAF scores that are above 70, most people with mental disorders have GAF scores that are below 70, reflecting at least mild impairment.
- Is the person experiencing one or more of the following?
  - Significant present distress (e.g., overwhelming sadness, suicidal ideation, agitation and anxiety)
  - Disability, or impairment in functioning (e.g., problems in concentration, impaired performance at work or home, emotional exhaustion)
  - Risk of suffering death, pain, disability, or an important loss of freedom (e.g., extreme restriction of food intake, criminal activity, suicidal ideation, use of harmful substances)

Meeting these criteria suggests that a mental disorder may well be present. However, clinicians must also consider the client's multicultural background before concluding that a mental disorder is present. People with symptoms that reflect what the *DSM-IV-TR* calls an "expectable and culturally sanctioned response to a particular event" (p. xxxi) should generally not be viewed as having a mental disorder. For example, many women from Hispanic cultural backgrounds present attitudes and behaviors that suggest a dependent personality disorder. However, if these women enjoy their traditional role, function well in that role, and have adaptive flexibility, they should not be viewed as having a mental disorder but, rather, as thinking and acting in ways that reflect the norms of their culture. Similarly, people from some Asian backgrounds have spiritual beliefs that include reincarnation and communicating with people who have died. Again, clinicians must consider the person's cultural background in order to determine whether apparent symptoms reflect an unfamiliar culture rather than pathology. Multicultural understanding, sensitivity, and competence are necessary for skillfulness in both diagnosis and treatment.

The 17 Categories of Mental Disorders

In addition to the multiaxial assessment format, the *DSM-IV-TR* includes 17 categories of mental disorders, allowing clinicians to identify, describe, and better understand the nature of people's difficulties. A thorough description of these categories is beyond the scope of this book, but this chapter presents a brief overview of these 17 categories to provide some understanding of the mental disorders included in the *DSM-IV-TR*.

Disorders Usually First Diagnosed in Infancy, Childhood, or Adolescence

This is the most heterogeneous category in the *DSM-IV-TR* because it is organized according to typical age at onset rather than similarity of symptoms. This section of the DSM is particularly important for school counselors, school psychologists, and other clinicians whose work focuses on the treatment of children, adolescents, and families. However, this category is also important for clinicians who only treat adults; although disorders in this category generally begin during the first 18 years of life, they may continue into and through adulthood, often in a somewhat altered form. In addition, many adults have a history of mental disorders in childhood or have children who have been diagnosed with mental disorders. Understanding the implications of these diagnoses for adults and families can be invaluable to clinicians.

Clinicians working with young people are most likely to encounter three disorders in this category: attention-deficit/hyperactivity disorder (ADHD), conduct disorder, and oppositional defiant disorder (ODD).

- **Attention-Deficit/Hyperactivity Disorder:** Difficulty in concentration and attention as well as impairment in social, academic, and occupational functioning characterize people with ADHD. Those with the hyperactive-impulsive type of this disorder tend to be in constant motion and often interrupt or intrude on others. Those with the inattentive type of ADHD tend to be careless and distractible and have difficulty with organization and careful listening. People with both types of ADHD usually have impaired executive functioning and, even if their hyperactivity declines and their concentration improves with age, that impairment may continue through adulthood.

- **Conduct Disorder:** Conduct disorder is reflected by a persistent pattern of violating laws, rules, and social norms. People diagnosed with conduct disorder typically engage in behaviors that are aggressive, destructive, deceitful, and severely disobedient (e.g., repeatedly running away from home overnight).
- **Oppositional Defiant Disorder:** ODD is often a precursor of conduct disorder and involves less serious violations of rules and norms. People with ODD typically are temperamental, argumentative, angry and vindictive, touchy, and deliberately disobedient. Their attitudes and behavior can present a challenge to their parents and teachers.

Other prevalent disorders included in this first section of the *DSM-IV-TR* are mental retardation, learning disorders, motor skills disorder, communication disorders, pervasive developmental disorders (e.g., autistic disorder, Asperger's disorder), tic disorders, elimination disorders, separation anxiety disorder, and reactive attachment disorder. Less common disorders in this section are feeding and eating disorders of infancy or early childhood, selective mutism (refusal to speak even though capable of speaking), and stereotypic movement disorder.

Delirium, Dementia, and Amnestic and Other Cognitive Mental Disorders

Disorders in this section reflect cognitive impairment (brain injury or malfunction), generally have an underlying medical cause (e.g., Alzheimer's disease, stroke, a neurological disease, head injury, HIV infection), and nearly always include memory impairment. Neurologists or psychiatrists rather than nonmedical clinicians usually diagnose these disorders, but treatment may be provided by both medical and nonmedical clinicians.

Mental Disorders Due to a General Medical Condition Not Elsewhere Classified

Disorders in this category reflect mental and emotional symptoms that are the physiological consequences of a medical condition. This category does not encompass people's emotional reactions to upsetting medical symptoms or diagnoses, but rather the direct physiological consequences of medical conditions. Like the previous category of disorders, a physician generally should diagnose these disorders.

Substance-Related Disorders

This important category in the *DSM-IV-TR* includes harmful use of drugs or alcohol (*substance abuse* and *substance dependence*) and the side effects and emotional symptoms stemming from that harmful use (substance-induced *disorders*). To make a diagnosis from this category, clinicians need to determine what substances are misused, whether the pattern meets the criteria for abuse or the more severe dependence, whether physiological dependence is present, and which secondary or induced disorders (if any) are present. Common induced disorders include intoxication, withdrawal, substance-induced mood disorders, and anxiety or psychotic symptoms. Misuse of drugs and alcohol is widespread in the United States and can be found in almost every setting, ranging from elementary schools to geriatric facilities. Consequently, knowledge of this category of the *DSM-IV-TR* is important for all clinicians.

Schizophrenia and Other Psychotic Disorders

Schizoaffective disorder, schizophrenia, delusional disorder, *brief psychotic disorder*, and other similar disorders are included in this category. These psychotic disorders are all characterized by impairment in awareness of reality. Symptoms commonly associated with these disorders include hallucinations, delusions, disorganized speech, and catatonic or disorganized behavior. Hallucinations are sensory experiences that are inconsistent with reality (e.g., hearing voices when no one is speaking, feeling insects crawling all over one's body when none are present, experiencing oneself incorrectly as emitting a foul odor). Delusions are beliefs that also are inconsistent with reality and can include a variety of extreme and inaccurate inferences about reality. Common delusions involve ideas of persecution, grandiosity, and imagined romantic relationships. Because medication is the primary treatment for most psychotic disorders, their diagnosis tends to fall to psychiatrists. However, nonmedical clinicians are often part of a treatment team for people with psychotic disorders.

Mood Disorders

Mood disorders are probably the most common disorders encountered by clinicians in both inpatient and outpatient settings. One or both of the following symptoms characterize mood disorders:

- *Depression,* reflected by such symptoms as sadness, excessive guilt, hopelessness, irritability, loss of pleasure in one's usual activities, impaired eating and sleeping, thoughts of death
- An abnormally elevated *mood* (mania or hypomania), typically reflected by such symptoms as grandiosity, anger and irritability, rapid and pressured speech, diminished need for sleep, and unwise and even dangerous decisions and behaviors (e.g., investing all one's savings in rejuvenating a long-abandoned oil well)

The nature, severity, and duration of the symptoms of depression and/or elevated mood determine whether the disorder is a major depressive, dysthymic, or bipolar disorder.

- **Major Depressive Disorder:** Characterized by at least two weeks of severe depression.
- **Dysthymic Disorder:** Characterized by moderate depression lasting for at least two years in adults and one year in youth.
- **Bipolar Disorders (e.g., bipolar I disorder, bipolar II disorder, cyclothymnic disorder):** Generally include a combination of elevated and depressed mood episodes, although a single manic episode may be sufficient to meet the criteria for the diagnosis of a bipolar disorder.

Determining the precipitant of an episode of a mood disorder can be especially informative; episodes can be caused by seasonal changes in available light, by hormonal changes experienced postpartum, by an actual or perceived rejection, and by many other factors.

Anxiety Disorders

Like mood disorders, anxiety disorders are a common reason for people to seek treatment, especially in outpatient settings. Symptoms of anxiety usually are both emotional (e.g., worry, hypervigilance, fear, apprehension) and physical (e.g., shortness of breath, heart palpitations, trembling, chills, intestinal discomfort). Clinicians should be sure to rule out a medical cause for these symptoms before diagnosing an anxiety disorder.

Anxiety disorders listed in the *DSM-IV-TR* include the following.

- **Panic Disorder:** The primary characteristic of this disorder is attacks of overwhelming panic, at least some of which are unexpected and have no apparent cause. This experience can lead people to worry about having additional attacks and to avoid places they believe might trigger such attacks (panic disorder with agoraphobia).
- **Agoraphobia Without History of Panic Disorder:** This disorder is characterized by avoidance of certain places or situations from fear of having panic-like symptoms, although the person has not met the criteria for a panic disorder. People with severe forms of agoraphobia may be housebound, relying on others for all their transactions with the outside world.
- **Specific Phobia:** This disorder is characterized by an excessive fear of a particular stimulus, leading to avoidance behavior that causes impairment. A strong anxiety response usually ensues if the person inadvertently encounters the stimulus. Common types of specific phobias include inordinate fear of dogs, insects, snakes, heights, thunderstorms, injections, and flying.

- **Social Phobia:** Like other phobias, social phobia involves an excessive fear; here, it is the fear of humiliation or embarrassment in social or performance situations. Fear of public speaking is a common type of social phobia.
- **Obsessive-Compulsive Disorder:** This disorder involves recurrent obsessions (intrusive thoughts) or compulsions (driven behaviors) that cause significant distress or impairment. Common obsessions focus on fear of contamination, persistent doubts, the need to have things in a particular order, and unacceptable sexual or aggressive urges. Common compulsions, including washing and checking, typically neutralize and counteract the obsessions. Although people generally are aware of the unreasonable nature of their obsessions and compulsions, they feel unable to curtail those symptoms.
- **Posttraumatic Stress Disorder (PTSD) and Acute Stress Disorder:** Both of these disorders involve maladaptive responses to traumatic experiences such as rape, physical or sexual abuse, a war experience, a natural disaster, or an accident. People with these disorders persistently reexperience the trauma in thoughts or dreams, avoid reminders of the trauma, withdraw from others, and experience anxiety symptoms. Acute stress disorder begins shortly after the traumatic experience and lasts no longer than a month, whereas PTSD typically lasts longer and may have a delayed onset.
- **Generalized Anxiety Disorder (GAD):** GAD involves pervasive and excessive anxiety and worry, lasting at least six months. Both emotional and physical symptoms of anxiety are present.

Somatoform Disorders

Somatoform disorders may be thought of as psychosomatic disorders, although clients tend to find that term offensive. In somatoform disorders, people believe they have a serious medical illness or physical symptom and may experience associated pain and disability. However, medical examinations and testing provide no evidence for the presence of the physical symptoms or disorder. Probably the best-known somatoform disorders include *hypochondriasis* (belief that one has a serious disease, based on misinterpretation of existing physical symptoms) and *conversion disorder* (reflected by a sensory or motor dysfunction such as blindness or paralysis). *Body dysmorphic disorder,* a somatoform disorder in which people are preoccupied with a slight or imagined defect in appearance, has received increasing attention in recent years and may well be on the rise.

Factitious Disorders

People with factitious disorders similarly present with unverified medical or psychological difficulties. However, the primary difference between people with somatoform disorders and those with factitious disorders is that people with factitious disorders are deliberately producing or pretending to have their symptoms, usually in order to assume a sick role and receive attention, care, and sympathy. In somatoform disorders, on the other hand, people genuinely experience and believe in the symptoms and concerns they report. In *factitious disorder by proxy*, a type of factitious disorder, people produce or feign symptoms in another person, typically a child or disabled person under their care, so that they can indirectly gain the benefits of being in the sick role.

Dissociative Disorders

Dissociative disorders are characterized by what the *DSM-IV-TR* (American Psychiatric Association, 2000) terms "a disruption in the usually integrated functions of consciousness, memory, identity, or perception" (p. 519). Probably the best known of these disorders is dissociative *identity disorder*, previously known as multiple personality disorder. Identity fragmentation and two or more distinct identities characterize this controversial disorder. Other dissociative disorders include dissociative amnesia, dissociative fugue, and depersonalization disorder.

Sexual and Gender Identity Disorders

This category includes three distinct groups of disorders.

- **Sexual Dysfunctions:** This group encompasses problems in sexual response (desire, arousal, or orgasm) as well as pain during sexual activities. Important to the accurate diagnosis of these disorders is information on the duration, circumstances, and medical or psychological causes of these disorders.
- **Paraphilias:** People with these disorders manifest harmful or self-destructive sexual responses, urges, or behaviors. Their sexual fantasies and desires focus on objects, suffering and humiliation, children, or others who do not consent to the sexual activity. Common paraphilias include pedophilia (sexual urges or actions involving children), voyeurism (sexual urges related to observing other people unclothed or engaged in sexual activities), sexual masochism, and sexual sadism.
- **Gender Identity Disorder (GID):** In this disorder, people have both a long-standing discomfort with their assigned gender and a strong identification with and wish to be the other gender. This is a controversial diagnosis. Many believe that GID, like homosexuality, is not a mental disorder and should be removed from the *DSM* as homosexuality was a number of years ago.

Eating Disorders

The two eating disorders in this category, anorexia nervosa and bulimia nervosa, are particularly common among adolescent and young adult women but are on the increase among both younger and older women as well as among men.

- **Anorexia Nervosa:** The primary characteristic of this disorder is a body weight that is less than 85% of the expected body weight for a person of that height, body build, and age. Anorexia nervosa may be characterized by either restricted eating or by binge eating with accompanying purging via self-induced vomiting or other means.
- **Bulimia Nervosa:** This disorder always includes recurrent episodes of binge eating and may or may not include compensatory purging. Both people with bulimia nervosa and those with anorexia nervosa may engage in binge eating and purging, but only those with anorexia have the symptom of low body weight.

Sleep Disorders

Increasing attention has been paid to sleep disorders over the past decade because of the growing awareness of the emotional difficulties that can cause and be caused by these disorders. Sleep disorders reflect a wide range of difficulties in achieving an adequate and restful sleep and include the following, listed along with their most characteristic symptoms.

- **Insomnia:** Persistent difficulty falling asleep or remaining asleep
- **Hypersomnia:** Persistent oversleeping
- **Narcolepsy:** Sudden attacks of sleep
- **Breathing-Related Sleep Disorder:** Abnormal respiration during sleep, which can cause fatigue and, in the long run, possible heart damage and other physical problems
- **Circadian Rhythm Sleep Disorder:** Incompatibilities between one's biological clock and one's lifestyle, such as recurrent jet lag
- **Nightmare Disorder and Sleep Terror Disorder:** Recurrent troubling dreams
- **Sleepwalking**

Diagnosis of these disorders often necessitates an evaluation of people's sleeping patterns in a medical facility where they can be monitored and assessed.

Impulse-Control Disorders Not Elsewhere Classified

Many disorders in the *DSM-IV-TR*, including eating disorders, substance-related disorders, and the disorders included in the "not elsewhere classified" category, are characterized by a buildup of tension or arousal discharged via some harmful or dysfunctional behavior that provides a sense of pleasure or relief. Although guilt may follow later, problems in impulse control lead to repetitions of the harmful behavior. Impulse-control disorders not elsewhere classified include the following, listed with their most characteristic symptoms.

- **Intermittent Explosive Disorder:** Typified by impulsive and aggressive outbursts

- **Kleptomania:** Impulsive theft of items that are not needed or that have little value
- **Pyromania:** Impulsive fire setting
- **Pathological gambling:** Gambling to a harmful extent
- **Trichotillomania:** Impulsive pulling out of one's own head or body hair

Adjustment Disorders

Adjustment disorders are among the mildest of the mental disorders. People with an adjustment disorder respond with distress and/or impairment to a stressor such as a developmental event (marriage, graduation from school), a negative event or experience (diagnosis of a serious illness, living in poverty), a disappointment (end of a romantic relationship, loss of a job), or another type of stressor. Symptoms of adjustment disorders are generally mild to moderate in severity, begin within three months of the stressor and, by definition, last no longer than six months after the termination of the stressor and its consequences. These are relatively common disorders that usually respond well to treatment and, with effective treatment, often lead to personal growth.

Personality Disorders

Personality disorders are long-standing, pervasive disorders that are evident by adolescence or early adulthood and sometimes much earlier. People with personality disorders tend to have poor coping skills, limited insight and empathy for others, and inflexibility. They have a persistent pattern of dysfunctional thoughts, emotions, and actions that typically cause impairment and distress in many or all aspects of their lives.

The *DSM-IV-TR* includes the following 10 personality disorders, listed along with their essential characteristics.

- **Paranoid Personality Disorder:** The hallmark of this disorder is distrust and suspicion of others.
- **Schizoid Personality Disorder:** Lack of involvement and interest in social relationships, as well as a restricted range of emotions, characterize people with schizoid personality disorders.
- **Schizotypal Personality Disorder:** Hallmarks of this disorder include distorted perceptions and thoughts, poor interpersonal skills and relationships, and odd or unusual behavior.
- **Antisocial Personality Disorder:** With conduct disorder as a precursor, this disorder is characterized by lack of concern for the rights and feelings of others and repeated violations of societal rules and norms, often manifested in criminal behavior.
- **Borderline Personality Disorder:** People with this disorder manifest self-destructive instability and impulsivity in behaviors, emotions, thoughts, and

relationships. They often have multiple co-morbid disorders such as eating disorders, substance-related disorders, and mood disorders.

- **Histrionic Personality Disorder:** A need to be the center of attention, volatile emotions, unstable relationships, and self-dramatization characterize this disorder.
- **Narcissistic Personality Disorder:** Like people with histrionic personality disorders, those with narcissistic personality disorders crave attention and admiration. They have an exaggerated sense of their own importance, along with feelings of entitlement, often masking underlying self-doubts.
- **Avoidant Personality Disorder:** People with this disorder tend to be socially isolated, like those with schizoid personality disorders. However, people with an avoidant personality disorder shun social activities because of their fear of rejection, their negative self-image, and their reluctance to risk embarrassment rather than from a lack of interest in relationships.
- **Dependent Personality Disorder:** People diagnosed with dependent personality disorder usually have a strong need for protection and nurturance, reluctance to take initiative or responsibility, and feelings of helplessness and dependency.
- **Obsessive-Compulsive Personality Disorder:** Rigidity, order, perfectionism, and need for control characterize people with this disorder and typically impair both interpersonal and occupational functioning.

Other Conditions That May Be a Focus of Clinical Attention

Problems named in this section of the *DSM-IV-TR* are not considered mental disorders, although they may be a focus of treatment. These conditions are used to describe concerns of people without mental disorders who seek treatment or to label prominent problems needing attention in people who also do have coexisting mental disorders. Categories of conditions include *psychological factors affecting medical condition, medication-induced movement disorders, relational problems, problems related to abuse or neglect,* and a miscellaneous group of additional conditions (e.g., *noncompliance with treatment, bereavement, academic or occupational problem, religious or spiritual problem, acculturation problem,* and *phase-of-life problem*).

Examples of Multiaxial Assessments

Most people need extensive study of and experience with the *DSM* before they can use this valuable tool with ease and accuracy. However, this introduction to the *DSM-IV-TR* provides some basic understanding of the multiaxial assessment format and the wide array of mental disorders.

Review the following brief descriptions of clients, along with their multiaxial assessments. You will probably find that this information is more meaningful to you now than it was before you read the preceding material. Using the Learning Opportunities at the end of this chapter, you can develop some preliminary multi-axial assessments. I strongly encourage you to take coursework or training in diagnosis using the *DSM* and to further your reading on this important topic via such books as *Selecting Effective Treatments* (Seligman & Reichenberg, 2007) and *Diagnosis and Treatment Planning in Counseling* (Seligman, 2004).

Case 1   Ralph is a firefighter who was present at the September 11, 2001, collapse of the World Trade Center. Although he was not injured, several of his colleagues were killed on that day despite Ralph's heroic efforts to rescue them. Since that experience, Ralph has had considerable anxiety, difficulty concentrating, and hypervigilance, as well as intrusive and recurrent images of the towers collapsing. He has found it difficult to fight fires in tall buildings and has become emotionally detached from his work. This has left him feeling isolated, because his colleagues at the fire station are his only friends. Ralph has been a loner as long as he can remember. Although he often fantasizes about having close friends, he fears that others would reject him if they knew him well and so he tends to reject others before they have the chance to reject him. He views himself as having poor social skills, and he rarely risks meeting new people.

Multiaxial Assessment of Ralph

Axis I 309.81: Posttraumatic stress disorder, chronic, moderate
Axis II 301.82: Avoidant personality disorder
Axis III Ralph reports no medical problems.
Axis IV Problems related to the social environment, other psychosocial, and environmental problems: Present at collapse of World Trade Center, deaths of colleagues
Axis V GAF = 60

Case 2   Wendy, age 8, was referred for counseling because she has refused to attend school for the past month. Her parents are currently separated, and Wendy tells her counselor that she needs to stay home to take care of her mother and make sure she is all right. Wendy fears that something awful will happen to her mother unless Wendy is with her. Wendy becomes upset when separated from her mother, even when her mother needs to take a shower. According to the history, Wendy's father had been verbally and physically abusive toward his wife and sexually abused Wendy. However, Wendy refuses to talk about this and changes the subject whenever she is asked about her father. Wendy's mother reports that Wendy has been diagnosed with asthma.

Multiaxial Assessment of Wendy

Axis I 309.21: Separation anxiety disorder, severe
     995.53: Sexual abuse of child

Axis II V71.09: No mental disorder on Axis II

Axis III Mother reports that Wendy has been diagnosed with asthma.

Axis IV Problems with primary support group: Reported sexual abuse by father; Wendy observed father's abuse of mother; parents' separation

Axis V GAF = 55

Case 3   Sara, age 15, was brought to therapy by her mother after Sara told her mother that she had ingested 15 aspirins in an effort to kill herself. Sara has been feeling very sad for the past eight months, since her older sister and only sibling left for college. (Sara has never felt this way before.) Sara reported that she could no longer bear being without her sister. Sara reports difficulty falling asleep almost every night and states that "nothing is fun anymore," even riding her beloved horse. Sara also reports feeling guilty and rejected because of her sister's decision to attend college on the other side of the country. Sara has a thin and frail appearance, with unusually heavy hair growth on her arms. Sara has lost more than 30 pounds in the past six months and now weighs only 75 pounds. Although Sara assists her mother in making dinner for the family and does the grocery shopping, Sara says that she wanted to have a "more athletic" appearance and so has been deliberately eating very little. Sara also is coping with severe acne. Sara's grades have dropped from an A− average to a C+ average, and she rarely spends time with friends, other than sending them instant messages.

Multiaxial Assessment of Sara

Axis I 296.23: Major depressive disorder, single episode, severe, without psychotic features, with melancholic features

    307.01: Anorexia nervosa, restricting type, severe

Axis II V71.09: No diagnosis on Axis II

Axis III Reports severe acne, appears markedly underweight

Axis IV Sister's departure for college

Axis V GAF = 20

Now that you have reviewed these diagnoses, think about how the multiaxial assessment organized information about each person and probably helped you understand them better. At the same time, you might have had some questions or concerns about these diagnoses. Despite its shortcomings, diagnosis using the *DSM* is an essential tool for clinicians.

Ethical and Professional Diagnosis of Mental Disorders

Some clinicians are uncomfortable with the process of diagnosis, fearing that they will label or stigmatize people in harmful ways or make errors in diagnosis. Such concerns are understandable. Diagnosis using the *DSM* is a powerful tool that can facilitate treatment and thereby help both clients and clinicians. However, it also can do harm if it is misused. The following guidelines are intended to maximize the benefits of making diagnoses.

- **Be accurate.** Clinicians sometimes give little thought to diagnoses and focus more on the circumstances of people's lives than on their symptoms. For example, clinicians may assume that a client has posttraumatic stress disorder because that person has experienced a traumatic experience. However, diagnoses should be based primarily on the client's inner experiences and symptoms. Making accurate diagnoses often requires both time and thought. If clinicians are uncertain about a diagnosis, they should consult with a colleague, ask the client questions to yield the needed information, and take time to understand the client more fully.

- **Avoid underdiagnosis or overdiagnosis.** Clinicians sometimes deliberately inflate people's diagnoses in an effort to obtain authorization for additional services or understate their diagnoses to avoid putting in the record the presence of severe pathology. Both of these approaches to diagnosis are unethical and can have significant negative consequences for both the client and the clinician, including malpractice suits against the clinician, ineffective treatment for the client, and inappropriate denial of security clearances and future insurance to a client who has been given an inflated diagnosis. Again, accuracy in diagnosis is essential.

- **Be sure to maintain multicultural sensitivity and competencies.** People who come from a culture other than that in which they are currently being treated may present with emotions, thoughts, and behaviors that seem unusual and even pathological even though these may simply be a reflection of the person's culture of origin and belief system. Clinicians should exercise particular care when diagnosing the symptoms of multicultural clients. Before making diagnoses, clinicians should be sure they have an in-depth understanding of their clients, their culture of origin, and their adjustment to the current culture. What may seem to be symptoms of a mental disorder in one culture may reflect appropriate coping, adjustment, attitudes, and beliefs in another culture.

- **Consider discussing the diagnosis with the client.** I believe that clinicians should avoid keeping secrets from their clients. That can undermine the therapeutic alliance, exaggerate the hierarchical nature and power differential in the client–clinician relationship, and curtail the client's learning and self-awareness. As long as clinicians present information with sensitivity and clarity, most clients are likely to benefit from knowing their diagnoses and understanding the implications of those disorders for their treatment and functioning. Particularly important is sharing with clients information that may be transmitted to insurance companies, so that clients can decide whether they want their insurance company to receive that information or whether they prefer to pay for their treatment themselves.

- **Protect people's confidentiality.** Keep in mind that diagnostic information, like all information on clients, should be kept confidential unless the client presents a danger or authorizes others to receive information about their diagnosis and treatment. Even under those circumstances, clinicians should share only the information that others need to know.
- **Use diagnoses to benefit clients.** The primary purposes of making diagnoses are to improve clinicians' understanding of their clients, to inform treatment planning, and to enable clinicians to provide the best possible help to clients. Those goals should be kept in mind when clinicians formulate diagnoses and should be used to accomplish those purposes rather than simply to label the client.

TREATMENT PLANNING

A multiaxial assessment using the *DSM* is essential information for developing an effective treatment plan. Also important, of course, is a clear understanding of the client's goals.

Sound treatment plans succeed in helping people resolve their difficulties, ameliorate their symptoms, and develop strengths and coping skills that will assist them in dealing with future concerns and challenges. Just as a map facilitates the journey during travel, reduces the likelihood of getting lost, enables us to get back on track after we have taken a detour, and successfully guides us to our destination, so does a clear and structured treatment plan accomplish the same goals for counseling and psychotherapy. Like diagnosis, treatment planning is an essential tool for clinicians. Treatment plans have the following benefits (Seligman, 2004, 2006).

- A carefully developed treatment plan, based on a sound understanding of the client, the client's goals, an accurate diagnosis, and knowledge of the research on treatment effectiveness, provides assurance that the counseling or psychotherapy has a high likelihood of success.
- Written treatment plans allow clinicians to demonstrate their accountability and effectiveness. Sound treatment plans can assist clinicians in obtaining funding for programs and in receiving third-party payments for their services. Treatment plans also can provide a defense in the event of allegations of malpractice.
- Use of a treatment plan that specifies goals and procedures can help clinicians and clients to plan their sessions and track their progress. They can determine whether goals are being met as planned and, if not, they can make appropriate revisions in the treatment plan.
- Treatment plans also provide structure and direction to the therapeutic process. They help clinicians and clients develop shared and realistic expectations for treatment and promote hope and optimism that progress can be made.

Formats for Treatment Plans

Treatment planning, like diagnosis, has become an essential tool for clinicians. However, no standard or universal format for treatment planning exists. Each mental health agency and each insurance company seems to have its own preferred format for treatment plans. These vary according to the nature and amount of information requested. I have developed a format for a treatment plan (Seligman, 2004), the DO A CLIENT MAP, presented here along with a sample of an abbreviated treatment plan similar to those used by some insurance companies (third-party payers).

The DO A CLIENT MAP

The DO A CLIENT MAP is a comprehensive 12-step format for treatment planning (Seligman, 2004). The first letters in the names of each of the 12 steps spell out DO A CLIENT MAP, thereby serving as a mnemonic device to facilitate recall of the elements of the treatment plan. The name CLIENT MAP also reflects the primary purpose of a treatment plan: to map out the clinician's work with a particular person or group of people.

The DO A CLIENT MAP consists of the 12 steps presented next. Following this list are guidelines that should be kept in mind for each step when developing a treatment plan. Information needed to complete the treatment plan comes from the client interview, the mental status exam (discussed in Chapter 6), and any relevant and available inventories or records.

The 12-Step DO A CLIENT MAP

1. Diagnosis
2. Objectives
3. Assessments
4. Clinician
5. Location of treatment
6. Interventions
7. Emphasis
8. Number of people seen in treatment
9. Timing
10. Medication
11. Adjunct services
12. Prognosis

Guidelines for Completing the DO A CLIENT MAP

1. Diagnosis
   - Be sure to complete all five axes of the multiaxial assessment for the client according to the format provided in the *DSM* and described earlier in this chapter.

2. Objectives

- Ideally, objectives should be formulated collaboratively, with the client and clinician working together to identify important treatment goals.
- Objectives should be specific, measurable, and achievable by the client. Breaking large goals down into small, realistic objectives maximizes the likelihood of success.
- All treatment plans should include short-term goals that can be accomplished in a few days or weeks. If treatment will continue longer than that, the plan also should include medium-term goals that can be accomplished within a few months. If treatment will be lengthy, long-term objectives also should be established.
- To avoid overwhelming the client, each group of objectives (short-term, medium-term, and long-term) should initially include approximately three to six items. Other objectives can be added as progress is made.
- When formulating objectives, consider the DSM diagnosis, presenting problems, both observable and reported symptoms, and client's strengths. Objectives may go beyond a person's diagnosis but should certainly address any identified mental disorders and their associated symptoms.
- Formulating objectives can be particularly difficult when clients have multiple diagnoses or problems. Determine choice of initial objectives primarily by three criteria:
  - Those that will reduce danger to the client and others
  - Those that can be readily achieved, promoting the client's hope, optimism, and involvement in treatment
  - Those that will be meaningful to the client, perhaps by reducing the person's pain or making a difference in the person's lifestyle and relationships

3. Assessments

- Identify any important missing information that might be obtained through assessment. Examples of such information include medical factors that might play a part in the client's emotional difficulties, the client's intellectual and academic abilities, and additional information on symptoms.
- Consider both outside sources of assessment (e.g., physicians, neurologists, gynecologists, school psychologists) and assessments that the clinician might administer (e.g., personality inventories, interest inventories, measures of learning style and ability).
- Determine those assessment tools and resources that are likely to provide the missing information and enable clinicians to develop a more effective treatment plan. Additional information on this process is provided in Chapter 6.

4. Clinician

   • Determine those clinician characteristics that are likely to contribute to the development of a sound collaborative therapeutic alliance with the client. Consider not only the clinician's skills and experience but also the clinician's gender, age, multicultural background, life experiences, and personality, as well as the interface of client and clinician characteristics.
   • Ascertain whether the client has a strong preference as to the characteristics of the clinician. Client preferences should be considered when selecting the clinician in order to increase client motivation and comfort.

5. Location of treatment

   • Evaluate the client's living situation, support system, self-care, and financial resources as well as the person's motivation to get help, contact with reality, and propensity toward harmful or aggressive behavior.
   • Based on this information, determine whether the client is currently in a safe situation and is likely to keep regular appointments at an outpatient treatment facility. If the client is not in a safe situation, presents a danger to self or others, or lacks personal resources or support systems, consider a treatment program that provides a higher level of care, such as a day treatment program or an inpatient treatment program in a psychiatric hospital.
   • Once the level of care has been determined, decide on the specific treatment program that is most appropriate for this client.

6. Interventions

   • Drawing on the current research on effective treatment of the client's problems or mental disorders, clinicians identify the treatment approach (e.g., psychodynamic, cognitive-behavioral, person-centered, integrative) that seems most likely to help this client reach the objectives that have been identified. Clinicians should keep in mind the importance of empirically supported treatments and integrative approaches (Prochaska & Norcross, 2003) and, whenever possible, select treatments that have been proven effective in treating symptoms and disorders similar to those of the client.
   • For each identified objective, determine specific strategies that are compatible with the treatment approach selected and that seem likely to achieve that objective. Begin with interventions designed to achieve short-term objectives and then develop a tentative list of interventions to address longer-term objectives. Examples of interventions are modification of distorted cognitions, reinforcement, and teaching new skills.

7. Emphasis

   • Consider both client and treatment approach to determine how the treatment process can best be adapted to and individualized for a particular client. For example, the clinician might think about whether

- Treatment will emphasize the past, present, or future.
- It will be structured primarily by the clinician or by the client.
- It will be exploratory or seek to accomplish specific tasks.
- It will be confrontational or reinforcing and supportive.

8. Number of people in treatment

- Understanding people in context (e.g., as part of a family system, a community, a classroom, a workplace) can help determine whether they are likely to benefit most from individual, family, or group treatment, or some combination of those. Assess whether the client's concerns are
  - Primarily individual and internal.
  - Intertwined with family dynamics and the attitudes and behaviors of family members.
  - Characterized by deficits in social skills and interpersonal relationships, a lack of support and positive role models, or limited understanding of what is healthy and normal behavior.
- Determine whether combining two or more modes of treatment (e.g., individual counseling and family therapy) is likely to be more powerful than either alone.
- Determine the client's readiness for group or family treatment. For example, people who are fragile and fearful, who have feelings of rage toward their families, or who have extremely poor social skills often benefit from an initial course of individual treatment before group or family treatment is added.
- Finally, decide whether and when individual, group, and family treatment will be part of the client's treatment.

9. Timing

- Determining the optimal timing for the treatment process involves making a series of decisions:
  - Decide whether standard 45- or 50-minute sessions are appropriate for this client or whether, because of the setting, the age of the client, the level of motivation, or the symptoms, a shorter or (occasionally) longer session may be preferable.
  - Determine whether the standard weekly appointment is appropriate for this client, whether the urgency or risk inherent in the person's situation suggests more frequent meetings, or whether the person is relatively high-functioning and able to make progress independently, perhaps needing less frequent sessions.
  - Determine the approximate total number of sessions you think will be needed to achieve the objectives that have been identified.
  - Determine the pacing of the treatment process. People with urgent concerns, those at risk, and those who are relatively healthy and motivated probably benefit most from a fairly rapid pace, whereas people who are apprehensive about treatment, vulnerable, or well defended usually require a gradually paced treatment.

10. Medication

- Based on current research, determine whether the client's mental disorder(s) and concerns are likely to benefit if medication is combined with psychotherapy.
- If medication seems likely to enhance the treatment process, determine the client's attitude toward the possibility of taking psychotropic medication.
- If medication seems indicated and the client is receptive to a medication evaluation, refer the client to a well-regarded psychiatrist who collaborates well with nonmedical clinicians.

11. Adjunct services

- Because treatment typically progresses more rapidly if people are engaged in positive and growth-promoting activities between sessions, clinicians should usually incorporate adjunct services into the treatment plan. To identify those adjunct services that are most likely to enhance the treatment process, assess the following dimensions of the client's life:
    - Basic survival needs (e.g., a safe environment, food, housing, warm clothing)
    - Legal and medical needs and resources
    - Health, weight, exercise, physical activity
    - Employment and finances
    - Use of drugs and alcohol
    - Relationships and leisure activities
    - Peer support and role models
    - Life skills (e.g., parenting, assertiveness), education, and information
    - Cultural, religious, and spiritual resources
- Identify interests, problems, or areas of unmet need.
- Determine adjunct services that can address these needs, such as the following:

  Basic survival needs: Government assistance, aid to dependent children, subsidized housing

  Legal and medical needs and resources: Legal aid, health insurance, low-cost medical and dental programs

  Health, weight, exercise, physical activity: Exercise classes, weight-control programs, Overeaters Anonymous or other relevant support groups, clubs focused on particular sports (e.g., hiking, surfing)

  Employment and finances: Assistance with résumé writing, job seeking, financial planning

  Use of drugs and alcohol: Alcoholics Anonymous, programs for adult children of alcoholics, other 12-step programs, Rational Recovery

Rewarding relationships: Leisure activities, support groups, workshops on communication skills, volunteer experiences, community recreation courses

Peer support and role models: Relevant peer support groups such as Parents Without Partners, Tough Love, professional organizations (e.g., American Psychological Association)

Life skills, education, and information: Classes on parenting skills, use of the Internet, college courses, community recreation classes

Cultural, religious, and spiritual resources: Involvement with a religious or spiritual community, meditation classes, reading on cultural background

12. Prognosis

- Review the literature to determine the usual prognosis for treatment of the client's mental disorders.
- Review information on the severity of this client's particular mental disorder(s) and the client's response to any previous treatment. Prognosis may be less positive if the client has more than one mental disorder or has not had a favorable response to previous treatment and more positive if this is the client's initial effort to change and the client has considerable motivation and assets.
- Consider the client's strengths, resources, support systems, motivation for treatment, source of referral, and the likelihood that the client will follow through on treatment recommendations, along with the probable effect of these on prognosis.
- Based on all this information, determine the prognosis for effective treatment of each of the client's problems or mental disorders.
- If the prognosis is positive (excellent, very good, good), move forward to implement the treatment plan, being sure to evaluate progress frequently.
- If the prognosis is questionable (fair, poor, guarded), consider revising objectives, interventions, or recommendation for medication to develop a more promising treatment plan.

A TREATMENT PLAN FOR EILEEN CARTER

The following treatment plan, developed for Eileen Carter, the client discussed throughout this book, illustrates the DO A CLIENT MAP format.

Diagnosis

Axis I 309.28: Adjustment Disorder with Mixed Anxiety and Depressed Mood
    300.04: Dysthymic Disorder, moderate
    304.80: Polysubstance Dependence, Prior History

Axis III 424.0: Mitral Valve Prolapse

Axis IV Problems with primary support group: Conflict with husband
   Educational problems: Barriers related to continuing education

Axis V GAF = 63 (current)

Objectives

Short-Term Objectives

1. Eileen will identify at least two plans for continuing her education while maintaining her commitment to her family, as measured by written descriptions of plans.
2. Eileen will achieve a reduction of at least three points in her level of depression as measured by the Beck Depression Inventory (BDI).
3. Eileen will achieve a reduction of at least three points in her level of anxiety as measured by the Beck Anxiety Inventory (BAI).
4. Eileen will achieve at least a one-point improvement in her self-esteem as measured by a 1–10 self-rating scale.
5. Eileen will report at least a one-point improvement in satisfaction with her interactions with her husband as measured by a 1–10 self-rating scale.

Medium-Term Objectives

6. Eileen will finalize and begin to implement plans for continuing her education as measured by self-report.
7. Eileen's score on the BDI will be in the normal mood range.
8. Eileen's score on the BAI will be in the normal range.
9. Eileen will report improved and at least satisfactory self-esteem, as reflected by a 1–10 self-rating scale.
10. Eileen will report improved and satisfactory skills in communicating with and interacting with her husband, as reflected in journal entries.
11. Eileen will report improved ability to make decisions, as reflected by a decision list in her journal.

Long-Term Objectives   Long-term treatment is not anticipated for this client, so long-term objectives are not needed at this time.

Assessments

- Beck Depression Inventory
- Beck Anxiety Inventory
- Informal 1–10 self-esteem self-rating scale
- Informal 1–10 self-rating scale of Eileen's satisfaction with her interactions with her husband
- Journal
- Strong Interest Inventory, to assess career interests

Clinician   Eileen expressed a strong preference for a female clinician about her age or somewhat older. She also thought she might feel more comfortable talking to an African American woman, but was willing to work with a clinician who was Caucasian. In addition, her clinician should be knowledgeable about family dynamics, have multicultural experience and competencies, and be able to provide information on sound parenting and career and educational development as well as support and affirmation to Eileen.

Location   Because Eileen is in a safe situation, has considerable emotional health, and is motivated to obtain help, an outpatient treatment setting is the preferred location. Eileen might feel especially comfortable in a treatment setting focused on helping women with their concerns.

Interventions

> **Treatment Approach:** Primarily cognitive-behavioral therapy
> **Specific Interventions:** (Numbers after each intervention link intervention to objective.)
>
> - Identification, assessment, and modification of distorted cognitions (2, 4, 7, 9)
> - Information gathering and brainstorming to generate possible ways for Eileen to continue her education (1, 4, 6, 9)
> - Teaching assertiveness and communication skills (2, 3, 4, 5, 7, 8, 9, 10, 11)
> - Role-playing of interactions with husband, other students, professors (1, 5, 10)
> - Relaxation and visualization (1, 3, 8, 9, 10, 11)
> - Identification of strengths and coping skills (1, 2, 4, 6, 7, 9, 11)
> - Decision-making training (11)
> - Clarification of interests and related and realistic career goals (1, 4, 6, 11)

Emphasis   Because treatment goals include empowering Eileen and developing her self-confidence, she will be encouraged to structure and take the lead in her own treatment as much as possible. Support and reinforcement from the clinician will facilitate that process. Although treatment will focus largely on Eileen's present concerns, some attention will be paid to past issues, to prevent resumption of drug and alcohol use and to help Eileen forgive herself for mistakes she made in the past.

Numbers   Most of Eileen's treatment will be individual therapy. However, some couples sessions with her husband might help them to understand each other better and to communicate more effectively. Important in determining whether her husband becomes involved in her therapy is Eileen's feelings about including him in that process. In addition, once she has made some progress, Eileen might benefit from group treatment, perhaps with women about her own age who are seeking to balance family, career, and individual goals. This could provide Eileen with affirmation, support, role models, new ideas and coping skills, and a sense of community.

Timing   Weekly sessions of 45 to 50 minutes seem appropriate for Eileen. The frequency of sessions can be increased if she needs to make some rapid decisions. A treatment duration of approximately 10 to 20 sessions is anticipated. Treatment can progress at a rapid pace because Eileen is eager to move forward with her life and because she seems relatively healthy at present.

Medication   Because of the nature of her diagnoses and Eileen's reluctance to take any drugs, a referral for medication is not indicated at present. In addition, helping Eileen take credit for her progress in treatment is important; a medication referral might lead her to credit the medication for her improvement instead of herself. However, if her depression does not respond to treatment fairly quickly, the question of a medication referral should be revisited.

Adjunct Services

- Exercise class to alleviate anxiety and depression and promote relaxation, self-esteem, and contact with others
- Involvement in a neighborhood baby-sitting co-op to increase free time and contact with others
- Possible involvement in church or other spiritual community
- Possible structured activities with other couples based on interests reported by Charles and Eileen

Prognosis   Because they are long-standing and deeply entrenched, dysthymic disorders and personality traits can be slow to respond to treatment. Adjustment disorders, on the other hand, typically have an excellent prognosis. Eileen is motivated, has many personal resources, and has already made many positive changes. Consequently, the prognosis for her successful treatment is at least good if not very good.

The treatment plan you have just read follows the DO A CLIENT MAP format. It is detailed and comprehensive, providing a clear and logical plan for Eileen and her clinician. Many clinicians prepare treatment plans of this nature to guide their work with their clients.

An Abbreviated Treatment Plan

Mental health agencies and insurance companies typically use shorter formats for treatment planning, often relying on checklists and brief questionnaires. The treatment plan shown in Figure 7–1 is typical of these. It has been adapted from those used by several third-party payers and has been completed with information on Eileen Carter.

FIGURE 7-1 Mental Health Outpatient Treatment Report

MENTAL HEALTH OUTPATIENT TREATMENT REPORT

Client name: Eileen Carter   **Date of birth:** 4/17/79
Therapist: Merle Young, Ph.D.   **Date of plan:** 6/3/03

Client's initial reason for seeking treatment and current clinical condition: Ms. Carter sought treatment because she was upset at her husband's request that she leave college. She presented with mild anxiety as well as moderate and long-standing depression. She successfully cares for herself and her family and has been attending college but otherwise is rather isolated. History of substance-related problems and unstable relationships contribute to depression, low self-esteem, and interpersonal difficulties.

Mental Status: Ms. Carter is oriented x 4. She appeared tearful and worried; emotions were appropriate to the topic. Some mild impairment in concentration and attention was noted. Judgment and decision making also reflect mild impairment.

Indicate presence of any symptoms below, manifested by this client:

_____ Danger to self
_____ Danger to others
_____ Thought disorder
_____ Potential for loss of impulse control
_____ Potential for decompensation into more serious illness
_____ Potential for decompensation into behaviors dangerous to self or others
_____ Perceptual disorder
_____ Disordered behavior
__x__ Disturbed affect
_____ Disorientation
_____ Impaired memory
__x__ Impaired judgment
_____ Current substance abuse or dependence

Client's strengths:

SOCIAL

_____ Supportive family
_____ Network of friends
_____ Use of community resource
_____ Leisure activities
__x__ Other—commitment to family

PHYSICAL

__x__ Good health
__x__ Good personal hygiene
__x__ Good grooming
__x__ Appropriate use of medical resources
_____ Other

EMOTIONAL:

_____ Good emotional control
_____ Copes well with stressors
__x__ Good reality testing
__x__ Other—highly motivated

BEHAVIORAL

_____ Adaptive flexibility
_____ Sound problem solving
_____ Seeks and uses help well
__x__ Other—no longer makes harmful use of drugs or alcohol

Diagnoses:

Axis I: 309.28 Adjustment Disorder with Mixed Anxiety and Depressed Mood
              300.06 Dysthymic Disorder, moderate
              304.80 Polysubstance Dependence, Prior History
Axis II: Dependent Personality Traits
Axis III: 424.00 Mitral Valve Prolapse
Axis IV: Problems with primary support group: Conflict with husband
              Educational problems: Barriers related to continuing education
Axis V: GAF = 63 (current)

Treatment Plan: Describe current treatment goals and focus of treatment—Goals of treatment include alleviation of depression and anxiety; improved decision making, family relationships, and self-esteem. Treatment will be primarily cognitive-behavioral in nature, modifying distorted cognitions and improving coping. Skill development will promote better communication and decisions. Some attention will be paid to past issues, particularly to prevent relapse of substance-related disorder.

Frequency, duration, and expected number of sessions until completion of treatment:

Approximately 20 weekly sessions, 50 minutes in length, are anticipated.

Medication: Not indicated at the present time.

Adjunct treatment: Exercise class, peer support group.

Prognosis: Describe client's anticipated level of functioning after treatment—Overall prognosis is good to very good. Considerable reduction in depression and anxiety is anticipated along with improvement in decision making, communication skills, self-confidence, coping skills, and relationships.

Source: Seligman, L. (2004). *Technical and conceptual skills for mental health professionals. Upper Saddle River, NJ: Prentice Hall.*

This chapter, together with Chapter 6, focuses on conceptual skills and formats to help clinicians think more clearly and accurately about their clients' concerns and strengths and about ways to succeed in helping them. These skills provide a focus and direction for treatment, promote client–clinician collaboration and hope, and contribute to a mutually rewarding outcome. This chapter has presented the following skills:

- Diagnosis using the *Diagnostic and Statistical Manual of Mental Disorders* (American Psychiatric Association, 2000)
- Treatment planning
- Using the DO A CLIENT MAP format for treatment planning
- Formulating brief treatment plans

The following exercises provide the opportunity to apply the skills you have learned in Chapter 7.

Discussion Questions

1. Diagnosis using the *DSM* has become an essential clinical tool. However, as recently as 25 years ago, nonmedical clinicians typically had little formal training in diagnosis, and many chose not to make diagnoses. How do you explain this great change? What advantages and drawbacks do you see in the establishment of diagnosis as a mainstay of clinical practice? What do you think clinicians can do to maximize the advantages and minimize the drawbacks of that process?
2. Treatment planning is another essential clinical tool. What do you see as the most challenging elements in the treatment planning process? What can you do to facilitate the process of treatment planning?
3. The DO A CLIENT MAP FORMAT is intended to guide the development of a clear and comprehensive treatment plan. What topics, if any, would you either add to or delete from the 12 steps of the CLIENT MAP and why?
4. Some agencies and clinicians emphasize the importance of sharing a multiaxial assessment and treatment plan with each client. What are your reactions to this policy? What advantages and disadvantages are inherent in this policy?

Written Exercises/Discussion Questions

1. In Chapter 3, pages 74–75, you were introduced to Rosa, a 22-year-old woman with emotional, academic, and family difficulties. Go back to Chapter 3 and review the information provided on Rosa. Formulate a tentative multiaxial assessment for Rosa.
2. Develop a treatment plan for Rosa, according to the steps in the DO A CLIENT MAP on pages 220–225 and 230–231.

Practice Group Exercise: Diagnosis and Treatment Planning

Although the practice group exercise in this chapter, like those in other chapters, involves role-playing, only one or two of the dyads will engage in role-plays here. The remaining time will be devoted to development of a diagnosis and treatment plan for the role-played clients. In this exercise, both the role-play and the subsequent discussion are important in solidifying your learning of the material in this chapter.

This exercise has the following purposes:

- To conduct an initial interview that provides the information the clinician needs to make an accurate diagnosis
- To develop an effective treatment plan for the role-played client, in light of the diagnosis that has been made and the information provided in the interview
- To make good use of your fundamental clinical skills so that the interview flows smoothly and does not seem like an interrogation

Only one or two of the dyads will engage in role-plays during this exercise. Based on the available time and the preferences of the group members, decide in advance whether to have one or two dyads present role-plays and the participants' respective roles during the role-play(s).

Because a diagnosis and treatment plan will be developed for the role-played client, people in the client role should not portray themselves in this exercise. Rather, they should take on the persona of someone unknown to the group or of an imaginary person.

The role-play should consist of a comprehensive interview, with necessary questions softened through the use of other interventions such as reflections of feeling and restatements. Following the interview and sharing of feedback for the clinician, all four members of the group should collaborate in developing a multiaxial diagnosis and treatment plan for the role-played client. The treatment plan should follow the DO A CLIENT MAP format.

Timing of Exercise

Allow approximately 20 to 30 minutes for the role-played interview. Following that, allow another 20 minutes for the group to discuss and decide on a diagnosis and treatment plan for the client. Feedback to the person in the clinician role will take approximately another 10 minutes and should focus on the categories in the accompanying Assessment of Progress form. In total, then, this exercise requires 50 to 60 minutes for one role-play, and double that amount of time for two role-plays.

Assessment of Progress Form 7

1. How successful was the clinician in obtaining the information needed to make an accurate diagnosis and develop an effective treatment plan? What

topics, if any, should have received more attention? What topics, if any, should have received less attention?

_____

_____

_____

Describe the flow of the interview. What interventions enhanced the flow of the interview? What interventions might have helped the interview to progress even more smoothly?

_____

_____

_____

2. Summary of feedback

   a. Strenths:

   _____

   _____

   b. Areas needing improvement:

   _____

   _____

Personal Journal Questions

1. Before reading this chapter, you probably had some preconceptions about diagnosis and treatment planning. What were they? Have they changed? If so, in what way?
2. What apprehensions do you have about learning and applying the skills of diagnosis and treatment planning? What can you do to reduce those apprehensions?
3. In what ways do you believe that diagnosis and treatment planning can enhance your work with your clients?
4. Identify a concern that you have and develop a treatment plan to help you address that concern, including objectives, assessments, hypothetical clinician, location, interventions, emphasis, numbers, timing, adjunct services, and prognosis. I encourage you to implement this treatment plan so that perhaps you can effectively resolve your concern.

SUMMARY

This chapter presented information on two of the most important clinical skills: diagnosis and treatment planning. These skills give structure to the treatment process and increase the likelihood that treatment will be effective.

Chapters 8 and 9 focus on conceptual skills associated with actions, the fourth element in the BETA framework. Included in Chapter 8 is information on generating solutions, referral and collaboration, structuring treatment, and writing progress notes.

Chapter 8

APPLYING CONCEPTUAL SKILLS TO ACTIONS FOR POSITIVE CHANGE

GENERATING SOLUTIONS, REFERRAL AND COLLABORATION, STRUCTURING TREATMENT, AND WRITING PROGRESS NOTES

OVERVIEW

Chapters 6 and 7 focused on conceptual skills related to thinking, the third element in the BETA model. Those chapters presented ways of thinking about people and their difficulties to help clinicians gain a full and deep understanding of their clients and develop effective treatment plans.

Chapters 8 and 9 focus on conceptual skills related to actions, the fourth element in the BETA framework. These chapters emphasize actions that clinicians take, in collaboration with their clients, to implement treatment plans and move treatment forward to a rewarding outcome. These chapters provide the remaining skills presented in this book. Knowledge of the skills described and illustrated throughout this text can enable clinicians to provide effective treatment to their clients.

This chapter covers the following topics:

- **Generating Solutions:** The treatment process is often replete with challenges, both those presented by clients and those encountered by clinicians. Having strategies for addressing and resolving those difficulties can accelerate the treatment process.
- **Referral and Collaboration:** Successful treatment often entails collaboration of the clinician with other professionals, including other clinicians, school personnel, psychiatrists, neurologists, other physicians, and even lawyers. Understanding when and how to make a referral to another specialist and knowing ways to work cooperatively with those other professionals can enhance the treatment process.
- **Structuring Interventions, Sessions, and the Treatment Process:** Each intervention and session has a pattern. The pattern may be random, evolving differently and haphazardly over the course of each session, or it may reflect the clinician's efforts to plan a productive session. Purposeful structuring of sessions for therapeutic benefit is another action that clinicians can

take to increase treatment effectiveness. Similarly, the treatment process it-self has a structure. Planning the overall structure of that process in a thoughtful way and then following that plan—with some flexibility, of course—is another way of enhancing treatment.

- **Progress Notes:** Progress notes help clinicians identify issues that need contin-ued attention, assess the strengths and weaknesses of the treatment process, de-termine the optimal structure of future sessions, modify the treatment plan as needed, and track progress toward goal attainment. Writing clear and concise progress notes is important in giving sessions a productive and smooth flow.

GENERATING SOLUTIONS TO CLIENTS' DIFFICULTIES

Most people seek treatment because of a dilemma that has probably left them feel-ing immobilized and confused. They may want to make changes but do not know how, they may feel unfulfilled and unhappy but do not know what to do to feel bet-ter, they may have a challenging decision to make, or they may be experiencing a conflict between themselves and others. Understanding people's presenting con-cerns and helping them with these problems are essential to building a sound ther-apeutic alliance and promoting client motivation and progress.

Treatment is most likely to be successful and empowering if the client and cli-nician work together to address the client's concerns. However, sometimes people ask clinicians to solve their problems for them or tell them what they should do. Such clients might ask:

- "My teacher picks on me. What should I do?"
- "My supervisor gives my colleagues credit for work I have done. What should I do?"
- "I feel overwhelmed and can't stop crying. What should I do?"
- "I'm pregnant and my boyfriend says the baby isn't his. What should I do?"

These are only a few of the innumerable requests for advice that clinicians receive from their clients. Because clinicians want to help their clients, because they proba-bly have some good ideas as to what the clients should do, and because it is gratifying to most clinicians to find solutions to problems that have stumped others, they may be tempted to reply with a suggestion: "You should talk to your teacher"; "You should inform your supervisor of the contributions you make"; "You need to plan more re-warding experiences and perhaps see a psychiatrist for a medication consultation"; or "You need to determine whether he is the father."

Pitfalls of Giving Advice

Whether or not these are useful and helpful ideas, clinicians should be extremely cautious about moving into an advice-giving role for several reasons.

- Self-determination is a core value in the mental health professions; when clinicians assume that they know what is best for their clients, it violates the client's right to self-determination.
- Telling clients what they should do can communicate a lack of confidence in their ability to solve their own problems.
- Even if the advice is helpful in the short run, telling people what is best for them does not teach them to solve their own problems; instead, they learn that asking another person what to do is the best strategy when they are confronted with a dilemma.
- Many people have a "yes, but . . ." reaction when others tell them what they should do: "Yes, but I have already talked to the teacher," or "Yes, but I know in my heart that he is the father of my child." Perhaps the client has already tried the clinician's suggestion, perhaps the advice is not right for the client, or perhaps the client does not really want to be told what to do. Often, one "yes, but . . ." response leads to another, until the clinician feels discouraged and drained of ideas, as in the following dialogue:

Client: My teacher picks on me. What should I do?
Clinician: You should try to discuss this with the teacher.
Client: Yes, but she's so busy, she never listens to me.
Clinician: What about scheduling an after-school appointment with her?
Client: Yes, but I have to catch the bus right after class.
Clinician: Can you arrange to meet with her on your lunch break?
Client: Yes, but she has lunch then, too.
Clinician: Can one of your parents pick you up so you can stay late at school one day?
Client: Yes, but it's hard for them to get time off of work.

As you can see, this is not a productive conversation.

- If the client follows the advice and it turns out not to be helpful, then the client may blame the clinician for providing harmful direction. This can lead the client to lose confidence in the clinician and the treatment process and can even lead to premature termination of treatment.
- Although some clients appear to want the clinician to give them advice and suggestions, they may not really want that sort of help and may undermine the help that is provided. There are several possible reasons for this sort of interaction. Perhaps the clients want to prove that therapy is not helpful to them, perhaps they need to be in control, or perhaps their self-doubts make it difficult for them to believe that anything can help them. For a variety of reasons, clients sometimes sabotage the treatment process and seek to demonstrate that it cannot help them. Giving clients advice makes it especially easy for them to demonstrate that treatment is not working for them.

Benefits of Giving Advice

Despite the risks in giving advice, this process can also have benefits. Some clients with multicultural backgrounds, particularly those with Asian roots, typically view therapy as a place where they will receive answers and direction. Failing to provide this, especially if the clinician becomes evasive and does not address the client's request directly, can jeopardize the treatment process and, worse yet, convince clients that therapy has nothing helpful to offer.

Rapidly assessing clients' backgrounds and their treatment needs, without overgeneralizing or stereotyping, as well as understanding their expectations for the treatment process, is essential to forming a sound therapeutic alliance and providing effective treatment. In addition, giving sage advice can enhance clinicians' credibility, help establish them as role models for clients, and mobilize clients enough so that they feel more empowered and begin to generate their own wise advice.

However, the manner in which clinicians deliver advice is critical to its effect. Unless clients present a danger to themselves or others, clinicians should not give them the message that the clinician has the one correct answer to the client's dilemmas or that choosing not to follow the clinician's suggestions will be harmful to the client and to the clinician's interactions with and perceptions of that person. Let's look at some effective ways to respond to clients' requests for and expectations that therapy is a place to receive advice and solutions.

Alternatives to and Modifications of Giving Advice

What, then, should a clinician do when a client requests advice? Three general principles should guide clinicians' thinking when they respond to clients' requests for advice.

- Build on strengths that the clients already have.
- Facilitate clients' efforts to solve their own problems, so they develop the confidence and skills they need to continue to resolve their own difficulties.
- Be sure that clients have both direction and relief by the end of the session. Especially for those clients who are not well informed about the treatment process, clinicians need to respect their requests and address them in ways that are both respectful and rewarding to the clients.

Many specific strategies are available to help clinicians implement these principles in their work. The growth and development of brief, solution-focused therapy has provided the basis for some of these (de Shazer, 1988; O'Hanlon & Weiner-Davis, 1989). The following lists strategies that clinicians can use when asked or tempted to give advice. These strategies are illustrated with responses to the following question posed by a client named Juan: "My wife leaves her crafts projects all over the house; the house is always a mess. What should I do?"

- Help people identify strategies they have used successfully to resolve past problems and concerns. Facilitate application of those strategies to the present problem.

Juan had a business colleague who annoyed him with loud music and distracting telephone conversations. Juan initiated a conversation about the problem, beginning with identification of his colleague's strengths and then collaborating with him to find a solution to the problem. They agreed that the music and telephone calls would be restricted to the afternoon, allowing Juan some quiet time in the morning for his most demanding work projects. Initiating a conversation with his wife, emphasizing the many strengths in their relationship, expressing his concerns in a nonblaming way, and then seeking a compromise reflected transfer to the present situation of the skills that Juan had used successfully in the past.

- Brainstorming solutions to the problem can be a creative and productive way to help people resolve their own difficulties.

In this approach, the client and clinician collaborate in developing a list of potential strategies to address a particular problem. Both viable and frivolous ideas should be included, to stimulate discussion and allow the client the opportunity to think about and evaluate the advantages and disadvantages of each suggestion. Juan and his therapist developed the following list of possible solutions:

1. I suggest that we turn the spare bedroom into a craft room for my wife.
2. I clean up after her each evening.
3. I talk to my wife about this problem and ask her for possible solutions.
4. I leave my woodworking supplies all over the house so that my wife can see how annoying it is when the house is a mess.
5. I buy my wife a dog so that she won't have so much time to spend on crafts.
6. I just live with this situation and focus on my wife's many strengths.
7. I offer to help my wife finish her craft projects so that she can put them away.

Clearly, not all of these solutions are good ideas. However, the goal of brainstorming is to stimulate thinking and generate possibilities that can then be evaluated and modified until a good solution emerges.

- Review what the client has already done to resolve the problem and encourage new approaches based on understanding what has and has not had a positive effect.

Before seeking advice from a clinician, people have usually made considerable effort to resolve their own difficulties. However, people's repertoire of strategies tends to be limited, and they typically do more of the same rather than seeking new solutions. Bringing a new perspective into a well-worn situation and interrupting repetitive and nonproductive sequences of behaviors can be therapeutic and can help people see new and hopeful possibilities.

Juan's usual way of dealing with his wife's tendency to leave her crafts projects around the house was to nag and criticize her for her sloppy behavior. Although she might put her projects away temporarily, she would inevitably fall back into her old behaviors. Juan responded to this by nagging more and becoming even more angry and critical. This not only failed to resolve the problem, it also escalated conflict and tension between Juan and his wife. At the clinician's suggestion that he consider a new approach, Juan decided that he would try to praise his wife whenever he saw a slight improvement in the organization of her crafts and withhold his criticism.

- Teach new skills or behaviors that clients can use to resolve their difficulties.

Sometimes, people simply lack the skills or knowledge they need to address their concerns successfully. Learning these skills can provide them with new and more effective strategies and also can help them feel empowered and optimistic about their ability to resolve their concerns.

Juan's usual way of operating was to take charge and to tell people what to do. He perceived this as an effective way to communicate and to get things done. However, this approach was not effective in changing his wife's behavior. Other ways of communicating seemed to Juan to reflect weakness and to give away power, stances that were unacceptable to him and conflicted with his view of himself as the head of his household. His therapist gave him some reading on win–win situations and assertive communication and practiced these skills with him in their sessions. Juan recognized that other styles of communication could maintain his sense of power and control and yet enable him to negotiate more successfully with others.

- Finding exceptions or times when problems seem improved can direct people's attention to viable solutions.

Most problems wax and wane in severity. If people can identify what circumstances and actions contribute to amelioration of the problems, they often can intensify or build on those improvements.

Juan noticed that his wife was particularly likely to keep her crafts projects organized when both of them were experiencing little stress at work and had more leisure time, particularly enjoyable time together. Juan made a deliberate effort to reduce the stress in both of their lives, to spend more rewarding time with his wife, and to avoid bringing his business worries home with him. Reducing stress and improving their relationship led Juan to become more tolerant of his wife's behavior and led her to pay more attention to her husband's requests.

- Reframing a problem or concern can help people see it in a new way; this, in turn, can enable them to develop solutions that might not have seemed possible before.

Juan very much valued the warmth and comfort of his home and had viewed his wife's crafts projects as detracting from the beauty of their home. However, when his clinician suggested that her projects reflected his wife's creativity and domestic leanings, Juan could see them in a more positive light.

Many alternatives to advice giving are available to clinicians. Helping clients to expect positive change can enhance the use of these alternatives. Clinicians can promote this attitude by using what solution-focused clinicians refer to as *solution talk* or *possibility language*. Juan's therapist, for example, asked questions that implied a successful resolution to the problem, such as "When this problem is solved, how do you think it will affect your relationship with your wife?" or "If you weren't feeling annoyed about the condition of your home, what different feelings do you think you would have instead?" Emphasizing clients' strengths and coping behaviors, focusing on actions rather than thoughts or emotions, and using words that suggest change, such as "different," "unexpected," "new," and "possible," all communicate the likelihood of change. Particularly powerful are interventions that are compatible with the client's worldview, that use images and metaphors to change perceptions, and that are indirect and empowering.

REFERRAL AND COLLABORATION

Effective use of referral and collaboration is another important way to promote positive change in people. Clinicians generally spend 45 or 50 minutes a week in face-to-face contact with a client. However, positive growth and change are ongoing processes that stem not only from therapy but from many factors in people's daily lives. If clinicians can help people build into their lives additional sources of help that enhance their development and coping skills, the treatment process is likely to be more effective and efficient. In addition, as powerful as counseling and psychotherapy are, clinicians and their treatment procedures have limitations that perhaps can be alleviated with additional sources of help.

Today, counseling and psychotherapy are increasingly collaborative procedures. For example, residents in a correctional setting where I served as a consultant were assigned to a treatment team, composed of the following members:

- A psychiatrist, who monitored and prescribed medication
- A counselor, who was responsible for individual psychotherapy
- A peer mentor, typically someone with a history of criminal behavior and drug or alcohol problems, who was now recovering and helping others with similar difficulties
- A clinical psychologist, who provided a deeper understanding of the client via psychological testing
- A life-skills trainer, who taught program residents to manage money and keep a budget, locate appropriate housing, and develop other basic skills needed to function effectively in society
- A job placement specialist, who helped people identify their work-related skills and interests, apply for employment, and successfully begin working as they made the transition from prison to community

In addition, residents of this correctional program had the opportunity to participate in Alcoholics Anonymous and other self-help programs, to engage in team sports, to exercise regularly, and to take classes in communication skills, relationship building, and parenting.

Of course, most programs and clinicians do not offer such an extensive array of services. However, clinicians are increasingly recognizing the advantages of a multifaceted treatment plan and so are collaborating with other programs and clinicians to enrich the services available to their clients. In addition, clinicians often refer clients to adjunct sources of help that may enhance their lives. Referrals may or may not involve collaboration, but in either case, the primary therapist should oversee the treatment process, follow up with the client on suggested referrals, and, when appropriate, contact those other sources of help with the client's permission.

Social workers have long engaged in collaborative professional relationships, particularly with psychiatrists, and many social work training programs continue to emphasize the importance of collaboration as well as referral. Similarly, school counselors often work closely with teachers, school social workers and psychologists, and others in the school environment, as well as with clinicians in the community. However, for mental health counselors, and especially for psychologists, operating independently has often been the norm, and partnering with other professionals may be a new and unfamiliar approach.

Determining the Need for Referral or Collaboration

When clinicians think about including another source of help in a client's treatment plan, they should consider the following questions:

1. Does this person need professional services that I cannot provide?

   - Should the person have an evaluation to determine whether medication is likely to enhance treatment?
   - Does the person need a psychological evaluation to clarify the diagnosis or determine whether a specific disorder is present (e.g., mental retardation, learning disorder, dissociative identity disorder)?
   - Does the person need a medical evaluation to determine whether physical conditions are contributing to symptoms?
   - Does the person need to be detoxified from drugs or alcohol, or does the person need frequent screenings to determine whether that person has been using drugs or alcohol?
   - Would the person benefit from family counseling, career counseling, or group therapy?
   - Are there other psychological services, such as eye movement desensitization and reprocessing, hypnotherapy, or biofeedback, that might enhance treatment?

2. Is the person likely to benefit from participation in a self-help or peer support group? Such groups are especially useful for people who have the following types of concerns:

   - Drug or alcohol problems
   - Eating disorders
   - Other impulse-control disorders
   - Chronic or life-threatening medical problems
   - Major life changes (e.g., separation/divorce, bereavement, suicide of a close friend or family member, having a child with a severe emotional or other problems)

- Traumatic experiences (e.g., combat and other war experiences, natural disaster, physical or sexual abuse, or severe family dysfunction)
3. Does the person need more friends and social contacts, and is the person ready to interact with others? If so, participation in groups that reflect the person's interests, such as book discussion groups, hiking clubs, karate classes, or quilting groups, can provide possibilities for interaction and friendship.
4. Does the person have a need for increased physical activity? If so, joining a health club or participating in a sport can have emotional and physical benefits as well as provide opportunities for interaction and creativity?
5. Does the person have a need for government or social services?

   - Does the person lack financial resources for basic needs?
   - Does the person need help in locating safe and affordable housing?
   - Is the person seeking to reenter the workforce but facing barriers such as discrimination, limited skills, a need for child care, or lack of appropriate clothing?
   - Does the person have a disability that limits mobility and employment?
   - Is the person an immigrant or from another culture, and might that person benefit from either a closer connection with representatives of that culture or from services designed to help people from diverse cultural backgrounds?
   - Is the person over the age of 65?
   - Does the person need legal assistance but is unable to afford a lawyer?
   - Does the person have medical problems but is unable to afford medical care?

6. Does the person need help in acquiring information and skills that cannot easily be provided during the course of counseling or psychotherapy? Training in such areas as effective parenting, nutrition, study skills, and self-defense, among others, can be beneficial to some people.

Planning the Referral or Collaboration

Once clinicians have determined that clients are likely to benefit from professional or other services that are not provided as part of counseling or psychotherapy, the clinicians can plan the integration of those services into the treatment process. This seems to be more acceptable to clients if they are involved in making relevant decisions; generally, the clinician suggests a referral and then discusses the benefits and possible disadvantages of the referral with the client. Unless clinicians believe that referral is essential to continuing treatment, such as a physical or medication evaluation, the final decision about whether to accept a referral belongs with the client.

The timing of referrals often is critical to the eventual outcome. Particularly risky are premature referrals, which may put clients in situations that are threatening and uncomfortable for them. Referrals generally should not be made until clients have developed a strong working alliance with their clinicians, as well as the self-confidence and coping skills that will enable them to manage any discomfort and to derive benefit from the referral. Unless clients have an urgent need for outside help, clinicians should not make referrals until they have taken the time to get to know their clients, establish and begin to implement a treatment plan, and become confident that referral will be a successful and helpful experience for the client. Failed referrals, especially if they raise clients' self-doubts, can actually harm clients and jeopardize the therapeutic relationship.

Determining whether to have direct contact with the referral source is another important decision for clinicians. Sometimes the answer is obvious. For example, a clinician is unlikely to establish direct contact with the director of a bridge club the client is joining, but would almost certainly contact the psychiatrist who is seeing a client for a medication evaluation. At other times, the answer may require considerable thought. For example, should the clinician contact the gynecologist of a woman who has been sexually abused and who has been apprehensive about her upcoming medical appointment? What about contacting the person who oversees workers' compensation benefits for a client who has had a traumatic work-related injury? Contact should probably be made with these people, but only after thought and discussion with the client.

Of course, disclosure of any information about clients, even the fact that someone is a client, requires the client's consent, unless ethical or legal standards mandate disclosure of information to prevent harm. When clients agree that the clinician and a referral source should be in communication with each other to facilitate collaborative work and shared decision making, clients should sign a written release that permits mutual disclosure of relevant information.

Close collaboration is especially important between the clinician and a psychiatrist or other physician. The two need to confer about the effects of medical treatment on emotional symptoms and whether any psychotropic medication that has been prescribed is ameliorating symptoms or causing side effects. Although the physician may be the expert on medication, the clinician usually has more contact with the client and is in a good position to monitor the effect of medication and determine whether it is helping the client and facilitating treatment. By maintaining communication with psychiatrists and other physicians, clinicians can help prevent clients from discontinuing medication in harmful ways, failing to comply with medical recommendations, and giving up hope that medication can benefit them. Finding a helpful medication for a client often entails a process of trial and error. Enabling clients to understand that process and keeping physicians informed of clients' emotional and physical reactions to a medication can contribute greatly to effective treatment.

Application

Now that you are familiar with some of the options and guidelines for referral and collaboration, you can use the following questions to conceptualize and guide the referral process.

- Would some type of referral enhance this person's treatment?
- If so, what type of referral or outside service should that be?
- How do I think the referral will enhance the client's treatment?
- When should the referral be made?

- Should I, the clinician, obtain the client's permission and contact the referral to establish a collaboration?
- What information do I need from the client or from the referral contact person to determine whether the referral is accomplishing what I hoped it would?

The following cases illustrate the application of these questions to specific clients.

Client 1   Sheila is a 69-year-old woman who has severe arthritis. She has driven little since her husband died six months ago and is concerned about transportation to her medical appointments. Her sadness about her husband's death has been exacerbated by her own medical condition. She knows that she needs to establish a more rewarding life for herself but feels hopeless about the future.

- *Would some type of referral enhance this person's treatment?*

Yes, Sheila is coping with many serious difficulties and probably would benefit from some outside sources of help. She needs more help than counseling or therapy alone can offer.

- *If so, what types of referrals or outside services are appropriate?*
    - A support group for people diagnosed with arthritis
    - Sources of information on arthritis and its treatment
    - Information about free or low-cost transportation to help people get to medical appointments
    - A bereavement support group
    - Classes or groups focused on activities of interest to Sheila
    - A medication evaluation for Sheila's depression

- *How do I think that the referral will enhance the client's treatment?*
    - It should increase Sheila's mobility.
    - It should provide support, information, social contacts, and rewarding activities.
    - It should improve her mood.

- *When should the referral be made?*

Referrals for medication, arthritis support and information programs, and low-cost transportation should be made almost immediately.

Referrals for the bereavement support group and activity group should be made later, once the immediate crisis has subsided and Sheila's motivation and energy are somewhat improved.

- *Should I, the clinician, obtain the client's permission and contact the referral?*

The psychiatrist should certainly be contacted, to promote collaboration and exchange of information. Depending on Sheila's preferences, the clinician might also contact the arthritis and bereavement support programs. Activity-group leaders probably need not be contacted unless Sheila would like the clinician to pave the way for her to begin the activity groups or classes.

- *What information do I need from the client or from the referral contact person to determine whether the referral is accomplishing what I hoped it would?*

    ○ Feedback from the psychiatrist about medication recommendations
    ○ Self-reports from Sheila on her participation in and reactions to the support, information, and activity programs

Client 2   Chantha is an 18-year-old woman who arrived in the United States from Southeast Asia about five years ago. Although language and cultural differences play a part in her difficulties, other concerns are also relevant. Chantha left high school in the tenth grade and has had a series of unrewarding and unsuccessful jobs since that time. She reports great difficulty in learning and concentration, dating back to her early childhood. She is living with her family and has few outside friendships or activities. She reports some experimentation with drugs, a source of great shame to her. In addition, she reports seeing deceased family members, especially when using drugs.

- *Would some type of referral enhance Chantha's treatment?*

Determining the nature of Chantha's difficulties, as well as ameliorating them, is challenging because they seem to be multidetermined. Outside sources of help are indicated, to provide a more comprehensive and powerful treatment package.

- *If so, what type of referral or outside service should that be?*

A thorough evaluation of Chantha's mental health, as well as her learning and intellectual abilities, is indicated. This should be done by a clinician with strong multicultural competencies and knowledge of Chantha's native language and culture. Particular attention should be paid to determining whether current drug use, an attention-deficit disorder, a learning disorder, and perhaps a psychotic disorder are present, although Chantha's visions of deceased relatives are probably culturally related rather than reflecting psychosis. In addition, the evaluation should pay considerable attention to identifying Chantha's strengths and abilities to facilitate helping her mobilize her resources and motivation toward positive change.

The evaluation might indicate the need for a medication referral because of attention-deficit/hyperactivity disorder and depression. Career assessment, as well as career counseling and job placement, are likely to be beneficial for Chantha.

In addition, Chantha needs help in regaining her once-strong connection to her culture of origin and also becoming part of her new culture. More active involvement in activities related to both cultures might be helpful to her. Particularly important is involving Chantha in rewarding activities with other young adults.

- *How do I think that the referral will enhance the client's treatment?*

A careful assessment of Chantha's strengths and abilities will facilitate effective treatment planning and identification of job possibilities and activities that might provide her with successful experiences. She needs to increase her involvement with her new culture and become more self-sufficient, while still making good use of her cultural background, inner strengths, and family relationships.

- *When should the referral be made?*

The assessment should be conducted as soon as Chantha is willing to invest time in the process and appreciates the value it might have for her. If a referral for a medication evaluation is needed, that, too, should occur early in the treatment process. Other sources of help can be phased in gradually; the clinician should be careful not to overwhelm Chantha with many new and possibly anxiety-provoking experiences. Chantha should control the timing and sequence of the referrals.

- *Should I, the clinician, obtain the client's permission and contact the referral?*

Contact should be made with the person who is conducting the assessment, to clarify the reasons for the assessment, and with the psychiatrist, if a medication referral is indicated. Contact probably should also be made with the person who will help to facilitate Chantha's career development. Contact probably need not be initiated with the other referrals.

- *What information do I need from the client or from the referral contact person to determine whether the referral is accomplishing what I hoped it would?*

A complete written report of Chantha's psychological assessment is needed. The psychiatrist should be contacted to share information on Chantha and for a report of any prescribed medications and their anticipated effects. A verbal assessment from the career counselor will probably be useful. Chantha's description of the benefits and drawbacks of the other referral sources will probably be sufficient.

STRUCTURING INTERVENTIONS, SESSIONS, AND THE OVERALL TREATMENT PROCESS

Make progress toward goals and solidify gains—These are the principles that guide the structure of the treatment process. If treatment is rushed forward in a haphazard way without moving toward goal attainment or reinforcing gains, both clients and clinicians are likely to feel that they are floundering or walking through a maze without end. On the other hand, treatment that focuses almost exclusively on maintaining gains can feel like running in place; it may be rewarding for a time, but it will ultimately feel limiting and unfulfilling.

Consider the following client statement and the three possible clinician responses that follow.

Amalia: That role-play we did on talking to my supervisor was really helpful. I did talk with her and made progress in resolving the billing problem, but then my computer crashed and I felt helpless and overwhelmed again.

Clinician 1: What did you do about feeling helpless and overwhelmed again?

Clinician 2: So you really felt good about your talk with your supervisor.

Clinician 3: So you were successful in problem solving with your supervisor but lost some of your confidence when your computer crashed. Let's look at both sides of that situation. What did you do that worked so well in talking to your supervisor?

As you can see, the first clinician response ignores the progress Amalia has made, while the second overlooks her subsequent loss of confidence. However, the third clinician attends to the effective skills that Amalia used as well as their fragility: She felt overwhelmed again when another crisis occurred. This intervention is most likely to help Amalia see that she did make successful use of new thoughts and behaviors and to facilitate her application of those new skills to other situations.

The guiding principle of *making progress toward goals and solidifying gains* can be used at all levels of intervention: a single statement, a segment of a session, an entire session, and the complete treatment process. This principle promotes hope and optimism in clients. It enables them to see that they are moving toward the goals they have identified; learning new ways of feeling, thinking, and acting; and achieving some success through these changes. This is empowering and encourages people to meet new challenges and continue to move forward toward their goals. Using this principle from the intake or initial session onward can increase people's motivation toward treatment and initiate a sense of accomplishment, even in the first hour of treatment. Chapter 9 discusses the application of this principle to the termination process.

When structuring interventions, sessions, and the overall treatment process, clinicians should keep the following two guidelines in mind:

- *Collaboration with the client is essential.* The client's presenting concerns and goals, accomplishments and disappointments, motivations and fears all should be considered as both client and clinician work together to determine the direction of the treatment process.
- *Clients and clinicians should have shared, clear, realistic, meaningful, and measurable goals.* Those goals should be reflected in the nature of the interventions that are used, the structure and content of the sessions, the progress that is made, and the gains that are reinforced.

Structuring the Intervention and Treatment Segment

Not all interventions will follow the format of *making progress toward goals and solidifying gains,* but keeping this principle in mind can help clinicians ensure that clients take pride in and learn from their accomplishments while continuing to move forward toward their goals. This principle can also provide a sense of closure at the end of the treatment process.

Let's consider Amalia, the client introduced earlier. During treatment, Amalia described herself as a person with many self-doubts, who blamed herself when anything went wrong. She avoided dealing with problems because she feared that confronting them would only reveal her inadequacies. She and her therapist had been addressing Amalia's distorted cognitions that contributed to her self-blame. In addition, her therapist had been teaching her communication and assertiveness skills to help her deal with problems more immediately and effectively.

Amalia's job involved processing, checking, and paying the bills for a large organization. In a previous incident, she had failed to back up her computer records and consequently had lost documentation substantiating the validity of bills submitted by a particular vendor. Amalia dealt with this by discarding bills from that vendor for nearly six months, until the vendor threatened to contact the president of the company. With help from her therapist, Amalia planned and role-played ways to present this situation to her supervisor; Amalia accepted responsibility for the problem and acknowledged her errors but avoided her usual pattern of excessive and generalized self-blame. In addition, she developed two possible solutions to the problem that she offered to her supervisor. She made a commitment to her therapist that she would contact her supervisor within two days to implement this plan.

Amalia successfully followed the plan she had developed with her therapist. She contacted her supervisor promptly, presented the problem clearly and concisely, took appropriate responsibility for the situation, and offered possible solutions. Although her supervisor was dismayed that Amalia had not addressed this problem sooner and strongly advised her to avoid situations like this in the future, the supervisor did not attack, humiliate, or fire Amalia as Amalia had feared. In fact, the supervisor commended Amalia for her creative solutions to the problem and for taking responsibility for her errors.

Although this was a powerful learning experience for Amalia, her long-standing self-doubts remained strong. When her computer crashed again, the anxiety associated with her previous computer problem rushed back. She lost sight of her accomplishments, at least temporarily, and reverted to her former pattern of feeling guilt, fear, and self-blame.

For most people, once they have made progress in overcoming a problem, it becomes easier for them to draw on their history of successes to rebound from a setback. Keeping this in mind enabled Amalia's therapist to reinforce Amalia's gains and sustain her forward movement. After identifying both Amalia's accomplishments with her supervisor and the deeply ingrained negative responses Amalia had to the second computer failure, the therapist began by collaborating with Amalia to reinforce and strengthen her gains. Discussion focused on Amalia's courage in finally addressing the initial problem, her follow-through on the plan she had developed, her use of assertiveness skills, her willingness to accept appropriate responsibility without making excuses or devaluing herself, and her ability to formulate tentative solutions to the problem. Rather than praising Amalia lavishly, the therapist enabled Amalia to identify her own strengths in this incident and take pride in her successful use of new skills.

Attention then shifted to the recent computer failure and Amalia's automatic reactions of self-blame and hopelessness. The therapist helped Amalia to recognize the relatively minor consequences of this situation and enabled her to transfer successful use of her new skills to this situation. Amalia recognized that she needed additional training and probably also a more powerful computer to help her accomplish her job. She planned and role-played a dialogue with her supervisor in which she would request both of these. Throughout the process, her therapist coached her on ways she could continue to use and build on her new skills. With plans in place for Amalia to talk to her supervisor, the session was concluded.

This segment of the session with Amalia included the following seven steps:

1. Follow-up on plans and new learning from previous session
2. Identification of new presenting concern
3. Reinforcement of accomplishments and application of new skills
4. Exploration of new presenting concern
5. Establishment of link between new skills and new concern
6. Application of new skills to current concern
7. Development of specific plans to address current concern

The interweaving of new learning and current concerns, the application of effective skills to those current concerns, and the development of plans to use the skills to resolve the current concerns make a powerful treatment package. Such a structure can characterize a single intervention, a segment of a session, an entire session, a series of sessions, or an entire therapeutic interaction. However, it probably lends itself best to structuring all or part of a treatment session.

Structuring the Session

Let's broaden our perspective and look at an entire treatment session. Whether it is a 20-minute meeting in a school counselor's office, a 50-minute session in a private practice or community mental health center, or a 90-minute group or family counseling session, all treatment sessions have a beginning, a middle, and an end. In addition, all sessions have a sense of flow or movement, perhaps smooth and productive, perhaps rocky and erratic. Having a prototype in mind for the format of a session increases the likelihood that the session will be a smooth and productive one.

Many outlines for clinical sessions have been developed. Two useful ones, developed by Judith Beck and Allen Ivey, are presented here. Clinicians can use these as a basis for developing their own session formats that take account of the nature of their clients, the clinical setting, the length of the sessions, typical client concerns, and treatment goals.

Judith Beck (1995), a cognitive therapist, advocates the importance of having a clear and consistent structure to treatment sessions. The following 10-step format is typical of Beck's sessions:

1. Collaborate with the client to establish a meaningful agenda for the session.
2. Determine and measure the intensity of the person's mood.
3. Identify and discuss current concerns.
4. Establish clear and meaningful goals for the session.
5. Embed the current concerns in context, focusing especially on similar concerns that the client has handled successfully.
6. Help the client to identify connections between current concerns and past difficulties.

7. Draw on past successes and promote development of new skills that will help the client resolve current concerns.
8. Suggest tasks to be completed between sessions.
9. Summarize the session.
10. Elicit client feedback on the session.

Allen Ivey and his colleagues (Ivey, Ivey, & Simek-Morgan, 1997), in a similar effort to develop a prototype for a clinical interview, suggest that a treatment session should include the following five steps:

1. Establish rapport and structure the interview.
2. Gather information on concerns, strengths, and resources.
3. Define desired outcomes.
4. Generate alternatives and address obstacles to successful resolution of difficulties.
5. Generalize and transfer learning.

Although Beck and Ivey have different theoretical orientations, with Beck advocating cognitive therapy and Ivey, a developer and proponent of developmental counseling and therapy (DCT), considerable similarity is evident in their session prototypes. Both include the following three stages:

1. Beginning

   - Development and strengthening of rapport, communicating a warm and welcoming presence as well as optimism and hope.
   - Review of previous session and outcome of homework tasks, which ease the client into the session and open the dialogue. Clinicians should take a stance of curiosity about homework tasks and avoid being judgmental. People often do not complete tasks as planned; nevertheless, learning can almost always be gleaned from their efforts and even from their avoidance of tasks.
   - Assessment of current mood: Improvement should be reinforced, and contributing factors underscored and strengthened, while a worsening mood may become the focus of the session and the clinician's interventions.
   - Presentation of immediate concerns and issues: Clients often want to review their week with their therapists; kept within limits, this can promote rapport and continuity of sessions. Honing in on the most important concerns so that the goals of the session can be established, however, is the primary task of this phase of the session.
   - Identification of desired outcomes—in other words, the learning and skills that would help the client deal effectively with the identified concerns while simultaneously enhancing that person's strengths.

2. Middle

   - Identification and reinforcement of accomplishments and new learning, with particular attention to helping clients recognize how they made good use of their strengths and abilities.
   - Exploration of immediate concerns and issues in greater depth.

- Linking of immediate concerns and issues to context (history, other concerns, accomplishments, and new learning).
- Development of ways to resolve and manage current concerns: This may involve clinicians helping clients to make shifts in thinking, feeling, and acting; using role-plays and other in-session learning and practice experiences; providing teaching and demonstration of new skills; as well as incorporating into the session brainstorming, relaxation, imagery, and other interventions.
- Reviewing, practicing, and clarifying application of relevant skills that can promote personal growth and resolution of current concerns.

3. End

- Consolidation of learning: This moves the session into a winding-down mode that prepares clients for the end of the session.
- Development of a detailed plan to continue addressing concerns, agreed on by both client and clinician, and written down for the client's reference and review.
- Suggestion of relevant between-session tasks, usually ones relevant to the concerns addressed during the middle section of the session, and agreement on tasks the client will undertake between sessions.
- Summarization of the session, generally begun by the client with additions from the clinician.
- Eliciting client feedback and wrapping up the session, setting the next appointment, and perhaps a final mention of gains made and agreed-on tasks.

Structuring the Treatment Process

Like a session, the treatment process has a beginning, a middle, and an end. The point at which one phase of treatment stops and another begins is usually unclear, and treatment often needs to dip back temporarily into an earlier phase. However, keeping the following three stages in mind can help ensure the success of treatment. Considerable progress needs to be made toward achievement of the goals of each stage before treatment can move successfully on to the next stage. The objectives and procedures of the three stages of the treatment process can be conceptualized as follows:

1. Beginning

- Provide information on the treatment process, including ethical guidelines, the clinician's training and theoretical orientation, school or agency policies, procedures (e.g., billing, scheduling, cancellations, emergencies), and the appropriate roles of client and clinician (role induction).
- Explore the client's immediate reasons for seeking treatment (referral source, precipitants for scheduling appointment), expectations for treatment, and presenting concerns.
- Begin to develop rapport and a positive therapeutic alliance. Use empathy, demonstrate warmth and caring, and convey hope and optimism from the first moment of contact. View the client as a partner and think in collaborative terms.

- Gather information on the client's history and cultural background, symptoms and difficulties, emotions, thoughts, and actions, usually via an intake interview.
- Develop a mental status examination as well as a diagnosis and case conceptualization.
- Help the client identify and clarify strengths and assets.
- Working collaboratively with the client, establish clear, specific, realistic, meaningful, and measurable treatment goals.
- Determine treatment approaches and strategies that are likely to promote client development and ameliorate the client's concerns, and organize treatment information into a clear treatment plan.

2. Middle

- Apply treatment approaches and strategies to client issues.
- Teach the client skills that can lead to growth and problem resolution.
- Enhance and build on the client's strengths, as well as feelings of empowerment and optimism.
- Track progress and revise the treatment plan as needed.
- Reinforce and promote generalization of learning and progress.
- Apply these steps to additional areas of concern as needed.

3. End

- Determine that the client has achieved adequate realization of goals.
- Determine that no new goals warrant treatment at present.
- Consolidate, reinforce, and generalize learning and new skills.
- Provide relapse-prevention strategies.
- Decide collaboratively when to terminate treatment, carefully planning that process and celebrating the accomplishment it reflects as well as any losses and disappointments. More will be said about termination in Chapter 9.
- Share feedback regarding the treatment process and conclude treatment, assuring the client that he or she can return at a later date if needed to address new concerns or issues of relapse.

PROGRESS NOTES

Growing emphasis on accountability, concern about malpractice suits, and especially the importance of clinicians' goals of providing the best possible treatment to their clients have combined to make progress notes an important component of the treatment process. Today's clinicians are expected to keep records of their diagnoses, their treatment plans, the process of their sessions, and the outcomes of their work. Having prototypes in mind for each session and for the overall treatment process, such as those presented in this chapter, facilitate the writing of progress notes (also known as process notes or session notes).

Clear, concise, and accurate progress notes have many advantages. They can

- Remind the clinician of the issues, content, and progress of previous sessions with a client.

- Remind the clinician of topics and tasks from a previous session that should be addressed in a future session.
- Facilitate assessment of treatment effectiveness.
- Allow the clinician to track the overall treatment process and determine whether adequate progress is being made.
- Facilitate communication with other mental health treatment providers. This is particularly important if the client is subsequently seen by another clinician.
- Help the clinician document the treatment process and demonstrate that appropriate treatment has been provided, in case legal or ethical questions are raised about the treatment.

Progress notes can be made in a chart, in a computer file (as long as confidentiality is maintained), or simply on a blank piece of paper, stored in a secure and locked file cabinet. Progress notes should include the date of the session, the name (and sometimes the birth date) of the client, information on the content and process of the session, and the signature of the clinician who wrote the progress notes. Progress notes should be brief and concise, containing essential information about the session. Paring down the rich content of a session to a brief but informative paragraph or two is usually the most challenging aspect of writing progress notes.

Formats for the content of progress notes vary. Some clinicians have developed their own structure for these notes; others follow formats used by their schools or agencies. Several standardized formats also have been developed.

SOAP Format

The SOAP format is widely used, especially in medical settings (Law, Morocco, & Wilmarth, 1981). The acronym SOAP represents four elements in the progress notes (Subjective, Objective, Analysis, Plans). Descriptions of these elements follow, along with a question that reflects the substance of that element. Answering the questions associated with each element can help clinicians develop a progress note for a given session.

Subjective: This section includes the clinicians' impressions of the client and the session, addressing such topics as the nature of the therapeutic alliance, the client's mood and level of functioning, and progress made since the prior session.

- **Question:** What were your impressions of the client during this session; particularly, what progress or backsliding was evident?

Objective: This section provides information on the content of the session and any important experiences or concrete changes in the client and the client's life (e.g., taking a new job, applying to college).

- **Question:** What was the focus of this session, and what new information did you learn about the client?

Analysis: In this section, clinicians make sense of the subjective and objective information presented, interpreting and commenting on the significance of the information.

- **Question:** What is the significance of your observations and the information provided during this session in terms of your understanding of the client and the direction of treatment?

Plans: In the last section of a progress note, clinicians develop short-term treatment plans. Particular attention should be given to suggested between-session tasks, important topics that need to be discussed further, other issues that need attention or follow-up, accomplishments that should be further reinforced, and plans for future interventions.

- **Question:** What tasks did you suggest to the client, and what are your plans for the next session with this person?

Example of a Progress Note Following the SOAP Format

December 2, 2007—7th individual session with Gregory O'Malley (D.O.B. 7/14/80)

Gregory arrived late for the session, avoided making eye contact, and seemed anxious and uncomfortable throughout the session *(Subjective)*. He reported that he had two drinks following an unsuccessful job interview, and he was disappointed that he had only maintained his sobriety for three months. Conflict with his wife escalated as a result of Gregory's drinking *(Objective)*. Despite some good initial use of stress management and other coping skills, Gregory was unable to maintain his abstinence from alcohol when confronted with stress and perceived rejection. He continues to need help in both understanding the risk of relapse and in strengthening his coping skills. I helped Gregory identify the triggers for his relapse and taught him to make better use of relaxation and stress management skills *(Analysis)*. Gregory agreed to practice the skills reviewed in this session and to attend an extra AA meeting each week. The next sessions should follow up on these plans and continue to strengthen his ability to remain alcohol-free. Attention should also be given to Gregory's interactions with his wife. Clinician: Diana Rodriguez, Ph.D., Licensed Psychologist

STIPS Format

Another format for progress notes is the STIPS format (Prieto & Scheel, 2002). Here, too, the acronym represents the five elements in the progress notes.

Signs and Symptoms (S): This first part of the progress note describes the client's current level of functioning, along with clinical symptoms and significant changes from the previous session. This is similar to a very brief mental status examination.

Topics of Discussion (T): The issues discussed in the session, as well as any changes in the client's symptoms, concerns, coping skills, and lifestyle, are recorded in this section.

Interventions (I): Here, clinicians describe the treatment approach, along with specific interventions, used in the session to address the client's concerns.

Progress and Plans (P): This section of the progress note describes indications of client improvement as well as difficulties encountered in the session and other obstacles to client progress. Plans for the next session also are included here.

Special Issues (S): New issues are included here, along with a description of critical client dynamics such as suicidal ideation, dangerousness, or loss of contact with reality.

Think about which of these models for progress notes you prefer and which seems most likely to help you in your work. Both the SOAP and STIPS formats are better suited to clinical than school settings, but they can be used in modified or abbreviated ways in all settings. Perhaps you will decide to revise one of these models or develop one of your own that is well suited to your clinical setting, or perhaps your school or agency has its own model for progress notes. The Learning Opportunities provide an exercise in which you are encouraged to write some progress notes.

LEARNING OPPORTUNITIES

This chapter focused on actions, primarily those that clinicians perform as part of their work. The action-oriented conceptual skills presented in this chapter include

- Helping clients generate solutions to their concerns
- Making referrals to and collaborating with other clinicians and helping professionals
- Structuring interventions, sessions, and treatment plans
- Writing progress notes

The following exercises provide the opportunity to apply the conceptual skills that have been presented in this chapter.

Written Exercises/Discussion Questions

1. Review the case of Rosa in Chapter 3, beginning on page 74—75. What types of referral sources, if any, do you think would be helpful to Rosa? What is the rationale for your recommendations?
2. Review the following progress note. Then rewrite it in the STIPS or SOAP format for progress notes.

   Rosa came to her session about 10 minutes late, looking upset and disheveled. Once she began talking, it was difficult to stop her. She had a great deal on her mind. She talked about her fear when her dog was lost for two days, her mother and stepfather's possible divorce, her discomfort with her stepfather, and the departure of her best friend for college. She also talked about her unsuccessful efforts to lose weight and how badly she felt when young men in her neighborhood called her "Two-Ton Mama." She seemed more anxious than depressed, but her mood shifted rapidly; positive feelings were evident only when she talked about the return of her dog. I tried to provide Rosa with considerable empathy and support, but that failed to slow her down and I wasn't even sure she heard me some of the time. Finally, we started to review her diet and exercise plan, but she really hadn't made any progress with that. My suggested tasks seem to have been too ambitious. She may need more time to vent, but that doesn't seem productive; I need to help her focus on realistic ways to make small changes and move forward.

3. This chapter provided information on the typical ingredients of the beginning, middle, and ending phases of the treatment process. Based on the case of Rosa, discuss or write down a list of goals and interventions for each of the three phases of treatment.

4. Although clinicians generally avoid giving clients direct advice, some clients and situations warrant advice giving as part of the treatment process. How would you decide whether to give a client advice? What client characteristics, problems, interactions, or elements in the therapeutic relationship make it likely that you would give a person advice? What client characteristics, problems, interactions, or elements in the therapeutic relationship make it unlikely that you would give a person advice?

Discussion Questions

1. What do you believe to be the ideal model for collaboration between a nonmedical psychotherapist who is providing counseling or therapy and a psychiatrist who is providing medication for the same client? What are the differences in the roles of these two people? What overlap is likely to exist? How would you handle the situation if a psychiatrist seemed to be doing therapy with a client whom you had referred only for medication?

2. The following examples illustrate clients requesting advice from their clinicians. Drawing on what you have learned about ways to help people generate solutions to their own problems, discuss how you would respond to each of these clients, if you were the clinician, and what strategies seem most likely to help each of them.

   - "I don't really enjoy my work but at least I feel comfortable with my colleagues and supervisor. I'm afraid that my disability will make it hard for me to find another job where I feel so well accepted. What do you think I should do?"
   - "I found a lump underneath my arm. Do you think I should ask a physician about it or just wait awhile and see if it goes away?"
   - "I was brought up with the philosophy, 'Spare the rod and spoil the child.' It worked with me, but my daughter just becomes angrier and more rebellious every time I spank her. What do you think I should do?"
   - "I've tried and tried to make my marriage work but nothing seems to help. Is it time to give up and move on?"
   - "I've been working hard at losing weight and I've got my weight down to 92 pounds. My parents say I look too thin but I'd like to lose another 10 pounds. I've stopped eating dinner. Do you think I should cut out breakfast as well?"

3. In your capacity as a college counselor, you are treating a client who tells you that she has been using cocaine to such an extent that both her work and her academic performance are seriously impaired. What decisions would you make about referring this client for other sources of help and about continuing your work with this client? What is the logic behind your decisions? How would you present your decisions to the client?

4. Assume that you referred the woman in the previous example to a substance use treatment program. However, the client told you that she would not take the referral and would not return to see you after this session. How would you use the remaining 30 minutes of your session with her?

5. What reaction do you have to the prospect of writing weekly progress notes on all of your clients? In formulating your response, think about the guidelines of your profession, the importance of accountability, your emotional reactions, and your thoughts on the benefits and drawbacks of progress notes.

Practice Group Exercise: Structuring the Session

In this exercise, you can both practice your conceptual skills and further refine your fundamental skills. As usual, divide into your practice groups and record both the practice session and the subsequent discussion. When in the client role, each person should present a problem behavior.

This exercise will encompass the following skills:

Fundamental Skills

- Open questions
- Restatement
- Goal setting
- Concreteness and specificity
- Suggesting homework tasks

Conceptual Skills

- Structuring the session

In this exercise, clinicians have the following goals:

1. Structure the session according to the 10-step model presented earlier in this chapter and restated here:

- Collaborate with the client to establish a meaningful agenda for the session.
- Determine and measure the intensity of the client's mood.
- Identify and discuss current concerns.
- Establish clear and meaningful goals for the session.
- Embed the current concerns in context, focusing especially on similar concerns that the client has handled successfully.
- Help the client to identify connections between current concerns and past difficulties.
- Draw on past successes and promote development of new skills that will help the client resolve current concerns.
- Suggest tasks to be completed between sessions.
- Summarize the session.
- Elicit client feedback on the session.

2. Make good use of fundamental skills such as open questions and restatement to establish goals for the session.
3. Make use of concreteness and specificity to obtain a clear picture of the client's problem behavior.
4. Suggest a task to be completed between sessions.
5. Bring appropriate closure to the session.

Observers can facilitate their efforts to provide feedback by dividing up the parts of this exercise to focus on during the role-play. For example, one observer might focus on the first goal listed, while the second observer focuses on the remaining four goals.

Timing of Exercise

Completing this exercise will require approximately 2 hours. Of course, reducing the number of role-plays from four to two will shorten time required. Each role-play should follow this schedule:

- Allow at least 20 minutes for each role-played interview.
- Allow 10 minutes for feedback and processing of each role-play.

Assessment of Progress Form 8

1. How well did the session follow the 10 steps in the format for structuring sessions? Which steps worked especially well? How might the process have been improved?

_____

_____

_____

2. Describe the process of goal setting. Were goals clear, relevant, and specific? How might the goal setting have been improved?

_____

_____

_____

3. Describe and assess the clinician's use of concreteness and specificity.

_____

_____

_____

4. Assess the appropriateness of the homework task that the clinician suggested to the client. Was the task clear, relevant to the client's problem behavior, and readily achievable? Was the client engaged in the process of formulating the homework task? How might the process of suggesting a homework task have been improved?

_____

_____

_____

5. Describe the strategies used to bring closure to the session and assess their effectiveness.

_____

_____

_____

6. Overall assessment

a. Strengths:

_____

_____

b. Areas needing improvement:

_____

_____

Personal Journal Questions

1. This chapter focused on actions and behaviors rather than background, emotions, or thoughts. How well did that mesh with your natural style of intervention? Which of the four areas of focus seems most compatible with your style as a clinician?
2. What aspects of this chapter appealed to you and came easily to you?
3. What aspects of this chapter were unappealing and presented you with a considerable challenge?
4. Many people enter the helping professions with the belief that they can give people good advice and help them in that way. Was that a belief you had? If so, how has that belief shifted? What was your reaction when you read, in this chapter, that giving clients advice is generally countertherapeutic? What changes, if any, do you think you will make in your treatment style as a result of this information?
5. This chapter places considerable emphasis on the importance of structure in the treatment process. What was your reaction to that? How does that fit with your preferred treatment approach? How do you think this information will affect the treatment you provide?

SUMMARY

This chapter focused on conceptual skills associated with actions. As in the previous chapter, most of the skills presented were designed for clinicians to use in better understanding and treating their clients. Particular attention was paid to generating solutions to clients' concerns; referral and collaboration; and structuring sessions, the treatment process, and progress notes.

Chapter 9 continues to focus on conceptual skills associated with actions. Areas of focus in Chapter 9 include concluding sessions, assessing and terminating treatment, and using research to enhance practice.

Chapter 9

APPLYING CONCEPTUAL SKILLS TO ACTIONS FOR POSITIVE CHANGE

ASSESSING AND TERMINATING SESSIONS AND TREATMENT AND USING RESEARCH TO ENHANCE PRACTICE

OVERVIEW

Chapters 8 and 9 focus on conceptual skills related to actions, the fourth element in the BETA framework. These chapters emphasize actions that clinicians can take, in collaboration with their clients, to move treatment forward to a rewarding outcome. Chapter 9 is the last chapter in this book in which new skills are introduced. This chapter covers the following topics:

- **Assessing and Terminating Sessions and Treatment:** Clinicians need to address treatment endings at various levels, including both the end of each treatment session and the conclusion of the treatment process. Bringing a successful and positive closure to both can enhance treatment. Treatment ends, sometimes because clients have achieved their goals and no longer have a strong need for help and sometimes for other reasons. Clinicians and clients need criteria for determining when termination is appropriate and, if it is, for making the termination process a beneficial ingredient in the overall treatment process.
- **Using Research to Enhance Your Practice and Your Professional Development:** Skilled clinicians constantly seek ways to learn promising new strategies and further develop their clinical abilities. Probably the most important way for them to accomplish this is through research, both by reading the professional literature and by researching the strengths and shortcomings of their own practice. This section presents ways for clinicians to benefit from involvement in research and to continue their professional development.

ASSESSING AND TERMINATING SESSIONS AND TREATMENT

Counseling and psychotherapy have many endings: the end of each session, the completion of work on a particular problem or issue, the premature ending of treatment, and the successful conclusion of a therapeutic relationship. These endings can be glossed over and ignored, they can be handled in troubling and destructive ways, or they can be made a rewarding part of the treatment process. Information presented here is intended to help make endings therapeutic and productive elements in treatment, just as earlier chapters provided guidelines to maximize the benefits of other ingredients in the treatment process.

Consider the following client statement and clinician responses.

Client: You know, I think I've gotten what I needed out of our work together. I feel ready to end treatment.

Clinician 1: I'm glad to hear that. Don't hesitate to call if you feel a need for help in the future. It's been a pleasure to work with you, and I wish you well.

Clinician 2: You've certainly made progress in addressing your career concerns, but we haven't addressed the difficulties you've been having with your sister. You really should do some work on that before you finish treatment.

Clinician 3: I can hear the pride in your voice when you say that. Let's go back to our original goals once more so that we can really pinpoint the progress you have made and what you have learned through this process. We can also think about what continuing goals you might have that you want to address, either in treatment or after we complete our work together.

The differences among these three clinician responses are probably evident. Only the third response considers the prospect of termination as a learning experience. The following hallmarks of the clinician's response facilitate that process:

- The clinician neither agrees nor disagrees with the client's perception that he is ready to conclude treatment.
- Rather, the clinician creates a situation that will enable the client to identify and solidify learning and accomplishments and to determine, in a thoughtful and careful way, whether this is indeed the right time for treatment to end.
- The conclusion of the treatment process is viewed as an opportunity for growth and positive change; it is seen as a transition, either to continued treatment with revised goals or to the client's independent efforts to maintain progress and continue positive development.
- Discussion of termination is a joint process that reflects a collaborative therapeutic alliance and a focus on learning, strengths, and successes.

Concluding Sessions

Similarly, the end of a session can be a learning experience or can miss important opportunities to help people make positive changes and progress toward achieving their goals. For example, suppose the last few minutes of a treatment session included this exchange:

> *Clinician:* We have just a few minutes before the end of our session.
> *Client:* But I haven't told you about an argument I had with my mother; that was another really stressful experience I had this week.

Now consider these possible clinician responses:

> *Clinician 1:* Unfortunately, our time is up for today. I'll see you next week at this same time.
> *Clinician 2:* Our sessions will be most productive if you bring up important issues early in each session. However, I do have a free hour following our session, so let's just talk for a few minutes about your argument with your mother before we wrap up.
> *Clinician 3:* It sounds like you are identifying a theme of stressful experiences as the focus of our session this week.

The differences among the three clinician responses are probably evident. The first clinician's response does maintain the time boundaries of the session, which is generally important in clinical work. However, the client may perceive the clinician as being abrupt and disinterested, and this can damage the therapeutic alliance. Clinician 2 seems more compassionate and flexible but, by allowing the client extra time, may inadvertently encourage the client's efforts to prolong sessions. Clinician 3 seeks to maintains the boundaries of the session but does so in a way that acknowledges the importance of the client's issues. Following is a continuation of the dialogue with Clinician 3.

> *Client:* Yes, it seems like everyone in my life is just out to give me a hard time.
> *Clinician 3:* Our time for today is nearly at an end, but this sounds like an important issue for you. How about, for next week, you jot down at least two stressful interactions you have with people between now and then and how you handled them. Then we can be sure to give this topic some more time next week.

Clients often bring up what has been referred to as "doorknob disclosures," new and apparently important material they mention for the first time at the end of the session. Although role induction and gentle feedback from the clinician can encourage clients to avoid this pattern and bring up important topics earlier in the session, dealing with such last-minute disclosures can be challenging for clinicians.

The response of Clinician 3 observes the following principles, which are closely related to those guidelines listed previously that should characterize the end of the treatment process:

- The clinician creates a situation that promotes new learning and accomplishments.
- The conclusion of the session is viewed as an opportunity for growth and positive change; it serves as a transition to both the next treatment session and to the client's independent efforts to maintain progress and continue positive development between sessions.

- The conclusion of the session is a collaborative process that maintains a positive and encouraging orientation to treatment.
- As always, the client and his or her concerns are treated with respect and caring.

Implementing Guidelines for Concluding a Session   The "doorknob disclosure" is only one of a variety of challenges that can arise at the end of a treatment session. Having a clear format for concluding the session that follows the previous guidelines will help both the client and the clinician to benefit from the end of a session, just as they should from all other parts of the session. In addition, a predictable format for bringing closure to the session usually is reassuring to clients, reduces awkwardness and ambiguity, and helps both the client and the clinician deal with that closure in ways that enhance the therapeutic alliance, contribute to the client's goal achievement, and leave the client with positive and empowered feelings about the session, the clinician, and the self.

Review the following discussion with another client, which creates a productive closure for the treatment session. Notice how the previously mentioned guidelines for concluding a session are incorporated into the dialogue. As you read the dialogue, try to identify what makes it effective.

Clinician: We have about five minutes until the end of this session. How would you summarize what you have learned from this session?

Client: I saw that, both with my colleague and with my daughter, I jumped to the conclusion that they had some bad feelings about me just because they weren't especially talkative. I didn't know that my daughter had a fight with her best friend that day and maybe my colleague had a bad day too, because she was fine the next day. I seem to be my own worst enemy sometimes.

Clinician: So you could see that you tended to make negative assumptions about what people were thinking about you. What did you learn about how you could change this pattern?

Client: I think being more aware of it will help. And if it's someone I'm close to, I can talk with him or her about what's going on.

Clinician: How would you feel about trying out these new strategies this week?

Client: That sounds like a good idea.

Clinician: Perhaps you could make some notes about one incident this week in which you became aware that you might have an inaccurate perception and took steps to check it out.

Client: Yes, I can do that.

Clinician: All right. I'll write that down on the back of our appointment card. What feedback do you have for me about our session today?

The conclusion of this session is consistent with the principles listed previously. The following clinician behaviors contributed to the success of this dialogue:

- The clinician reminded the client that the session had only a few minutes remaining.
- The clinician encouraged the client to take primary responsibility for identifying learning during the session.

- The clinician used summarization to verify what had been said and reinforced the client's perceptions.
- Emphasis was placed on the client's acquisition and application of new thoughts and actions.
- Learning was reinforced via repetition.
- A between-sessions task was suggested to build on and solidify new learning.
- The clinician checked out the client's willingness to complete the suggested task; the task would be modified if it were not acceptable to the client.
- The task was written down to encourage completion.
- Although client–clinician collaboration was emphasized, the clinician maintained control of the session; the clinician asked for feedback and moved toward ending the session on schedule.

The Learning Opportunities at the end of this chapter will enable you to practice using these guidelines to end a treatment session.

Concluding Treatment

Bringing the entire treatment process to a productive and rewarding conclusion is generally more complex and challenging than concluding a treatment session. The two ingredients that are key in bringing a positive end to treatment are

1. A clear and up-to-date statement of treatment goals.
2. An open, trusting, and collaborative treatment alliance between client and clinician.

Reasons for Termination   Termination of treatment typically occurs for one of four reasons (Seligman, 2006).

- **Clinician's Choice:** Clinicians may be changing jobs or retiring and so may need to conclude treatment with their clients. Alternatively, the agency or school where treatment occurs may be changing its mission, may have experienced financial and staff cutbacks, or may have changed the managed care plans with which it is affiliated. These circumstances may require clinicians to end their work with some or all of their clients.
- **Client's Choice:** Clients sometimes terminate treatment before clinicians believe they are ready to end their work. Most premature terminations occur early in the treatment process, before the development of a sound therapeutic alliance and clear and meaningful goals. Following are some common reasons why clients end treatment prematurely:
  - Clients believe that the treatment process or the clinician cannot help them.
  - They find it threatening or upsetting to take an honest look at their concerns.

- ○ Clients have financial, logistical, or other obstacles that make it difficult for them to continue treatment.
- ○ They believe they have gotten what they need from treatment, even though their clinician may not share that perception.

- **Mutual Agreement/Negative Outcome:** Occasionally, clients and clinicians agree that treatment should end because it is ineffective. This may occur when the clinician cannot provide the sort of treatment the client needs, when the client-clinician match is not a positive one, or when all efforts to engage the client in productive treatment have been unsuccessful. Referrals to other agencies or treatment providers should be offered to the client in cases such as these.
- **Mutual Agreement/Positive Outcome:** The ideal culmination of the treatment process occurs when both clients and clinicians agree that treatment has been successful, that the clients have achieved their goals, that the therapeutic alliance has been a positive one, and that the clients are ready to complete treatment. Often clients telegraph their readiness to end treatment. They may cancel sessions for unimportant reasons. They may have little to talk about in sessions. Or the focus of the sessions may shift from a presentation of troubling emotions and painful experiences to talking about interpersonal successes and rewarding activities. Clues such as these suggest that clinicians might broach the topic of termination and begin to explore whether the time is right to end treatment.

Determining Whether the Time Is Right for Termination   Before introducing the idea of concluding treatment, clinicians should ask themselves the following questions.

- Have the clients achieved most or all of their goals?
- If new issues have been introduced that were not incorporated into the clients' initial goals, have the clients made satisfactory progress in resolving those issues?
- Have the clients developed a repertoire of adaptive, coping, communication, problem-solving, decision-making, self-care, and other life skills they can use to resolve future concerns?
- Have the clients established healthy sources of gratification and pleasure in their lives?
- Have the clients established healthy, rewarding, and compatible relationships?
- Do the clients have a sense of well-being and awareness of their strengths and assets?
- Are they practicing strategies and habits that will continue to enhance their physical and emotional well-being?
- Are the clients giving messages that they may be ready to complete treatment?

If all or most of these questions are answered affirmatively, then the clients are probably ready to complete their treatment.

Effecting a Successful Termination Regardless of whether treatment has been successful or unsuccessful, and regardless of who is initiating the end of treatment, termination should be viewed as a process, not an event. Facilitating clients' completion of treatment and making that a positive experience for them can make a big difference in their ability to use what they have learned in treatment and to create rewarding lives for themselves. Clinicians are encouraged to use the following procedures to help make the ending of treatment a positive process.

- *Allow ample time* to discuss whether termination is appropriate and to complete the termination process. If possible, three or more sessions should be allocated to the process of concluding treatment.
- *Facilitate clients' expression of thoughts and emotions about the idea of terminating treatment.* Typically, clients have a mixture of positive and negative responses at the conclusion of their treatment. They may feel apprehensive about their ability to maintain gains without the clinician's help, and they may feel sad at the loss of contact with the clinician. They may feel angry that treatment is ending, even if it is their choice. On the other hand, they may also feel proud of their accomplishments, relieved to be free of the commitment of time and money that treatment entails, and eager to move forward with their lives. Clinicians should be sure to normalize these mixed reactions and give clients permission and opportunity to express both positive and negative thoughts and emotions.
- *Clinicians should take the time to identify and process their reactions to the termination process,* either on their own or with a supervisor or colleague. Clinicians, too, often have strong and conflicted responses to the termination of a client's treatment, especially if treatment has not been fully successful or if it has been long-term treatment that has culminated in considerable client growth and development. If the treatment process has been a disappointing one, clinicians may fault themselves for not having been more helpful to their clients and may even doubt their abilities as clinicians. On the other hand, if a strong bond between client and clinician has developed in the context of successful treatment, clinicians may regret that they will probably not have the opportunity to see their clients blossom and make effective use of all they have learned in treatment. Just as parents have mixed emotions when they see their grown children leave home for college, an important relationship, or employment, clinicians too can have bittersweet reactions to the launching of a client. As long as clinicians are aware of their responses to the termination process and deal with those feelings in appropriate and professional ways, these mixed reactions can be viewed as a normal and understandable aspect of termination and reflective of the caring and closeness clinicians often feel toward their clients.
- *Collaborate with the client in identifying and listing the client's accomplishments during treatment.* This process usually is most meaningful to clients if their perceptions of accomplishments are elicited first and are written down. Once clients have finished their report of their accomplishments, clinicians can suggest additional gains and, if accepted by the clients, these can be added to the list. Reviewing the list later can remind clients of all they have gained through treatment, and it can remind them of their strengths when they encounter personal challenges after the end of treatment.

- *Compare accomplishments with goals.* This can help clients to see even more clearly the progress they have made since entering treatment. Even people who are leaving treatment prematurely usually find they have made some progress; the process of identifying difficulties and seeking help can be an important accomplishment in itself. People who are concluding successful treatment often discover that they have achieved many but not all of their original goals and that they also have made gains that they had not anticipated at the inception of treatment. Rather than viewing this as a failure, clinicians can emphasize that having ongoing goals is a normal and healthy part of life and can be growth-promoting as long as people have effective ways to move toward goal achievement.

- *Facilitate clients' efforts to look forward to the future.* Discussion might focus on ways in which clients can continue to use and build on their improved skills to accomplish new goals, as well as those goals that may not have been completely realized during treatment. Writing down these goals, along with strategies to address them, can help clients keep them in mind and continue the positive changes begun during treatment.

- *Ask clients for feedback on the treatment process and the work of the clinician.* Learning more about themselves as clinicians and about what clients perceive as the successful and unsuccessful components of treatment can help clinicians understand their strengths and limitations as well as those of the treatment they provide. Clinicians then can use that information to research their practice (discussed in the next section of this chapter) and focus their efforts to improve their knowledge and skills.

Once these procedures have been completed, usually over the course of several sessions, it is time to say good-bye to the client. A handshake, or even a hug, is often appropriate, along with congratulations to the client for hard work and successes. In addition, clinicians should remind clients that counseling and psychotherapy are resources that can be helpful to them again in the future if they run into difficulties they cannot handle effectively on their own. Ending the treatment process on a positive note and, if appropriate, leaving the door open for future contact can be reassuring to clients and help them terminate treatment with feelings of confidence, pride, and hopefulness.

Example: Eileen Carter   Eileen Carter, an African American woman who was having considerable difficulty balancing her own needs and those of her husband and son, has been used throughout this book to illustrate many of the skills and concepts. A dialogue between Eileen and her therapist is presented here as an example of part of the termination process. Assume that Eileen and her therapist have agreed that she has achieved most of her goals and is now ready to conclude her treatment. The following illustrates part of a session and reflects the guidelines and principles for termination listed previously.

Therapist: Now that we've decided to end our work together for the foreseeable future, I'd like us to take a look at the results of your treatment.

Eileen: That sounds like a good idea.

Therapist: How about if you start by describing some of the accomplishments you see yourself as having made through treatment, and I'll write them down.

Eileen: Most important, I found ways to continue my education while still meeting the needs of my husband and son. I got some financial aid from the college, and I'm using the day care there for my son when I am in class.

My husband and I understand each other better. He finally realizes how important college is to me, and I can understand why he was worried that my taking college classes might jeopardize our marriage.

I feel more like I belong at college. Before, I felt like an impostor, hiding my background from the other students, who all seemed so young and innocent. Now I have been using some of my experiences in my writing. People have been really interested in what I went through and how I got myself on track.

I feel more confident about myself as a mother and wife, too. I seem to be less caught up with my own feelings and issues and more tuned into my husband and son. I'm able to relax more with both of them, and we have more good times together.

I feel like I've forgiven myself for all those mistakes I made when I was younger. I wish I hadn't gone through all that, especially the abortions, but I don't feel the hatred I had toward myself in the past. In fact, I value myself and have come to appreciate my strengths. That's about all I can think of.

Therapist: You have come up with quite a few positive changes. There are a few additional successes that occur to me. Let me tell you what they are, and you can decide whether to include them in our list.

- You seem much less depressed and anxious. We saw a big change when we compared the depression and anxiety inventories you took at the beginning of treatment with the ones you took last week.
- You have made some women friends, both at college and in your neighborhood.
- Your college grades have improved now that you have become more open and comfortable in your writing. Having a clearer career direction has also helped you to be more successful in your courses.
- You've begun an exercise program and have been trying to eat more healthfully. That's another way to show that you value yourself.
- You've also started to reestablish contact with your family of origin and visited your mother when she was ill.

Eileen: Yes, you're right, I have done all of that and you can add those accomplishments to our list, but I'm still not where I want to be in terms of my relationship with my mother and in getting regular exercise.

Therapist: We can talk about that in a few minutes, but first I'd like to compare your goals with the ones we wrote down when you began counseling. Here's a copy of the list we developed together.

Eileen: Wow, some big changes. I didn't even know if I wanted to stay married then, and now I am committed to my marriage. I can see I had many doubts about myself and was pretty sure I would have to give up college, or at least put it off for years. My mood is much better and I have become more confident in myself as I had hoped. But when we wrote up these goals, I was so focused on the immediate problems, I didn't even think about dealing with my past or making new friends or improving my health. We've accomplished even more than I had hoped.

Therapist: You must feel very proud to see all you have accomplished.

Eileen: I really am. But it seems like I have new goals now. Does that mean I'm not really ready to finish counseling?

Therapist: Let's talk about that. What are those new goals?

Eileen: I'm not exercising as much as I would like, and I'm just beginning to deal with my family of origin. Then pretty soon I have to make a final decision on my major at college. This is a never-ending process.

Therapist: That's true. We always have new goals and issues to address, but that doesn't necessarily mean you need to continue counseling at this time. How do you feel about your ability to handle those issues yourself?

Eileen: I can certainly try. I have narrowed down my choice of major. And my exercising is going in the right direction. Dealing with my mother is another issue, though.

Therapist: That seems like the most challenging concern for you. What do you think you could do to improve your relationship with her?

Eileen: I could analyze my thoughts like we did here and make sure I was thinking clearly about the situation. I could use some of those communication skills I used so well with my husband. And I could talk to my best friend Betty about the situation; she has problems with her mother, too.

Therapist: So it sounds like you have quite a few strategies to help you achieve your goals without counseling.

Eileen: Yes, I can see that I do. If I really get stuck, can I come in for a few more sessions?

Therapist: Yes, of course you can call me for an appointment, but I hope that first you'll remember and use all those skills you already have. Before we finish our session today, I'd like us to talk about the counseling process and our work together. It would help me to hear about what was especially useful to you and also how we might have improved on our work.

Eileen: It's hard to say Counseling has certainly helped me. I always felt that you were there for me and your support meant a lot, but you wouldn't really tell me what to do. You'd just help me figure it out for myself. I liked that decision-making strategy you taught me, and practicing new ways to talk to my husband really helped.

Therapist: So you learned quite a few new skills from our work together. What would have made our work together even better?

Eileen: I can't really think of anything.

Therapist: Let's see if I can help you identify a few things that might have improved our work. During our first few sessions, you seemed uncertain about whether counseling would be helpful. Can you remember what triggered those feelings?

Eileen: Yes, I guess so. I was really in a crisis when I first came to see you, and I wanted you to jump right in and tell me what to do. I felt that you didn't understand how urgent my situation was.

Therapist: So it felt like you needed more direction at that time?

Eileen: Yes, that's it. Also, I wasn't sure about how you reacted when I told you about my abortions. I was crying then, and all you did was hand me a tissue.

Therapist: What would have helped you at that time?

Eileen: Maybe a pat on the shoulder or more acknowledgment of how bad I was feeling.

Therapist: I can understand how that would have been helpful to you. Thank you for giving me that feedback. What other ways can you think of for improving our counseling?

Eileen: I can't come up with anything else.

Therapist: We have talked before about the differences in our backgrounds and your initial concern that I couldn't really understand you because I was Caucasian and had more education than you did. Those feelings became especially strong after I returned from vacation. What thoughts do you have now about that aspect of our work together?

Eileen: You're right. That was a barrier between us, especially after I heard you had gone to Africa on your vacation. I thought, there you were spending lots of money to see animals but not really understanding the African culture. That did bother me.

Therapist: So initially the differences between us did present an obstacle in our work together and it sounds like you felt distant from me and maybe even angry with me. What happened to those feelings?

Eileen: You seemed to sense how I was feeling, and we talked about it. You really did seem to accept and understand me as an individual and didn't just stereotype me. Eventually those feelings became less important and I felt good about how open I could be with you. Maybe our getting past the differences between us even helped me to relate to some of those college students who seemed so different from me.

Therapist: So what started out as a barrier wound up being helpful, although it was important that we did talk about our differences.

Eileen: Yes, that's true.

Therapist: As we planned, our next session will be our last session. How would it be if, during the week, you review the list of accomplishments and write down some of those future goals that we began to discuss? You can add to or change any of the items on those lists and we can discuss them in our last session.

Eileen: That sounds fine.

Therapist: I'll write that down on your appointment card. And if you have any further thoughts about the strengths and weak areas in our work together, I'd be interested in hearing more about that, too.

Eileen: All right, see you next week.

Now that you have read this dialogue once, go back over it, keeping in mind the guidelines for concluding treatment beginning on page 267. See if you can find the lines of dialogue that reflect each of those guidelines. If you discover that any of them were not addressed well, think about how you might have improved this dialogue.

USING RESEARCH TO ENHANCE YOUR PRACTICE AND YOUR PROFESSIONAL DEVELOPMENT

Now that you have learned about ending the treatment process, you are almost ready to conclude your learning of new skills from this book. However, you have one more step to take, which is self-evaluation.

Counseling, social work, and psychology are vital and evolving fields. They are rich with exciting research, informative professional journals, and stimulating local, national, and international conferences and training opportunities. You might already feel overwhelmed by all there is to learn about your profession and the constant challenge of acquiring important new knowledge and skills.

In order for clinicians to provide excellent service to their clients and take pride in their work, they must become lifetime learners, always excited about the advances in their field. At the same time, of course, clinicians cannot become knowledgeable about all of the new developments. How, then, can clinicians continue to enhance their knowledge and skills in meaningful ways without becoming overwhelmed? The following guidelines can help you to answer this question for yourself.

Developing Your Professional Specialization

Finding your niche, your area of specialization in your profession, is an important step. Probably your area of specialization will evolve as you gain experience and discover new interests and opportunities, so you do not need to regard your current interests as fixed. However, identifying a circumscribed area of interest will help you to focus your learning, develop strong skills, clarify your professional roles and identity, and build a reputation in your field.

My own areas of specialization have evolved considerably over the years. After college, I became a high school English teacher and collaborated with school counselors to educate students about harmful drugs and provide help to those students who were already misusing drugs or alcohol. This led me to seek a master's degree in school counseling.

However, by the time I finished my master's degree, I also had become interested in career development and family dynamics. Those interests led me to enter a doctoral program so that I could learn more, not only about my continuing interest in substance-related disorders and their treatment, but also about career development and family therapy. While pursuing doctoral study, I developed an interest in multicultural counseling; my first publications focused on two areas, multicultural counseling and career counseling (Seligman, 1977, 1979, 1980). These interests grew out of learning that had been emphasized in my doctoral studies.

After finishing my doctorate, I combined teaching and practice, training graduate students in psychology and counseling while concurrently providing treatment in a program for troubled children, a correctional facility, and later a private practice. These experiences led me to develop a strong interest in understanding mental disorders and developing effective treatment plans. Those areas have become my most enduring and important areas of specialization, reflected in six books (Seligman, 1986, 1990, 1996a, 1998, 2004; Seligman & Reichenberg, 2007) and many articles and presentations on those topics. Finally, issues in my own family as well as concerns of my clients led me to develop a special interest in helping people cope more effectively with serious illness (Seligman, 1996b). At present, my primary professional interests include diagnosis and treatment planning, education of mental health professionals, helping people cope with chronic and life-threatening illnesses, treating people who have had traumatic experiences, theories and strategies of counseling and psychotherapy, and multicultural counseling.

Your professional development will probably follow a similar pattern. Your interests will evolve and change over time, with some interests enduring and others fading. Your interests will be sparked by many experiences, both personal and professional, and you will continue to relish the excitement of our stimulating and always changing profession.

Identifying Your Professional Specialization

Think about what you currently view as your areas of professional specialization. These specializations can be defined in many ways:

- *Age* (e.g., children in elementary school, adolescents, people over 65)
- *Presenting problems* (e.g., infidelity, career concerns, anger and aggression, drug and alcohol misuse, bereavement, chronic and life-threatening illnesses)
- *Mental disorders* (e.g., personality disorders, mood disorders, anxiety disorders, attention-deficit/hyperactivity disorders, conduct and oppositional defiant disorders, dissociative disorders)
- *Type of treatment setting or facility* (e.g., middle school, community mental health center, university, rehabilitation facility, women's center, or private practice)
- *Treatment approaches* (e.g., cognitive-behavioral therapy, psychoanalysis, eye-movement desensitization and reprocessing, play therapy, or person-centered therapy)

Researching Your Own Practice

Once you have identified one or more areas of specialization, you can begin to conduct research on your own practice and interests. The first step is to assess the present status of your work.

- Determine what you do that is effective and successful.
- Determine what you do that is not usually effective.

- Determine what important unanswered questions you have about your work, your clients, and their difficulties.

Many tools and approaches are available to help you research your practice (McLeod, 1994). These include

- **Structured Inventories:** Inventories have been developed to help clinicians assess the effectiveness of their work. Administered to clients at predetermined points in the treatment process, these self-report inventories yield a quantitative measure of clinical outcome. Alternatively, you can develop your own questionnaire, asking clients to provide structured and specific feedback on your work. The journal *Counselor Education and Supervision*, as well as Internet and print resources listing tests and inventories, are good sources for such inventories.
- **Single-Subject Design:** Empirical research also can be conducted on a single client, following principles established for single-subject design. Tracking the progress of one client can give you insight into the nature and quality of your practice.
- **Qualitative Research:** Structured or semistructured interviews, conducted with a small number of clients, can yield useful qualitative information about the nature, strengths, and weaknesses of your clinical work. This approach to research can be individualized to yield the sort of information that is especially useful to you.
- **Goal Attainment Scaling:** In this process, clinicians obtain data on their success in helping clients achieve their goals (Cytrynbaum, Ginath, Birdwell, & Brandt, 1979; Zaza, Stolee, & Prkachin, 1999). Once goals have been selected, they can be weighted based on their relative importance. Expected outcomes and an anticipated time frame for goal attainment are then determined. Finally, attainment of each goal is rated by client or clinician on a −2 to +2 scale, reflecting how the actual outcome compares with the anticipated outcome. A composite score reflects overall treatment effectiveness (empirical information on effectiveness).
- **Informal Assessment:** Unstructured discussions, incorporated into the treatment process, also can yield valuable information on clinician and treatment effectiveness. Many cognitive-behavioral therapists, for example, elicit client feedback at the conclusion of each session. Patterns in feedback can point to strengths as well as areas needing improvement.

Example   Thomas, an African American man who was a counselor in a middle school, believed it would enhance his work to conduct a systematic evaluation of his effectiveness. He used a checklist for self-evaluation, qualitative interviews with students whom he had counseled, and an informal assessment inventory he had created to research his practice. He came up with the following evaluation of his work.

- *Determine what I do that is effective and successful.* I generally think I do a good job, but I seem to work especially well with African American boys. I am direct and straightforward with them, drawing on Glasser's reality therapy to help them assess whether their behaviors are helping or hurting them. I make sure to follow up with them, once they have made a commitment to make some changes. I confer with their teachers and parents and think holistically about the young people with whom I work. All of these procedures seem helpful.

- *Determine what I do that is not usually effective.* I don't do as well forming a therapeutic alliance with students who are not motivated to succeed at anything, whether it is academics, athletics, or friendships. Reality therapy doesn't seem to work as well with them either. I may be missing some underlying depression and may be expecting too much from them. I also have more difficulty building rapport with the girls than I do with the boys.

- *Determine what important unanswered questions I have about my work, my clients, and their difficulties.*

  - Have I made an accurate assessment of my strengths and weaknesses as a counselor?
  - How does depression look in young people in early adolescence?
  - What approaches seem effective in reducing their depression and increasing their motivation?
  - What does the literature say about using reality therapy with young people who are depressed?
  - What can I do to learn more about the development of girls in early adolescence, especially their interests, values, and cognitive abilities, as well as ways to connect with them better?
  - How do the teachers and parents regard my work? Would they benefit from even more contact with me?

Thomas can now move onto the next phase of researching his practice, gathering additional information to support or refute his conclusions and provide some answers to his questions. He can go about this in a variety of ways:

- He might interview small groups of teachers and parents to elicit their perceptions of his work and how he might be even more helpful to them.
- He might ask his colleagues and supervisor about their perceptions of his work.
- He might complete a brief checklist each time he meets with a student, listing the student's concerns, the strategies Thomas used to help the student, and his impression of the effectiveness of his work. He could later compare this information with the student's attendance record and grades. This could help Thomas determine whether his hypotheses about the quality of his work are accurate and obtain further clarification of his strengths and weaknesses as a counselor.
- Thomas might do some additional reading, specifically on diagnosis and treatment of depression in adolescents, on the developmental stages and needs of girls in early adolescence, and on the use of reality therapy to address depression in young people.

- Thomas might identify teachers and counselors who seem to work especially well with girls in middle school and talk with them about their understanding of the girls and ways they build rapport with them. He might also try out some new approaches to working with the girls in his case load, based on these discussions and his reading.

Turn to the Literature

Over the past 15 years, researchers in social work, counseling, and psychology have produced a substantial body of literature, clarifying the nature of people's difficulties and mental disorders and identifying effective ways to treat them (Seligman & Reichenberg, 2007). Particularly important has been the research conducted by the American Psychological Association's (APA's) Task Force on Empirically Supported Treatments (Waehler, Kalodner, Wampold, & Lichtenberg, 2000). Empirically supported treatments have been defined as "specified interventions designated as having demonstrated efficacy for individuals with specific psychological disorders" (p. 657). The APA task force conducted meta-analyses of large numbers of empirical research studies and identified more than 50 treatment strategies that had convincingly demonstrated their effectiveness. Clinicians should become skilled in those strategies that have proven value and that are relevant to their practice in order to maximize their effectiveness in their work.

Clearly, the professional literature is an important source of information for clinicians interested in improving the power and value of their work. However, the large body of literature available to clinicians is overwhelming to most. How can you make good use of available information to better your work? The following guidelines should help you to narrow your focus.

- Join one or more national professional associations such as the American Psychological Association, the American Mental Health Counselors Association, the National Association of Social Workers, and the American Counseling Association.
- Join divisions or special-interest groups offered by these national professional associations that reflect your identified areas of specialization.
- Read the relevant journals and newsletters issued by the professional associations you have joined.
- Attend national conferences in your field, listen to the keynote speakers as well as those of special interest to you, browse through the bookstore at the professional conference to discover professional literature of interest to you, and network with colleagues who share your interests. If time and finances allow, also attend local, state, and regional conferences.
- Become familiar with the names and concepts that are especially important to your work and seek out additional relevant information and training.

This book is only a beginning in your development into a clinician with strong fundamental and conceptual skills. Participating actively in your profession, becoming familiar with the literature that is pertinent to your areas of specialization, and continuing your professional development through training, reading, researching your practice, and conferring with your supervisors and colleagues can help you become a clinician who makes a positive difference in people's lives and who finds great rewards in your professional work.

LEARNING OPPORTUNITIES

This chapter, like Chapter 8, focused on actions, primarily those that clinicians perform as part of their work. The conceptual skills presented in this chapter include

- Bringing sessions, as well as the overall treatment process, to a positive conclusion.
- Using research to enhance your practice.

The following exercises provide the opportunity to apply the conceptual skills that have been presented in this chapter.

Written Exercises/Discussion Questions

1. Chapters 3 and 8 provided information on Rosa Ishak and her treatment. (See pages 74–75 and 256.) Assume that Rosa has satisfactorily completed her treatment. Write or role-play a dialogue with Rosa that brings her treatment to a close. Follow the principles presented on pages 267–268 for concluding treatment.
2. Assume that you have had a lengthy and positive therapeutic relationship with a client. You have come to like the client personally, and you look forward to your sessions. The client is someone you could envision having as a friend. Now it is time to terminate your successful work together, and you are feeling sad about that. How would you deal with your reactions to the termination process? What, if anything, would you say to the client about your feelings? Describe the thinking that led you to these conclusions.
3. Clients sometimes want to conclude treatment before their clinicians believe they are ready to take that step. Consider the following scenarios, in which clients suggest premature termination. Discuss how you would handle each of these situations if you were the clinician or, alternatively, role-play your discussion with each client, focusing on the decision of whether to end treatment. Feel free to add information on each person, as long as it is consistent with the information already provided.

- Client 1 has made some progress but has not achieved most of his goals. The client has recently received a promotion at work and tells you that he is too busy to continue treatment.
- Although Client 2 has made some progress, it has been slow. The client tells you that treatment is not helping and wants this to be his last session.

- You have had difficulty building a therapeutic alliance with Client 3 because of her limited motivation. The client now tells you that you lack good listening skills and understanding of her concerns, and that this will be the last session the two of you will have together because she is beginning treatment with another clinician.
- Although you have only had three sessions with Client 4, he tells you that all his problems have been solved, he has met his "soul mate," and thanks you profusely for your help. He reports wanting to stop treatment because everything is now "just perfect."

4. What obstacles are clinicians likely to face as they begin to research their practices? What can they do to minimize these obstacles and facilitate the process of researching their practices?

Practice Group Exercise: Concluding the Practice Group Experience

The members of your practice group have probably gotten to know each other very well through the many role-played interviews you have done over the course of the training experiences presented in this book. This exercise provides the opportunity to use the skills you have learned in this chapter to bring closure to your work together.

The clinician in this role-play has the following goals:

- To bring a positive close to your work with your partner
- To identify and reinforce the clinical and other strengths and gains that your partner has made over the course of this training experience
- To determine two skills that your partner wants to improve, along with ways for your partner to continue bettering these skills
- To explore your partner's feelings about the end of the role-plays
- To express your own feelings about the end of the role-plays in an appropriate professional way
- To say good-bye

This should be an exploratory session rather than a problem-solving one. Although the person in the clinician role should, as usual, be in charge of the session, collaboration is important in this exercise, as it nearly always is when treatment ends. The clinician is primarily a facilitator in this exercise, promoting the client's expression of thoughts and feelings in reaction to the end of this training experience. A high level of clinical skills should be maintained throughout this process, with participants applying what they have learned throughout the training.

Practice group members in the client role should be themselves for this session, talking about their learning in the practice sessions and processing their reactions to the end of the learning experience, with emphasis on strengths and progress. This session should provide an opportunity to reinforce the partner's gains, further growth, and provide closure. It also is a transition, as participants move onto other training experiences or into the practice of counseling and psychotherapy.

Timing of Exercise

The role-plays should follow this schedule:

- Allow 15 minutes for each role-play.
- Following the interview, the entire group should contribute to developing a list of the strengths and challenges of the person who has just been in the clinician role. This should take approximately 10 minutes. For this role-play, be sure that all group members have the opportunity to be in both client and clinician roles, so that they can receive feedback on their skills and process the end of the group experience.

Assessment of Progress Form 9

1. List the strengths and gains that you, your partner, and your group observed in you over the course of this training experience. This list should be compiled after you have been in the clinician role.

   _____

   _____

   _____

2. List two fundamental or conceptual skills that warrant your continued attention.

   _____

   _____

3. How successful were you at bringing a positive closure to your work with your partner and facilitating that person's expression of feelings and identification of strengths and areas needing improvement? What made this session as successful as it was? What would have further enhanced the session?

   _____

   _____

   _____

Personal Journal Questions

1. What sorts of treatment terminations do you think will be most difficult for you? What challenges do you think you will face overall during the termination process? What steps can you take to overcome those challenges?
2. What reactions do you usually have when dealing with endings and closure? How do you think you will generally react to ending treatment with a client? Which of your usual reactions to endings and closure do you think will be repeated when you terminate treatment with clients?
3. What do you currently view as your areas of specialization? Have they evolved over time, remained stable, or are you only now beginning to think about your areas of specialization? How do feel about your progress in identifying an area of specialization?

4. If you were to research your practice, how would you go about doing that? Assess your current practice (even if this has included only role-played interviews) according to the following steps:

- Determine what you do as a clinician that is effective and successful.
- Determine what you do as a clinician that is not usually effective.
- Determine what important unanswered questions you have about your actual or anticipated work, your clients, and their difficulties. What steps can you take to find answers to those questions?

SUMMARY

This chapter focused on two conceptual skills: concluding sessions and the treatment process, and using research to enhance your own practice. These topics and this chapter bring a close to the new skills you will learn through this book.

Chapter 10 provides an opportunity to review and apply much of what you have learned during the course of this training experience. Chapter 10 will also enable you to synthesize and integrate the feedback you have received, as well as your own perceptions of your clinical skills, so that you can continue to develop into an outstanding clinician.

Chapter 10

SOLIDIFYING CONCEPTUAL SKILLS

REVIEWING, INTEGRATING, AND REINFORCING LEARNING

OVERVIEW

This final chapter will help you accomplish the following goals:

- Review the learning you have acquired through the information and exercises provided in this book.
- Raise your awareness of how much you have learned through your study of this material.
- Enhance and increase the learning you have acquired.
- Provide another opportunity for you to practice your conceptual and other skills.
- Reinforce your learning.

The first section of this chapter presents an intake interview with a young woman who enters treatment at the insistence of her parents. Following that interview is a series of Learning Opportunities that will enable you to review and apply to this case many of the skills presented in this book. Included in the Learning Opportunities are written exercises/discussion questions and a comprehensive self-evaluation based on the Assessment of Progress forms you have used throughout this book. Here you will find another opportunity to assess your skills, identifying strengths as well as areas that continue to need attention. Completing these forms should give you an even clearer picture of yourself as a clinician and help you focus your continuing efforts to improve and refine your skills. Finally, a series of personal journal questions concludes the Learning Opportunities, enabling you to further reflect on and synthesize the material you have studied and learned.

INTAKE INTERVIEW WITH SUMMER HARRIS

Clinician: Summer, what brings you in for some help?
Client: It was my mother's idea, well, not so much her idea as her requirement. And my real name isn't Summer.

Clinician: It sounds like we need to back up and have you fill me in on some background. Just start anywhere and tell me what you think is important for me to know about you.

Client: I suppose I might as well tell you what's going on rather than just wasting time for both of us, since I do have to be here. The forms I filled out said that whatever we talk about is confidential. Is that right?

Clinician: Yes, that's right, unless you present a danger to yourself or someone else.

Client: I might like to present a danger to my mother. I guess I shouldn't joke about that. You might take me seriously. No, I don't present a danger to anyone.

Clinician: You sound very angry at your mother, though.

Client: Yeah, I am. I guess I should start at the beginning so you won't be so confused. I was born in Korea; from what I know, my real mother was Korean and my father was African American and in the U.S. military. I don't know whether he knew my mother was pregnant, but he apparently left Korea before I was born. Sounds like that opera, Madame Butterfly. Anyhow, having a mixed-race child out of wedlock was a big disgrace, so my mother put me in an orphanage. I lived there until I was about a year old and then George and Stephanie came along and adopted me. I usually call them George and Stephanie because they don't feel like my parents, at least not how I think parents should be.

Clinician: So you had the challenge of being placed in an orphanage for a year and then being adopted by people who sound like they have been a disappointment to you.

Client: Yeah, big time! George and Stephanie already had two biological sons when they adopted me; I was supposed to be the trophy child, the sad little waif who nobody wanted who would show the world how wonderful they were. George was in the state senate and had big dreams of running for national office and Stephanie was playing the role of the politically correct stay-at-home mom who baked brownies and home-schooled her children. I was supposed to complete the picture, be the cute little girl who would reward them for being so magnanimous by being perfect in every way. I suppose I also helped George to get the African American and Asian vote, because he really talked up my ethnic and cultural background. Of course, they didn't teach me much about my background; I've had to learn about that on my own.

Clinician: It sounds like you feel used, and maybe even cheated of the opportunity to learn about your background and become your own person.

Client: That's how I feel now, but when I was younger, I bought into the story and tried to be everything George and Stephanie wanted me to be. My brothers didn't have to do anything to get their love but not me, I only got praised when I did everything they wanted me to do. One of my brothers had a drinking problem and even wrecked his car and got a DWI. George paid off the judge or something, told my brother to stop drinking, and that was the end of it. If I had done that, I would have been grounded for life. But of course I wouldn't have done that. I just studied hard, got all A's, played the piano in the school orchestra, did well on the school soccer team, and did everything I could to make George and Stephanie proud of me. I think George really was; he would give me a hug sometimes and tell me how well I was doing. Not Stephanie, though. She'd listen for every mistake I made when I played the piano, she'd ask me why I wasn't captain of the soccer team, and she'd tell me about her friend's daughter who was taking four advanced placement courses when I was only taking one. Nothing was ever good enough for her, but I just kept trying to please her.

Clinician: It sounds like you were running in a race you didn't think you could ever win. How did all this make you feel?

Client: I didn't realize it at the time, but I think I've been depressed for years, probably since elementary school. I feel sad and tired lots of the time, I don't feel good about myself, and for years it just felt like I was walking down a dark hallway without any end. I never have much appetite, I didn't really enjoy what I was doing or have close friends like the other kids. I just did what I thought George and Stephanie wanted me to do. I guess I did it pretty well, because I got into a top college. George and Stephanie made a big party for me when I graduated from high school last year and invited all their friends. I thought that I had finally made them happy, but even then Stephanie was talking about her friend's daughter who got advanced standing at an Ivy League school, which I hadn't even tried to do.

Clinician: So you felt like you did everything that your adoptive parents wanted you to do, but you still felt like a failure and were struggling with depression. What did you do to try to help yourself feel better?

Client: Nothing really. I didn't even know I was depressed then; I just thought this is how people feel.

Clinician: So you didn't know how sad you felt. What has the past year been like for you?

Client: I did go off to college, lived in the dorms with a roommate, and started out studying hard and getting good grades just as I had always done. Then it was like something snapped and suddenly I was fed up with it all and didn't want to be that way anymore. My roommate partied a lot and I started going out with her and her friends. They would drink and use drugs when they could get them. They'd go to bars and hook up with guys they just met there. For the first time in my life, I felt excited and energetic. I was doing things that I knew were dangerous and that would have been devastating to George and Stephanie, but I just kept doing them. The problem was George and Stephanie kept me on a tight leash, didn't give me much money to spend, and I couldn't explain why I needed more money. So I stole a credit card and used it to pay for dinners for my roommate and her friends and for drinks for everyone. I wanted to dress differently and so I used the credit card to buy clothes that were more stylish. I worried about using one credit card too much, so I threw it away and stole another one and then another one. Finally, somebody checked the card and I got caught. The police got called, I was charged, and the school called George and Stephanie. They came rushing out to the college to clear up the "mistake." They nearly passed out when I told them it was all true, that I had stolen three credit cards and run up five or six thousand dollars in charges.

Clinician: What was it like for you to be caught and to have George and Stephanie find out what you had done?

Client: I know this sounds pretty strange, but in a way I was glad. I showed them I wasn't their perfect little girl anymore. The more upset they got, the happier I felt. I used to feel guilty if I got a grade on a paper that wasn't an A, but now somehow I didn't feel guilty that I had broken the law. I sort of felt proud of what I had done.

Clinician: So even though you had broken the law, you finally felt like you had some independence and were able to be something other than what you believe your adoptive parents had programmed you to be.

Client: Yes, that's true. I felt like finally I was me, not just an extension of George and Stephanie. Of course, the consequences of my actions have been pretty bad. George was able to pull some strings, and between that and my clean record, I didn't have to go to jail, but I'm on probation for a long time. I have to make restitution to the people whose credit cards I used, and I have to do community service. George and Stephanie put up the money for the restitution, but they put all sorts of conditions on me too. I have to pay the money back to them, I have to live at home, attend college part-time, and get a job to earn money for the restitution and for my room and board, and I have to get some counseling. So here I am.

Clinician: Your life has changed dramatically again. How has this been for you?

Client: It's been three months since I was arrested. I've been back with George and Stephanie since then, I have a part-time job as a receptionist in an office, and next month I'll be starting two courses at the local community college. The hardest part has been living with George and Stephanie. George is pleasant enough; he just doesn't seem to know what to say to me. My arrest made the local papers, and I'm sure this was a big embarrassment to him, but he's playing the role of the forgiving and magnanimous father. He even talked to a parents' group about dealing with behavioral problems in adolescents and went to a Tough Love meeting. Anything to protect his political career, but at least he doesn't seem to hate me. Stephanie is another story. She treats me like I'm something you'd find in the toilet bowl. All she can talk about is how much they did for me, how ungrateful I am, and how disturbed I must be to have acted like this. I think she sees counseling as a sort of punishment, a place where you'll tell me what a terrible person I am and how I need to shape up and appreciate my wonderful parents. What a joke!

Clinician: Living with your parents again has been difficult for you, and you've had quite a few challenges since your arrest. I wonder what your idea of counseling is and how you think it might help you.

Client: Actually, I have been thinking about that. I know that stealing was a mistake, and yet it showed me that I could feel differently and that I need to find a better way to figure out who I am and make a life for myself away from George and Stephanie. I've been doing quite a bit of reading about Korea and about the culture there. If I'd stayed there, I might have been a Buddhist and probably would have been poor and wouldn't have been able to go to college or have any of the so-called advantages I have now. Or maybe if my birth father had stuck around, he would have taken me back to the United States with him and I would have been brought up as an African American; maybe I would have been a Baptist. There are so many directions in which my life could have gone. Instead, I was brought up in a Caucasian family with plenty of money and status, but I've been miserable. I need to figure out who I am and who I want to become. I just feel so confused right now; I don't even know what race or religion I am. I don't know if I really want to go to college or what I want to study. I started out as a music major because of my years of studying the piano, but I'm not going to be a great pianist. So then what? Do I want to be a music teacher? Not really, but I don't know what else I could do. Maybe you could help me to figure some of this out.

Clinician: Yes, that is certainly something we could work on together. I wonder how your mood has been in the past few months and if that could use some attention too.

Client: I guess so. I felt great for awhile when I had the credit cards and could buy whatever I wanted, but it was like I was buying friends and popularity. I don't really have any friends who just like me for me, and being back home is pretty depressing. Stephanie makes me feel guilty for breathing; I can't seem to do anything right in her eyes and sometimes I buy into that and think I'm pretty worthless. Yeah, I guess my mood could use some attention.

Clinician: So that's something else we could work on together. We've talked about some of the difficulties you have had over the years, and especially the situation you've been dealing with for the past few months, but I think you also have many strengths that we could draw on in our work together. What do you see as your strengths?

Client: It's hard for me to see myself as having any strengths.

Clinician: And yet you have had many successes in your life that do reflect your strengths.

Client: I guess so. I do have to study pretty hard to do well at school, but if I apply myself I can get good grades. I'm fairly athletic and I was the pianist for the school orchestra, so I guess I'm at least a competent musician.

Clinician: So your academic abilities, your music, and your athletic abilities are all strengths. I think along with that is your determination to do well in school and to keep up your grades in high school. Maybe another strength is your curiosity about your background and yourself and your wish to sort of reinvent yourself in a way that is rewarding to you and is true to who you really are.

Client: How is that a strength? It just seems to be confusing me.

Clinician: And yet you haven't run away from that confusion. You have been reading and learning and trying to figure out who you are. That takes courage.

Client: I guess you're right; I never thought about it that way. You know, I said to you that Summer wasn't even my real name. George and Stephanie gave me that name because I was supposed to bring sunshine into their lives. How insipid! They told me I had a Korean name when they adopted me but they had trouble pronouncing it so they just changed it. I think I'd like to take back my Korean name as a start to figuring out who I really am. It must be in my adoption papers, and I can find out how to pronounce it.

Clinician: So that would be a first step for you in figuring out who you are and who you want to become.

Client: Yes. Do you think it would be a good idea for me to change my name?

Clinician: I wonder how it would feel to you and what you see as the pros and cons of doing that.

Client: I don't think George and Stephanie would like the idea, but maybe that will start to give them the message that I am no longer going to fit the mold they have created for me. I don't have to break the law to give them that message; I can find other ways to do that. I think it would feel good for me to take back my Korean name; it's a symbol for me that I can be the person I want to be.

Clinician: So it sounds like that would be a rewarding step for you. Perhaps there are also other ways for you to continue to figure out who you are and build on your strengths.

Client: I do want to continue learning about my background. I thought I might go to a Korean grocery and see what the food is like and what it feels like to be there. I also wanted to find out more about Korean and African American music, and I thought I might get some piano music from both of those cultures.

Clinician: So you have quite a few ideas about initial steps you could take to become more familiar with the cultures in your background while also getting to know yourself better. We have just a few minutes left before the end of our session. How have you felt about our first meeting?

Client: Much better than I thought I would. I was angry that Stephanie insisted that I get some counseling. I thought this was just for people who are really sick, and that's probably what Stephanie thinks I am, but I can see ways that this could help me. And you didn't tell me what a terrible thing I had done or make me feel worse about myself. In fact, you really seemed to listen to me and to appreciate some things about me.

Clinician: So perhaps counseling can be helpful to you after all. What did you learn from this session that you can take away with you today?

Client: I learned that it's not crazy for me to want to figure out who I am and try to build a more rewarding life for myself. I could see that I have been depressed for a long time and maybe I could find some healthy ways to feel better. And I learned that maybe I do have some strengths, even more than I knew I had.

Clinician: How about if we write these down so you will remember them? Also, I wonder if we could write down some of the plans you have, such as changing your name and learning more about Korean and African American cultures.

Client: That sounds like a good idea. These things are fresh in my mind right now, but I do want to be sure I remember them.

Clinician : How do you feel about our scheduling another meeting?

Client: That sounds like a good idea. Stephanie said I had to meet with you at least 10 times, but I think I might want to meet again even if I didn't have to do that. Can I come next week at this same time?

Clinician: Yes, that works fine for me.

LEARNING OPPORTUNITIES

Written Exercises/Discussion Questions

Drawing on the conceptual skills presented in this book will help you to understand Summer Harris, introduced in the preceding interview. The following exercises, organized according to the sequence of chapters in this book, can help you review the skills and concepts presented in this book. You can focus on those questions and exercises that are particularly relevant and interesting to you, on those that have been assigned in your class or other learning experience, or you can work your way systematically through all the questions and exercises as presented.

Chapter 1: Establishing the Foundation for Developing Conceptual Skills

1. Chapter 1 introduced the BETA (background, emotions, thoughts, actions) framework. Which of these areas is emphasized in this interview? Which are deemphasized? Would you have changed this emphasis? If so, how and why?

2. Briefly list relevant information about Summer Harris according to the four components of the BETA model:

   a. Background
   b. Emotions
   c. Thoughts
   d. Actions

3. Respond to the following questions about Summer.

   a. In what ways can Summer's strengths be mobilized and maximized?
   b. How can a positive and collaborative therapeutic alliance best be developed with Summer, especially in light of her having been adopted, her limited experience with positive relationships, and her mistrust of her adoptive parents?
   c. What is the connection between Summer's background experiences and her emotional, cognitive, and behavioral difficulties?
   d. Which of these three areas (emotions, thoughts, actions) reflects her most prominent or troubling symptoms?
   e. Which of the three areas reflects the symptoms that are most amenable to change?
   f. What is Summer's preferred means of relating to the world?

Chapter 2: Using Conceptual Skills to Understand, Assess, and Address Background: Bloom's Taxonomy, Context, Multiculturalism, and Interpretation

1. Provide an in-depth picture of Summer using the framework of the modified Bloom's taxonomy, outlined here. For additional information about this process, see Chapters 2 and 3.

   Content (What are the facts?)
   Process

   - Comprehension (What do I know and understand about the facts?)
   - Organization (What principles, categories, and generalizations help me to understand this information?)
   - Analysis/Synthesis (How are these facts related, and what inferences can I draw about their connections?)
   - Interpretation (What does all this mean, and what sense does all this make?)

- Application (What approaches seem most likely to be effective in building a sound therapeutic relationship with Summer and helping her achieve goals?)
- Evaluation (How would I assess the effectiveness of my treatment of Summer?)

2. In what areas would Summer benefit from having greater insight? Create two interpretations that might help her gain that insight, being sure that the interpretations reflect the guidelines presented in Chapter 2.
3. Develop clinician statements that reflect the following types of interpretations and that might be helpful to Summer:

   a. Gender-based interpretation
   b. Developmental interpretation
   c. Multicultural interpretation
   d. Interpretation based on a particular theory of counseling or psychotherapy

4. Discuss the context in which Summer presents for treatment, addressing the follow eight areas. If information is missing, you may add information to what we already know about Summer:

   a. Demographic characteristics of the client
   b. Source of referral
   c. Choice of clinician
   d. Treatment facility
   e. Precipitant for seeking services
   f. Motivation
   g. Presenting problem(s)
   h. Strengths and assets

5. What multicultural variables are most important in understanding Summer? What information do they provide about her? How do multicultural factors such as gender, age, religion, ethnicity, and others affect Summer and her view of the world? Summer's multicultural background is complex; what skills seem especially important to use with this client so that her counseling reflects multicultural competence?

Chapter 3: Using Conceptual Skills to Understand, Assess, and Address Background: Eliciting Information, Intake Interviews, Transference and Countertransference

1. How would you describe the quality of the intake interview conducted with Summer? What skills did the interviewer use that contributed to the quality of the interview? What were the most important topics that were explored? How might the interview have been improved? Were there gaps in the interview or areas that should have been explored in greater depth in this initial session? If so, what were they and how might the interviewer have explored them further?
2. What sort of transference reaction do you think that Summer is most likely to develop in relation to her clinician? What difference would it make, in her transference reactions, if her clinician were a man? A woman? Close to her own

age? Close to the age of her adoptive parents? Korean? African American? Caucasian? How do you think the clinician could make sound therapeutic use of any transference reaction that Summer may have?

3. What sort of countertransference reaction do you think a clinician is most likely to develop in relation to Summer? How should the clinician address and make use of that reaction?

Chapter 4: Using Conceptual Skills to Make Positive Use of and Modify Emotions: Therapeutic Alliance, Role Induction, Clinician Self-Disclosure, Clinicians' Reactions to Clients

1. What emotions does the client manifest at the beginning of the session? At the end of the session? If you see a change, how do you explain that change?

2. What emotions, if any, are manifested by the clinician during the interview with Summer? Do you think the clinician should have expressed more emotion? Less emotion? If you would recommend a change, why and what would the nature of that change be?

3. The following list includes 10 ways in which clinicians can promote development of a positive therapeutic alliance. Which of these do you observe in this session and how are they communicated? Which of these do you think are most important in building a positive therapeutic alliance with Summer?

   a. Empathy
   b. Good listening skills
   c. Trustworthiness, reliability, and ethical behavior
   d. Caring and concern
   e. Genuineness, sincerity, and congruence
   f. Persuasiveness and credibility
   g. Optimism
   h. A sense of structure and direction
   i. Support, encouragement, reassurance, and affirmation
   j. Ability to address problematic client behaviors and attitudes

4. The following list reflects client characteristics that can make an important contribution to treatment effectiveness. Which of these were demonstrated by Summer and how did she convey those characteristics?

   a. Maturity—being responsible, well informed, and reasonably well organized
   b. Capacity to trust others and form caring and stable relationships
   c. Ability to establish appropriate interpersonal boundaries, being neither too dependent on others nor too isolated from others
   d. Capacity for introspection and insight
   e. High frustration tolerance and ability to delay gratification
   f. Motivation toward accepting help and making positive changes in oneself
   g. Positive but realistic treatment expectations
   h. Good self-esteem and feelings of empowerment

5. The counselor who is interviewing Summer makes little use of self-disclosure. In light of what you have learned about Summer, do you think this was a wise

choice, or do you think the clinician should have used more self-disclosure? If so, what sort of self-disclosure would have been helpful? Give two examples of clinician self-disclosures that might enhance Summer's treatment? Assume that Summer's clinician had been adopted. Do you think the clinician should share that information with Summer? Why or why not?

6. At one point, Summer asks the clinician for advice as to whether she should change her name. What is your assessment of how the clinician responded to this request? Would you have handled this differently? If so, why and how?

Chapter 5: Using Conceptual Skills to Make Positive Use of and Modify Emotions: Addressing Strong Client Emotions and Variations in Client Readiness for Treatment

1. Summer expresses some strong emotions during her intake interview, particularly anger at her adoptive mother. What part does anger seem to play in Summer's difficulties? Drawing on the guidelines presented in Chapter 5, how would you go about helping her understand, reduce, and redirect her anger, and replace that feeling with more constructive emotions?

2. Especially at the beginning of the intake interview, Summer is not eager to become involved in treatment. Looking at the five stages of change in the model developed by Prochaska and Norcross (1999),

   - Precontemplation
   - Contemplation
   - Preparation
   - Action
   - Maintenance

   what stage of change does Summer seem to be in when she begins treatment? What is your evidence for this conclusion? What implications does this have for her treatment?

3. What stage of change is Summer in at the end of the intake interview? If her stage has shifted, how do you explain the shift? What strategies would you use at this point to help her to engage in treatment?

Chapter 6: Using Conceptual Skills to Enhance Thoughts: Assessment, Mental Status Examination, Defining Memories, and Case Conceptualization

1. Prepare a brief mental status examination of Summer, including information on the following 12 categories (described in greater detail in Chapter 6):

   a. Appearance
   b. Behavior
   c. Speech
   d. Emotions and overall affect
   e. Orientation to reality
   f. Concentration and attention
   g. Thought processes
   h. Thought content

      i. Perceptions
      j. Memory
      k. Intelligence
      l. Judgment and insight

2. Develop a case conceptualization for Summer using one of the following models presented in Chapter 6:

- Concept mapping
- Clinical factor analysis
- The modified Bloom's taxonomy
- Inverted pyramid heuristic

Chapter 7: Using Conceptual Skills to Facilitate Diagnosis and Treatment Planning

1. If you have sufficient familiarity with diagnosis, prepare a multiaxial assessment for Summer, based on the categories and diagnostic format suggested by the *Diagnostic and Statistical Manual of Mental Disorders* and described in Chapter 7. Otherwise, review the 17 categories of diagnosis presented in Chapter 7. Identify one diagnosis that might reflect Summer's difficulties, and provide your rationale for this diagnosis.
2. Develop a treatment plan for Summer, based on what you have learned about her from the intake interview. Your treatment plan should follow the format for the DO A CLIENT MAP described in Chapter 7 and should include a rationale for your overall plan.

Chapter 8: Applying Conceptual Skills to Actions for Positive Change: Generating Solutions, Referral and Collaboration, Structuring Treatment, and Writing Progress Notes

1. Assume that Summer is debating whether to continue living with her adoptive parents or to move in with a roommate. Discuss how you would go about helping her make this decision and what strategies you would use in this process.
2. Do you think that any referrals or professional collaborations would be useful to Summer? Why or why not? If yes, what sort of interactions do you think her clinician should have with the referrals? How would you go about making the referral to increase the likelihood that Summer will respond well to the referral?
3. How would you describe the flow and structure of the initial interview that was conducted with Summer? What seems to have been effective about that structure? Are there ways in which you might improve on the structure of the session? If so, what are they?
4. Develop a plan for the second session with Summer, following the intake interview. The 10-step format beginning on page 250 suggests a prototype for this process. What elements do you think will be most important in the beginning, middle, and ending phases of the second session with Summer?
5. Write a brief progress note for the initial interview with Summer, following either the SOAP (subjective, objective, analysis, plans) or the STIPS (signs and

symptoms, topics, interventions, progress and plans, special issues) format presented in Chapter 8.

Chapter 9: Applying Conceptual Skills to Actions for Positive Change: Assessing and Terminating Sessions and Treatment, Using Research to Enhance Practice

1. Assume that Summer completes her treatment successfully. List at least five goals that you would expect her to achieve by the end of her counseling, as well as two or three additional goals that she might want to work on after termination of her treatment.

2. On the other hand, assume that, after a few sessions, Summer tells her counselor that she does not think her treatment is helping her. What might be a probable reason for this response? How would you recommend that her counselor address this?

3. What sorts of research do you think would help Summer's counselor to better understand her and provide her with more effective treatment?

4. As you reflect on your analysis of Summer and her concerns, which sections of these exercises were comparatively easy for you? Which presented the greatest challenge? What can you learn from this about what you need to focus on in your continued reading and study?

Comprehensive Self-Evaluation

This section presents again all the Assessment of Progress forms that have appeared throughout this book. This material can be used in the following ways.

- As you learn the material and complete the exercises in earlier chapters, you can look ahead to this section for a preview of the learning and exercises to come. This can help you put in context the information presented in earlier chapters and anticipate learning in later chapters.

- You can use these forms for a final class exercise and skill review. Divide into your usual practice groups. Ample time should be allowed for this exercise so that each person has the opportunity to role-play both client and clinician. Allow at least 30 minutes for each role-play plus at least 15 minutes for processing. If necessary, the processing time can be shortened by ensuring that each session is recorded for later review and analysis. If that is done, participants in the exercise can then complete their self-evaluation forms alone, with their role-played clients, or with the entire group either outside of class time or in a subsequent class session.

    The role-played session should represent an initial meeting between client and clinician, with clients presenting different concerns or issues than they addressed in earlier role-played sessions. Other than that, the focus of the session should be determined by each client. The session simulates an actual treatment session in that clinicians may have

little or no information about their clients and their concerns at the initial meeting.
- A third approach to using these evaluation forms is as a stimulus for reflecting on the growth in clinical skills you achieved while you engaged in the learning provided in this book. Review your initial self-evaluations in earlier chapters and think about improvements you have made in your skills. Also identify those skills that you recognize as still needing improvement. Recalling specific examples of both growth and weaknesses in your skills can help you to prepare specific and meaningful self-evaluations. Based on your reflections, complete this second set of forms, providing a written record of your progress.

Now you should be ready to complete the Assessment of Progress forms again, based either on a final role-played exercise or on your perceptions of your overall clinical skills.

Assessment of Progress Form 1

1. Identify at least two strengths demonstrated by the clinician, indicating the interaction with the client or the intervention that exemplified each strength.
   a. _____
   b. _____
2. What efforts did the clinician make to initiate a positive therapeutic alliance with the client? How effective were they?

   _____

   _____

3. Describe how the clinician approached the process of obtaining information from the client. Consider the types of interventions the clinician used (e.g., open question, closed question, encourager), the pacing of the session, the mix of interventions used by the clinician, and nonverbal communications. How successful was the clinician in obtaining the information in the questions provided for this role-play?

   _____

   _____

   _____

   _____

4. List two ways in which the clinician might have improved upon his or her use of clinical skills and the process of the session:
   a. _____
   b. _____

Assessment of Progress Form 2

1. Describe the types of interventions the clinician used during this interview.

   _____

   _____

   _____

   _____

a. Should a particular type of intervention have been used more or used less?

_____

b. How effective was the balance of open and closed questions?

_____

c. How well were other interventions integrated with the questions?

_____

2. What was the flow of the interview like? What made it flow well? What would have made it flow more smoothly?

_____

_____

_____

_____

3. How effective were the clinician's efforts to gather information on:
   a. The client's presenting concerns?

_____

   b. Important multicultural variables in the client's life?

_____

4. What might have made the clinician's efforts to gather that information more successful?

_____

_____

_____

_____

5. What interventions or clinician attitudes demonstrated multicultural competencies? What improvements, if any, might the clinicians have made in how he or she elicited and addressed multicultural characteristics?

_____

_____

_____

_____

6. Did the clinician make at least one interpretation? If so, comment on the timing and effectiveness of that interpretation.

_____

_____

_____

_____

7. Summary of feedback, including identification of at least two strengths and one area needing improvement:
   a. Strengths:

_____

_____

   b. Areas needing improvement:

_____

Assessment of Progress Form 3

1. How well did the clinician succeed in conducting a comprehensive intake interview that would facilitate an in-depth understanding of the client? What topics, if any, were omitted or discussed too briefly? What issues, if any, received too much emphasis?

   _____

   _____

   _____

   _____

2. What interventions contributed to making the interview effective? How might the interview have been even more effective?

   _____

   _____

   _____

   _____

3. Describe the types of interventions the clinician used during this interview. How effective was the clinician's use of questions? How well were other interventions integrated with the use of questions?

   _____

   _____

   _____

   _____

4. What was the flow of the interview like? What made it flow well? What would have made it flow more smoothly?

   _____

   _____

   _____

   _____

5. Summary of feedback, including identification of at least two strengths and one area needing improvement:
   a. Strengths:

   _____

   _____

   b. Areas needing improvement:

   _____

Assessment of Progress Form 4

1. a. What strategies and clinician characteristics were used to initiate the session and build a positive treatment alliance?

   _____

   _____

   _____

b. Which of these seemed particularly successful? What made them effective?

_____

_____

c. What else might the clinician have done to further develop the treatment alliance?

_____

_____

2. What is your overall assessment of how the clinician conducted the role induction? What were the strengths of this process? How might it have been improved?

_____

_____

_____

3. How well did the clinician handle the client's questions? Were different strategies used to respond to personal questions than were used to address professional questions? What were the strengths of this process? How might it have been improved?

_____

_____

_____

4. How successful was the clinician at integrating a variety of interventions into the interactions with the client? What strengths did you observe in the clinician's use of interventions? How might the clinician's use of a variety of interventions have been improved?

_____

_____

_____

5. Summary of feedback
   a. Strengths:

_____

   b. Areas needing improvement:

_____

Assessment of Progress Form 5

1. What interventions and strategies were used to initiate the session and build a positive treatment alliance?

_____
_____

_____

     a. Which of these seemed particularly successful? What made them effective?

     _____

     _____

     b. What else might the clinician have done to further develop the treatment alliance?

     _____

     _____

2. Which of the clinician's interventions (e.g., encouragers, open questions, reflection of feelings) seemed particularly successful?

     _____

     _____

3. How might the clinician have improved on his or her interventions?

     _____

     _____

4. What was the clinician's strategy in dealing with the client's strong emotions?

     _____

     _____

     a. What interventions were especially effective in helping the client understand and modify his or her unhelpful emotions?

     _____

     _____

     b. How might the clinician have dealt even more effectively with this client?

     _____

     _____

     _____

5. Summary of feedback
     a. Strengths:

     _____

     _____

     b. Areas needing improvement:

     _____

     _____

Assessment of Progress Form 6

1. What strategies were used effectively to enhance the therapeutic alliance and conduct a productive session?

   _____

   _____

   _____

2. Describe ways in which the clinician elicited and explored the defining memory.

   _____

   _____

   _____

3. Which interventions seemed particularly successful?

   _____

   _____

   _____

4. How might the clinician have improved on the use of these interventions?

   _____

   _____

   _____

5. Summary of feedback
   a. Strengths:

   _____

   _____

   b. Areas needing improvement:

   _____

   _____

Assessment of Progress Form 7

1. How successful was the clinician in obtaining the information needed to make an accurate diagnosis and develop an effective treatment plan? What topics, if any, should have received more attention? What topics, if any, should have received less attention?

   _____

   _____

   _____

2. Describe the flow of the interview. What interventions enhanced the flow of the interview? What interventions might have helped the interview to progress even more smoothly?

   _____

   _____

   _____

3. Summary of feedback
   a. Strengths:

   _____

   _____

   b. Areas needing improvement:

   _____

   _____

Assessment of Progress Form 8

1. How well did the session follow the 10 steps in the format for structuring sessions? Which steps worked especially well? How might the process have been improved?

   _____

   _____

   _____

2. Describe the process of goal setting. Were goals clear, relevant, and specific? How might the goal setting have been improved?

   _____

   _____

   _____

3. Describe and assess the clinician's use of concreteness and specificity.

   _____

   _____

   _____

4. Assess the appropriateness of the homework task that the clinician suggested to the client. Was the task clear, relevant to the client's problem behavior, and readily achievable? Was the client engaged in the process of formulating the homework task? How might the process of suggesting a homework task have been improved?

   _____

   _____

   _____

5. Describe the strategies used to bring closure to the session and assess their effectiveness.

   _____

   _____

   _____

6. Overall assessment
   a. Strengths:

   _____

   _____

b. Areas needing improvement:

_____

_____

Assessment of Progress Form 9

1. List the strengths and gains that you, your partner, and your group observed in you over the course of this training experience.

_____

_____

2. List two fundamental or conceptual skills that warrant your continued attention.

_____

3. How successful were you at bringing a positive closure to your work with your partner and facilitating that person's expression of feelings and identification of strengths and areas needing improvement? What made this session as successful as it was? What would have further enhanced the session?

_____

_____

_____

Personal Journal Questions

This final set of personal journal questions is designed to help you further synthesize your learning from this book and your reactions to the process of skill development presented here.

1. Describe your overall reactions to the information and learning experiences provided in this book.
2. What were the most important skills this book provided to you?
3. How will you use these skills in your professional work?
4. What parts of this book were especially challenging for you? How do you explain that? How did you deal with those challenges?
5. What parts of this book were least interesting or least important to you? How do you explain that?
6. In no more than three sentences, describe the positive changes you have made in your skills as a result of your work with this book.
7. What have you learned about yourself through your work with this book?

SUMMARY

This final chapter included

- An intake interview with Summer Harris.
- Written exercises/discussion questions based on that interview, reflecting the learning that has been presented in this book.
- A comprehensive self-evaluation based on the Assessment of Progress forms included in the Learning Opportunities for each chapter, gathered here to enable you to do a final review and rating of your skills or a final role-playing exercise.
- A final series of personal journal questions.

The information and exercises in this book were designed to help you build on the fundamental clinical and counseling skills you have already learned and to develop advanced conceptual skills. Although, of course, time and practice are needed before you can master these skills, the learning you have gained from this book should enable you to think like a clinician, to understand your clients at deeper and more complex levels, and to make effective use of a broad range of clinical tools such as diagnosis and treatment planning so that you are knowledgeable and prepared for the challenging and rewarding role of the mental health professional. I wish you much success as you continue your learning and further develop your professional skills in our exciting field!

REFERENCES

Acosta, F. X., Yamamoto, J., Evans, L. A., & Skilbeck, W. M. (1983). Preparing low-income Hispanic, African American, and Caucasian patients for psychotherapy: Evaluation of a new orientation program. *Journal of Clinical Psychology, 39,* 872–877.

Adler, A. (1931). *What life should mean to you.* Boston: Little, Brown.

American Psychiatric Association. (2000). *Diagnostic and Statistical Manual of Mental Disorders (DSM-IV-TR).* Washington, DC: Author.

Arredondo, P. (1999). Multicultural counseling competencies as tools to address oppression and racism. *Journal of Counseling and Development, 77,* 102–108.

Arredondo, P., Rosen, D. C., Rice, T., Perez, P., & Tovar-Gamero, Z. G. (2005).Multicultural counseling: A 10-year content analysis of the *Journal of Counseling and Development. Journal of Counseling and Development, 83,* 155–161.

Bachelor, A. (1995). Clients' perception of the therapeutic alliance: A qualitative analysis. *Journal of Counseling Psychology, 42,* 323–337.

Beck, A. T. (1999). *Prisoners of hate: The cognitive basis of anger, hostility and violence.* New York: Harper Collins.

Beck, J. S. (1995). *Cognitive therapy: Basics and beyond.* New York: Guilford.

Bloom, B. L. (1981). Focused single-session therapy: Initial development and evaluation. In S. H. Budman (Ed.), *Forms of brief therapy* (pp. 167–216). New York: Guilford Press.

Bloom, B. S., Engelhart, M. D., Furst, F. J., Hill, W. H., & Krathwohl, D. R. (1956). *Taxonomy of educational objectives: Cognitive domain.* New York: McKay.

Bowlby, J. (1978). Attachment theory and its therapeutic implications. *Adolescent Psychiatry, 6,* 5–33.

Bowlby, J. (1988). *A secure base: Parent-child attachment and healthy human development.* New York: Basic Books.

Burns, D. D. (2007). *The feeling good handbook.* New York: Penguin.

Carney, J. V., & Hazler, R. J. (1998). Suicide and cognitive-behavioral counseling: Implications for mental health counselors. *Journal of Mental Health Counseling, 20*(1), 28–41.

Cochrane-Brink, K. A., Lofchy, J. S., & Sakinofsky, I. (2000). Clinical rating scales in suicide risk assessment. *General Hospital Psychiatry, 22,* 445–451.

Constantine, M. S., & Ladany, N. (2000). Self-report multicultural counseling competence scales: Their relation to social desirability attitudes and multicultural case conceptualization ability. *Journal of Counseling Psychology, 47,* 155–164.

Cowan, E. W., & Presbury, J. H. (2000). Meeting client resistance and reactance with reverence. *Journal of Counseling and Development, 78,* 411–419.

Cytrynbaum, S., Ginath, Y., Birdwell, J., & Brandt, L. (1979). Goal attainment scaling: A critical review. *Evaluation Quarterly, 3,* 5–40.

Deffenbacher, J. L., & McKay, M. (2000). *Therapist protocol: Overcoming situational and general anger.* Oakland, CA: New Harbinger.

de Shazer, S. (1988). *Clues: Investigating solutions in brief therapy.* New York: W. W. Norton.

DiGiuseppe, R. (1996). The nature of irrational and rational beliefs: Progress in rational emotive behavior therapy. *Journal of Rational-Emotive and Cognitive-Behavior Therapy, 14,* 5–28.

Duys, D. K., & Hedstrom, S. M. (2000). Basic counselor skills training and counselor cognitive complexity. *Counselor Education and Supervision, 40,* 8–18.

Edwards, C. E., & Murdock, N. L. (1984). Characteristics of therapist self-disclosure in the counseling process. *Journal of Counseling and Development, 72,* 384–389.

Eells, T. D. (2007). Comparing the methods. In T. D. Eells (Ed.), *Handbook of psychotherapy case formulation.* New York: Guilford Press.

Ellis, A. (1977). *Anger: How to live with and without it.* New York: Institute for Rational Living.

Emmerson, G. J., & Thackwray-Emmerson, D. (1992). Clinical case conceptualizations using clinical factor analysis. *Counseling Psychology Quarterly, 5,* 403–409.

Fein, M. L. (1993). *A common sense guide to coping with anger: Integrated anger management.* Westport, CT: Praeger.

Goh, J. (2005). Cultural competence and master therapists: An inextricable relationship. *Journal of Mental Health Counseling, 2005,* 71–81.

Granello, H. (2000). Encouraging the cognitive development of supervisees: Using Bloom's taxonomy. *Counselor Education and Supervision, 40,* 31–46.

Hinkle, J. S. (1994). The *DSM-IV*: Prognosis and implications for mental health counselors. *Journal of Mental Health Counseling, 16,* 174–183.

Horvath, A. O., & Symonds, D. D. (1991). Relation between working alliance and outcome in psychotherapy: A meta-analysis. *Journal of Counseling Psychology, 38,* 139–149.

Ivey, A. E., Ivey, M. B., & Simek-Morgan, L. (1997). *Counseling and psychotherapy.* Boston: Allyn & Bacon.

Juhnke, G. A., & Hovestadt, A. J. (1995). Using the SAD PERSONS Scale to promote supervisee assessment knowledge. *The Clinical Supervisor, 13,* 31–40.

Kivlighan, D. M., Jr., & Shaughnessy, P. (2000). Patterns of working alliance development: A typology of clients' working alliance ratings. *Journal of Counseling Psychology, 47,* 362–371.

Knox, S., Hess, S. A., Petersen, D. A., & Hill, C. E. (1997). A qualitative analysis of client perceptions of the effects of helpful therapist self-disclosure in long-term therapy. *Journal of Counseling Psychology, 44,* 274–283.

Kottler, J. A., & Brown, R. W. (2000). *Introduction to therapeutic counseling: Voices from the field* (4th ed.). Belmont, CA: Brooks/Cole.

Kroeger, O., & Thuesen, J. M. (1988). *Type talk.* New York: Dell.

Lambert, M. J., & Bergin, A. E. (1994). The effectiveness of psychotherapy. In A. E. Bergin & S. L. Garfield (Eds.), *Handbook of psychotherapy and behavior change* (4th ed., pp. 143–189). New York: Wiley.

Law, J., Morocco, J., & Wilmarth, R. R. (1981). A problem-oriented record system for counselors. *AMHCA Journal, 3*(1), 7–16.

Lerner, H. G. (1985). *The dance of anger.* New York: Harper & Row.

Loganbill, C., & Stoltenberg, C. (1983). The case conceptualization format: A training device for practicum. *Counselor Education and Supervision, 22,* 235–241.

Mayfield, W. A., Kardash, C. M., & Kivlighan, D. M., Jr. (1999). Differences in experienced and novice counselors' knowledge structures about clients: Implications for case conceptualization. *Journal of Counseling Psychology, 46,* 504–514.

McLeod, J. (1994). *Doing counselling research.* London: Sage.

Miller, D. A., Sadler, J. Z., Mohl, P. C., & Melchiode, G. A. (1991). The cognitive context of examinations in psychiatry using Bloom's taxonomy. *Medical Education, 25,* 480–484.

Miller, W. R., & Rollnick, S. (1991). *Motivational interviewing: Preparing people to change addictive behavior.* New York: Guilford Press.

Motto, J., Heilbron, D. C., & Juster, R. P. (1985). Development of a clinical instrument to estimate suicide risk. *American Journal of Psychiatry, 142,* 680–686.

O'Hanlon, B., & Weiner-Davis, M. (1989). *In search of solutions: A new direction in psychotherapy.* New York: W. W. Norton.

Orlinsky, D. E., Grawe, K., & Parks, B. K. (1994). Process and outcome in psychotherapy-noch einmal. In B. A. Garfield & S. L. Garfield (Eds.), *Handbook of psychotherapy and behavior change* (4th ed., pp. 270–376). New York: Wiley.

Patterson, W. M., Dohn, H. H., Bird, J., & Patterson, G. A. (1983). Evaluation of suicidal patients: The SAD PERSONS Scale. *Psychosomatics, 24,* 343–349.

Pfeiffer, A. M., Whelan, J. P., & Martin, J. M. (2000). Decision-making bias in psychotherapy: Effects of hypothesis source and accountability. *Journal of Counseling Psychology, 47,* 429–436.

Potter-Efron, R. T. (1994). *Angry all the time: An emergency guide to anger control.* Oakland, CA: New Harbinger.

Potter-Efron, R. T., & Potter-Efron, P. S. (1991). *Anger, alcoholism and addiction: Treating individuals, couples and families.* New York: W. W. Norton.

Prieto, L. R., & Scheel, K. R. (2002). Using case documentation to strengthen counselor trainees' case conceptualization skills. *Journal of Counseling and Development, 80,* 11–21.

Prochaska, J. O., & Norcross, J. C. (1999). *Systems of psychotherapy.* Belmont, CA: Brooks-Cole.

Prochaska, J. O., & Norcross, J. C. (2003). *Systems of psychotherapy: A transtheoretical analysis.* Pacific Grove, CA: Brooks-Cole.

Robinson, T. L. (1997). Insurmountable opportunities. *Journal of Counseling and Development, 76*(1), 6–7.

Rogers, C. R. (1967). The conditions of change from a client-centered viewpoint. In B. Berenson & R. Carkhuff (Eds.), *Sources of gain in counseling and psychotherapy.* New York: Hold, Rinehart & Winston.

Rogers, C. R. (1980). *A way of being.* Boston: Houghton Mifflin.

Rothman, A. D. & Nowicki, S. (2004). A measure of the ability to identify emotion in children's tone of voice. *Journal of Nonverbal Behavior, 28,* 67–92.

Schwitzer, A. L. (1996). Using the inverted pyramid heuristic in counselor education and supervision. *Counselor Education and Supervision, 35,* 258–267.

Seligman, L. (1977). Haitians: A neglected minority. *Personnel and Guidance Journal, 55,* 409–411.

Seligman, L. (1979). Understanding the black foster child through assessment. *Journal of Non-white Concerns in Personnel and Guidance, 7,* 183–191.

Seligman, L. (1980). *Assessment in developmental career counseling.* Cranston, RI: The Carroll Press.

Seligman, L. (1986). *Diagnosis and treatment planning in counseling.* New York: Human Sciences Press.

Seligman, L. (1990). *Selecting effective treatments.* San Francisco: Jossey-Bass.

Seligman, L. (1994). *Developmental career counseling and assessment.* Thousand Oaks, CA: Sage.

Seligman, L. (1996a). *Diagnosis and treatment planning in counseling* (2nd ed.). New York: Plenum.

Seligman, L. (1996b). *Promoting a fighting spirit: Psychotherapy for cancer patients, survivors, and their families.* San Francisco: Jossey-Bass.

Seligman, L. (1998). *Selecting effective treatments: A comprehensive systematic guide to treating mental disorders* (Rev. ed.). San Francisco: Jossey-Bass.

Seligman, L. (2001). *Systems, strategies, and skills of counseling and psychotherapy.* Upper Saddle River, NJ: Merrill/Prentice Hall.

Seligman, L. (2004). *Diagnosis and treatment planning in counseling* (3rd ed.). New York: Kluwer Academic/Plenum.

Seligman, L. (2006). *Theories of counseling and psychotherapy: Systems, strategies, and skills.* Upper Saddle River, NJ: Pearson Merrill/Prentice Hall.

Seligman, L. (2008). *Fundamental skills for mental health professionals.* Columbus, OH: Pearson Merrill Prentice Hall.

Seligman, L., & Reichenberg, L. (2007). *Selecting effective treatments* (3rd ed.) San Francisco: Jossey-Bass.

Seligman, M. (1999). Teaching positive psychology. *APA Monitor on Psychology, 30*(7). Available from www.apa.org.

Simone, D. H., McCarthy, P., & Skay, C. L. (1998). An investigation of client and counselor variables that influence likelihood of counselor self-disclosure. *Journal of Counseling and Development, 76,* 174–182.

Smith, E. J. (2006). The strength-based counseling model: A paradigm shift in psychology. *The Counseling Psychologist, 34,* 13–79.

Srebalus, D. J., & Brown, D. (2001). *A guide to the helping professions.* Boston: Allyn & Bacon.

Stevens, M. J., & Morris, S. J. (1995). A format for case conceptualization. *Counselor Education and Supervision, 35,* 82–94.

Stosney, S. (1995). *Treating attachment abuse.* New York: Springer.

Strean, H. S. (1994). *Essentials of psychoanalysis.* New York: Brunner/Mazel.

Sue, D. W., Arredondo, P., & McDavis, R. J. (1992). Multicultural counseling competencies and standards: A call to the profession. *Journal of Counseling and Development, 70,* 477–486.

Tavris, C. (1989). *Anger: The misunderstood emotion.* New York: Simon & Schuster.

Teyber, E. (1997). *Interpersonal processes in psychotherapy.* Pacific Grove, CA: Brooks/Cole.

Waehler, C. A., Kalodner, C. R., Wampold, B. E., & Lichtenberg, J. W. (2000). Empirically supported treatments in perspective: Implementations for counseling psychology training. *The Counseling Psychologist, 28,* 657–671.

Walborn, F. S. (1996). *Process variables.* Pacific Grove, CA: Brooks/Cole.

Westefeld, J. S., Range, L. M., Rogers, J. R., Maples, M. R., Bromley, J. L., & Alcorn, J. (2000). Suicide: An overview. *The Counseling Psychologist, 28,* 445–510.

Williams, R., & Williams, V. (1993). *Anger kills.* New York: Harper Perennial.

Yakushko, O., & Chronister, K. M. (2005). Immigrant women and counseling: The invisible others. *Journal of Counseling and Development, 83,* 292–298.

Zaza, C., Stolee, P., & Prkachin, K. (1999). The application of goal attainment scaling in chronic pain settings. *Journal of Pain & Symptom Management, 17,* 55–64.

INDEX

clinicians' understanding of, 71–72
context for seeking treatment, 39–46
demographic characteristics of the client, 40–41, 42
empowering, 115
engaging in treatment, 105
health of, 49, 205, 208
intelligence of, 172–173, 176
interests of, 49, 176
motivation for seeking services, 41, 42
negative emotions of, 125–126, 142–151, 168
precipitants for seeking services, 41, 42
problematic attitudes of, 105
problematic behaviors of, 105
readiness for treatment, 151
relationship experiences of, 49
relationship status of, 49
reluctance of, 68, 156–163, 168
resistant, 105
self-awareness of, 71–72
strengths and assets of, 42
suicidal ideation and, 126–135
treatment-enhancing characteristics, 107
clinical disorders, 204
clinical factor analysis, 192
clinicians. *See also* client–clinician relationship
characteristics for treatment planning, 222
choice of, 41, 42
effectiveness of, 12
enhancing practice, 261, 272–277
ethical behavior of, 99–100
feelings toward clients, 118–120, 124
immediacy of, 109–118
listening skills of, 99
multiculturally skilled, 49–50, 58–59
professional development of, 261, 272–277
professional specialization of, 272–277
providing information about, 113–114
research and, 261, 272–277
self-disclosure of, 109–118
treatment planning and, 222
understanding of clients, 71–72
Cochrane-Brink, K. A., 128
cognitive-behavioral therapy, 6. *See also* cognitive therapy
cognitive impairment, 208
cognitive mental disorders, 208
cognitive therapy, 6, 250–251

collaboration, 235, 241–247, 260
communication disorders, 208
competencies, multicultural, 47–59
concentration, 172–173
concept mapping, 187–192
conceptual skills, 27
actions and, 235–280
background and, 29–65, 67–92
books on, 3–4
clarifying with Bloom's taxonomy, 30–34
context and, 39–46
diagnosis and, 203–219, 232–234
emotions and, 93–168
foundation for, 1–27
fundamental skills and, 2–4
solidifying, 281–301
thought-enhancing, 169–201
thoughts and, 169–201
treatment planning and, 219–234
concern, demonstrating, 100–101
conduct disorder, 207, 208
confidentiality, in practice group exercises, 23–24
congruence, 101
Constantine, 48
constructivist therapy, 6
content, in Bloom's taxonomy, 31
context, 39–46, 65
applying conceptual skills to, 39–46
choice of clinician, 41, 42
client strengths and assets, 42
demographic characteristics of the client, 40–41, 42
historical context, 49
motivation for seeking services, 41, 42
multicultural, 47–59
political context, 49
precipitants for seeking services, 41, 42
presenting problems, 41–42
social context, 49
source of referral, 41, 42
treatment facility, 41, 42
conversion disorder, 211
coping mechanisms, assessing, 129
counseling. *See also* treatments
developmental counseling and therapy (DCT), 251–252
person-centered counseling, 6